# MY FIRST MRCP BOOK

## 2nd Edition

**HUGH MONTGOMERY**
Professor of Intensive Care Medicine
*University College London (UCL), UK*

Consultant Intensivist
*Whittington Hospital, London, UK*

Director
*UCL Institute for Human Health and Performance, London, UK*

**NEIL GOLDSACK**
Consultant Respiratory and General Physician
*Kent and Canterbury Hospital, Canterbury, UK*
*Queen Elizabeth The Queen Mother Hospital, Margate, UK*

**VICTORIA CAMPBELL**
Haematology Registrar
*St Mary's Hospital, London, UK*

**DOROTHY IP**
Acute Medicine Trainee
*Barnet General Hospital, London, UK*

**VIVEK SIVARAMAN**
Cardiovascular Research Fellow
*Hatter Cardiovascular Institute, UCL, London, UK*

REMEDICA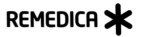

## EDITORS

### HUGH MONTGOMERY

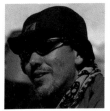

Hugh Montgomery, MBBS, BSc, FRCP, MD, FRGS, is a professor of intensive care medicine at University College London (UCL), a consultant intensivist at Whittington Hospital, London, and the Director of the UCL Institute for Human Health and Performance. He qualified at the Middlesex Hospital Medical School in 1987, and has since worked in London, Reading, and KwaZulu-Natal, and (briefly) as an air ambulance doctor. He is accredited in general medicine, cardiology, and intensive care medicine, and has had more than 160 peer-reviewed scientific articles published. Hugh has written, contributed to, and edited a number of medical books including the 'Puzzling Out…' series (in which the whole undergraduate medical curriculum is taught in puzzle book format) and *Surviving Prescribing*, a guide to practical prescribing. He is also author of two works of fiction for all ages (*The Voyage of the Arctic Tern* and *Cloudsailors*), and gave the televised 2007 Royal Institution Christmas Lectures.

Photo courtesy of Caudwell Xtreme Everest

### NEIL GOLDSACK

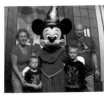

Neil Goldsack, MBBS, BSc, MRCP, FRCP, is a consultant respiratory and general physician based at both Kent and Canterbury Hospital in Canterbury and the Queen Elizabeth The Queen Mother Hospital in Margate. He has always enjoyed teaching and has considerable experience in doing so both for the MRCP and at undergraduate level. Outside work Neil enjoys fishing, playing cricket, and watching Liverpool football club. He is married with two children and enjoys taking his family to Florida each year to meet Mickey Mouse.

# Authors

## Victoria Campbell

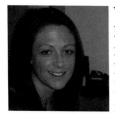

Victoria Campbell, MBBS, BSc, MRCP, is a haematology registrar. She graduated in 2004 from Imperial College School of Medicine and became a Member of the Royal College of Physicians in 2007. Whilst her long-term goal is to become a haematology consultant, she enjoys teaching medical students and junior doctors for finals and fellowship exams. She keeps mind and body active through art (both her own and admiring the works of others) and sport (athletics, hockey, tennis, squash and skiing).

## Dorothy Ip

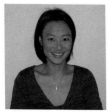

Dorothy Ip, MBBS, BMedSci, MRCP, graduated from Nottingham Medical School in 2003. After her nomadic life in various medical specialties, she decided that she enjoys working in all of them! She is currently a registrar in acute medicine in north London, and has an active interest in medical education: she has been involved in organising courses for junior doctors and teaching MRCP candidates.

## Vivek Sivaraman

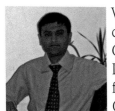

Vivek Sivaraman, MBBS, MRCP, is a cardiovascular research fellow at the Hatter Cardiovascular Institute at University College London. He gained his medical degree in 2001 from India, and became a Member of the Royal College of Physicians in 2005. Vivek has been a fan of *My First MRCP Book* ever since the first edition helped him pass his exam! He is currently researching myocardial preconditioning and protection.

## A NOTE ON THE SECOND EDITION

Welcome to the second edition of *My First MRCP Book*. In some ways, not much has changed: the ethos of the book, and its style, remain the same. However, two things are new. Firstly, fresh young authors have assisted the original old crusties, who are now generally occupied with spooning spilt custard from their cardigans. Secondly, the content has changed slightly. The book was always intended to provide a 'process of learning' as well as the key facts required to pass 'The Test' and not to be yet another book of practice questions. However, the MRCP examination style has changed, and it seemed sensible – where possible – to adapt some text to reflect this. Beyond that, expect the same juvenile sense of humour and a constant reminder that studying for examinations can be painless. Indeed, we hope that you continue to have as much fun with the new book as your predecessors did with the last.

## ACKNOWLEDGEMENTS

We would like to thank Dr David White, Consultant Radiologist from University Hospital Aintree, Liverpool, for the images that he provided for our radiology questions.

# INTRODUCTION

Gaining membership of the Royal College of Physicians (MRCP) is, in many ways, like a first sexual experience: most even modestly attractive people tend to get around to it in the end (think surgeons); peer pressure makes many try when they aren't quite ready; those that haven't are unsure what it's like; those who plan to have often been fed a variety of myths about how to; first attempts are often embarrassing and short lived; and those who have been successful always claim to have sweated over it for hours, obtaining high scores first time. The very elderly can't remember how and some don't even know if they ever did.

On the other hand, MRCP is generally a more expensive business by far.

This book hopes to dispel some of the myths and to teach you all you need to know in an enjoyable and informative way. It is, if you will, 'The joy of membership' – a hands-on guide. We recognise, of course, that the MRCP examination format changes. However, the basic knowledge required does not, and nor has the approach that can be used. This book, therefore, remains truly 'Your First MRCP Book'. Its use is not restricted, however: all students of medicine (including those who practice!) can use it to hone their diagnostic skills.

Whatever. Too much foreplay.

Starting from page 1, we shall teach you in a step-by-step fashion, in the privacy of your own room. By the time you reach the end, we hope that you will have all of the skills that you need. However, we would still advise you to go and buy other books in the field and practice what you have learned.

We hope that this book will give pleasure, as much to the student as to the more qualified reader, and, whoever you are, we hope that you will enjoy your lessons. But remember – don't leave your room smiling. Maintain the myth of the tortured youth.

## How to use this book

This book is **not** just another compilation of questions, and you should not treat it as such. It is a complete and structured course. If you start on page 1 and work steadily through to the end, you will have learned not just the facts that you need but also a strategy of attack. Dipping into the book randomly in search of questions will, we promise, be a pretty unrewarding business.

We have put a great deal of time and effort into the preparation of this book.

- We have assumed reasonable background knowledge. If you hit upon a diagnosis about which you remember little then look it up elsewhere.
- We have emphasised the subject matter that commonly appears in the examination.
- We are, however, aware that it may be difficult for you to accumulate adequate information on some of the more obscure topics and we have attended to these in more detail. Short texts on these subjects are given where knowledge may be thin.
- We have structured the text so that you build on knowledge. You will need facts learned early in the book to be able to answer questions later on.

We have also tried to use a little sensible educational theory. We all learn in different ways and sticking to one way is tedious, so we have provided a variety of tools: historical vignettes, mnemonics, pictures, poems, puzzles, tables, and equations. Intermittently, you will come across a puzzle, joke, or other form of amusement. Please do not rush over these – they are designed to reinforce facts that you have already learned. They are also spaced so as to give your brain a rest between more intensive bouts of cramming.

Once you have read and learned then every other book on the market becomes a practice ground for you. We strongly encourage you to buy a generous selection of these, as ultimately there is no substitute for practice.

So off you go. Slow and steady from start to finish.

Do learn.

And, please, do enjoy too.

# Contents

# 1

# THE STRATEGY

Are you sitting comfortably? Then let us
begin. Start by having a go at this first
question. Don't look anything up – just
make a stab at it. All will be revealed when
you turn the page.

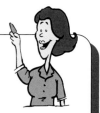

**Q1** A 12-year-old girl of Nigerian origin lives with her parents and grandparents. She has a 5-year-old brother who has recently suffered an acute coryzal illness. Her mother is a primary school teacher, while her father is in the diplomatic service; the family move biannually to different countries. The family returned to the UK from Peru only 3 months ago, having spent their final month visiting ancient Inca tombs. The girl now presents to her local emergency department with a 10-day history of fever and general malaise. Twenty days before her presentation she had received a 1-week course of antibiotics from her GP for a throat infection. The family kitten (an adopted and unvaccinated stray that was smuggled through customs) died of an unknown infection 3 weeks earlier. In addition to her fever, the girl complains of several days' pain and swelling in both wrists, plus her left knee and right ankle, which she attributes to a recent hockey training session. Her mother can remember no history of joint problems.

## ON EXAMINATION

- Temperature = 39.4°C
- Pulse = 98 beats/min regular
- Blood pressure = 105/70 mmHg
- JVP not elevated
- Mouth clear
- No rashes or LAN
- Chest clear
- Heart sounds 1 + 2 + soft ESM left sternal edge
- Abdomen soft, no HSM
- Painful, hot, and swollen wrists, knee, and ankle (see above)

## INVESTIGATIONS

- Haemoglobin = 10.5 g/l
- U&E = normal
- Urinalysis:
  normal dipstick
  no casts/cells
  negative cultures
- Mean corpuscular volume = 89 fl
- Bilirubin = 8 μmol/l
- White cell count = 13 × 10⁹/l
- Neutrophils = 85%
- Platelets = 450 × 10⁹/l
- ESR = 130 mm in first hour
- Aspartate aminotransferase = 70 IU/l
- C-reactive protein = 76 mg/l
- Chest X-ray = normal
- ECG = sinus rhythm (see **Figure 1**), PR interval 0.3 s, QRS 0.12 s, QT 0.4 s, normal axis

ECG: electrocardiogram; ESM: ejection systolic murmur; ESR: erythrocyte sedimentation rate; HSM: hepatosplenomegaly; JVP: jugular venous pressure; LAN: lymphadenopathy; U&E: urinalysis and electrolytes.

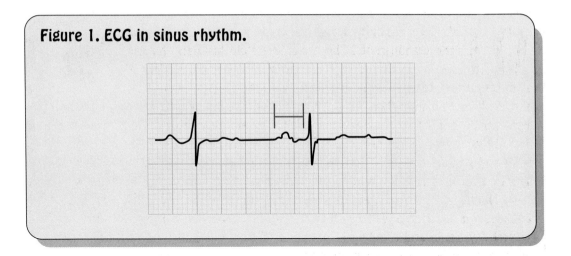

**Figure 1. ECG in sinus rhythm.**

### a) What is the most likely diagnosis?

i)   polyarticular Still's disease

ii)  acute rheumatic fever

iii) coccidioidomycosis

iv)  toxocariasis

v)   toxoplasmosis

### b) Which investigation will confirm your diagnosis?

i)   rheumatoid factor

ii)  *Toxocara* antigen ELISA

iii) toxoplasmosis serology

iv)  acute and convalescent serum anti-streptolysin O (ASO) titres

v)   blood cultures

### c) What is the appropriate management?

i)   corticosteroids

ii)  acetylsalicylate

iii) opiate analgesia

iv)  pyrimethamine and sulphadiazine

v)   mebendazole

The first stage in answering a 'grey case' such as this is to recognise the examiners' tactics. Invariably, they have marred the clarity of any story with 'smoke and mirrors' – extraneous facts that just cause confusion. Some are in there as meaningless bulk, while others are there as malicious red herrings. But then again, this pretty much emulates real life!

The key, then, is to positively ignore the waffle and *seek out only those features of the examination and investigations that you know are always pathological*. Is the fact that the cat died always pathological for the patient? No. Is the fact that she is Nigerian? No. Is the fact that they were recently in Peru? No! And Inca graves? Nonsense! These factors might later be helpful in confirming a diagnosis, but not in making it: at the moment they are nothing more than white smoke. Or tear gas. So what *are* the findings that are always pathological? They are:

- fever
- polyarthropathy
- normochromic normocytic anaemia
- elevated white cell count with leucocytosis
- elevated aspartate aminotransferase level
- elevated erythrocyte sedimentation rate (ESR) and C-reactive protein (CRP) level
- prolonged PR interval

Of these, some are quite nonspecific, such as fever. In fact, you can dismiss most of these findings as nonspecific. Fever, elevated ESR, raised CRP level, raised white cell count... Hmmm. She is suffering an acute inflammatory condition. Well, no s**t, Sherlock! So now identify which of these has only a limited list of potential causes and hone in on those. Finally, write down the list of causes for each abnormal feature that you have identified.

In this case, the features that are always pathological and that have a limited list of causes are *polyarthropathy* and *first-degree heart block*.

The causes of polyarthropathy are principally rheumatological, infectious, and haematological...

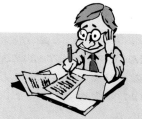

## CAUSES OF POLYARTHRALGIA

*Joint attacks are done by three –*
*RA, Still's, and HSP*
*Pyrophosphate, SLE*
*And seronegativity*

*Parvo, clap, group A, TB,*
*Germans, chicken pox, hep B*
*Spread by ticks (and not by fleas)*
*Is the dreaded Lyme disease*

*Sarcoid, i/c, SBE*
*Hep A, B, C*
*Coming over sickle-y*
*With widespread malignancy*

*FMF and Behçet's do*
*Chronic hepatitis, too*
*Crohn's and Whipple's, never fear!*
*UC shall bring up 'the rear'!*

Behçet's: Behçet's syndrome; clap: gonorrhoea; Crohn's: Crohn's disease; FMF: familial Mediterranean fever; Germans: German measles (rubella); group A: group A β-haemolytic *Streptococcus*; hep: hepatitis; HSP: Henoch–Schönlein purpura; i/c: immune complex disease; parvo: parvovirus; RA: rheumatoid arthritis; SBE: subacute bacterial endocarditis; SLE: systemic lupus erythematosus; Still's: Still's disease; TB: tuberculosis; UC: ulcerative colitis; Whipple's: Whipple's disease.

Remember that seronegative joint inflammation may be due to osteoarthritis as well as reactive arthritis (Reiter's syndrome), Poncet's disease (tuberculous rheumatism), ankylosing spondylitis, ulcerative colitis, and Crohn's disease. Haemochromatosis is an example of a metabolic cause, and leukaemia in children is an example of a malignant cause, often of monoarthritis but also of polyarthritis. In addition, remember the haematological causes, such as sickle cell disease, which can give rise to hand-and-foot syndrome. In addition, septic polyarthritis can occur when joints are seeded with organisms such as *Neisseria gonorrhoeae* or *Staphylococcus*.

How many of these are associated with a long PR interval? You probably don't even have to remember a list, as three come almost immediately to mind: acute rheumatic fever, sarcoidosis, and Lyme disease. It is likely to be one of these three. Now you return to the history. It is unlikely to be Lyme disease as she has not been wandering around the New Forest. She does not have the characteristic erythema nodosum or bilateral hilar lymphadenopathy of sarcoidosis. She has, however, had a recent sore throat. Which fits best? Evidently, acute rheumatic fever, and this is where you put your money.

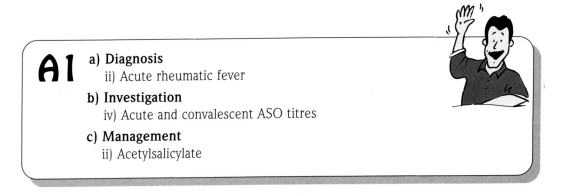

**A1**   a) **Diagnosis**
           ii) Acute rheumatic fever
       b) **Investigation**
           iv) Acute and convalescent ASO titres
       c) **Management**
           ii) Acetylsalicylate

Did you know the causes of a long PR interval? If not, come up with a list and a way to remember them. Jot them down here.

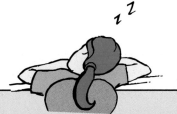

## REVISION ZONE

**Revised Duckett Jones criteria for acute rheumatic fever**

MAJOR     Pancarditis
Polyarthropathy
Sydenham's chorea
Erythema marginatum
Subcutaneous nodules (Aschoff nodules)

MINOR    Prolonged PR interval
Arthralgia (not applicable if polyarthropathy is used as a major criterion)
Elevated ESR/CRP level
Past rheumatic fever
Leucocytosis

The diagnosis of acute rheumatic fever rests on evidence of a recent streptococcal infection (acute and convalescent ASO titres; positive throat cultures for group A *Streptococcus*; streptococcal antibodies) and at least:

- two MAJOR criteria
- or one MAJOR and two MINOR criteria

The patient in the case history has one major and three minor criteria: polyarthropathy + prolonged PR interval, elevated ESR/CRP level, and leucocytosis.

Now, check that you have learnt the causes of a long PR interval, the causes of polyarthropathy, and the diagnostic criteria for rheumatic fever. When you are absolutely confident that you can write out the lists, you may move on!

## A QUICK JOKE

Talking of PRs, the tale is told of a rather quick-witted but lazy house surgeon. After a long night on the beers, he had clerked a patient in somewhat of a rush, and was now presenting him on the ward round. "Abdomen soft and nontender," he said. "No LK2S or nodes. PR NAD." The professor went puce. "PR NAD?" he howled. "NAD? This man has had an abdomino-perineal resection! What do you mean, PR NAD?" The house officer looked the professor straight in the eye. "No anus detected," he replied.

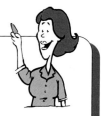

**Q2** A 14-year-old girl presents to her local emergency department with a 10-day history of fever and malaise, which have prevented her from going to school. She is of European origin and lives with her parents and her 5-year-old brother, who has been in complete remission from acute lymphoblastic leukaemia for 1 year. Her mother is a primary school teacher while her father is in the diplomatic service, necessitating the family to make biannual moves abroad. They now live near the 'Elaphos Priory' outside Southampton. Ten days before the onset of her symptoms, the girl's GP gave her a 1-week course of antibiotics for a throat infection. In addition to her fever, she complains of several days' pain and swelling in both wrists, her left knee, and right ankle. She mentions an annular rash on her right arm, which she noticed a few weeks ago but which now appears to be fading.

## On examination

- Temperature = 39°C
- Pulse = 98 beats/min regular
- Blood pressure = 105/70 mmHg
- JVP not elevated
- Mouth clear
- No LAN
- Chest clear
- Heart sounds 1 + 2 + soft ESM left sternal edge
- Abdomen soft, no HSM
- Painful, hot and swollen wrists, left knee, and right ankle
- Annular erythema on right arm

## Investigations

- Haemoglobin = 12 g/l
- U&E = normal
- Urinalysis:
  normal dipstick
  no casts/cells
  negative cultures
- Mean corpuscular volume = 89 fl
- Bilirubin = 8 μmol/l
- White cell count = 13 × 10⁹/l
- Neutrophils = 85%
- Platelets = 450 × 10⁹/l
- ESR = 130 mm in first hour
- Aspartate aminotransferase = 45 IU/l
- C-reactive protein = 76 mg/l
- Chest X-ray = normal
- ECG = sinus rhythm, PR interval 0.3 s, QRS 0.12 s, QT 0.4 s, normal axis

ECG: electrocardiogram; ESM: ejection systolic murmur; ESR: erythrocyte sedimentation rate; HSM: hepatosplenomegaly; JVP: jugular venous pressure; LAN: lymphadenopathy; U&E: urinalysis and electrolytes.

## a) What is the most likely diagnosis?

i)     polyarticular Still's disease

ii)    acute rheumatic fever

iii)   hand-and-foot syndrome of sickle cell disease

iv)    Lyme disease

v)     juvenile rheumatoid arthritis

## b) Which one investigation will confirm your diagnosis?

i)     rheumatoid factor

ii)    haemoglobin electrophoresis

iii)   anti-*Borrelia burgdorferi* immunoglobulin M antibodies

iv)    acute and convalescent serum ASO titres

v)     X-ray of the joints

## c) What is the appropriate management?

i)     intravenous ceftriaxone

ii)    penicillamine

iii)   opiate analgesia

iv)    acetylsalicylate

v)     immunosuppressive agents

The case history here is similar to the previous one, and similar lists for polyarthropathy and a prolonged PR interval can be used to aid with finding the diagnosis. As before, the history is important in determining the most likely diagnosis and allows a diagnosis that is different to that of the first case to be reached. It is the *annular* rash that is the clue. This is designed to suggest erythema chronicum migrans rather than erythema marginatum, making Lyme disease the most likely diagnosis.

Bonus points for any Greek scholars: *elaphos* is Greek for 'deer'. Out of interest (but don't bother to learn it!), Lyme disease is tick-transmitted by *Ixodes dammini* in the USA, *I. ricinus* in Europe, and *I. persulcatus* in Asia. Lyme disease was first described in 1977 in Old Lyme, Connecticut, USA.

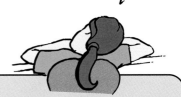

**A2**   **a) Diagnosis**
      iv) Lyme disease

    **b) Investigation**
        iii) Detection of antibodies to *B. burgdorferi* in serum

    **c) Management**
        i) Intravenous ceftriaxone (or cefotaxime)

Note that in the presence of the characteristic rash and fever alone, i.e. without any of the joint/cardiological/neurological complications, oral tetracycline (doxycycline) or penicillin would be sufficient. Note the similarities to syphilis, another spirochaetal disease.

## REVISION ZONE: LYME DISEASE

There are three main phases:

1) **EARLY LOCALISED DISEASE (within days)**
   **Erythema chronicum migrans**
   **Associated symptoms:** malaise, fever, arthralgia, stiff neck

2) **EARLY DISSEMINATED DISEASE (within weeks)**
   **Cardiological:** myocarditis or pancarditis with conduction disturbances
   **Neurological:** lymphocytic meningitis, encephalitis, cranial nerve palsies, Bannwarth's syndrome, mononeuritis
   **Musculoskeletal:** polyarthritis
   **Renal:** microhaematuria
   **Hepatic:** hepatitis
   **Ocular:** iritis, conjunctivitis
   **Dermatological:** erythema nodosum
   **Lymphadenopathy**

3) **LATE DISSEMINATED DISEASE (within months to years)**
   **Musculoskeletal:** migratory polyarthritis
   **Neurological:** chronic neuroborreliosis, dementia
   **Dermatological:** acrodermatitis chronica atrophicans *(Borrelia afzelii)*

**Q3** A 43-year-old woman presents with headaches. Until 3 years ago she was an airline stewardess, but she now works at a ticket desk at the airport. She is married with three children, all of whom are in good health. She was well until 2 weeks ago when she developed severe headaches that started waking her up in the early hours of the morning. The headaches are pounding in nature, characteristically starting behind her right eye, and she says that her husband mentioned that her eye had gone red on one occasion. She has also noticed that the headaches are associated with a feeling of having a blocked nose and this tends to occur with a runny eye. Her medical history is unremarkable. She has suffered from irritable bowel in the past, but this has settled over the last 6 years. She is not taking any medication.

| ON EXAMINATION | INVESTIGATION |
| --- | --- |
| • Unremarkable | • CT scan of the head: NAD |

CT: computed tomography; NAD: no abnormality detected.

### a) What is the most likely diagnosis?

i) chronic paroxysmal hemicrania

ii) trigeminal neuralgia

iii) migraine variants

iv) migrainous neuralgia

v) chronic sinusitis

Whoops. The answer here is easy to tease out, although all of the choices seem likely. This is one of those questions that you either recognise as a 'classic textbook description' or you haven't a clue and, therefore, get no marks. It's not at all fair, although the MRCP examination does unfortunately love questions like this. However, there aren't that many of them, and we'll try to cover most of them as we go along. Shy–Drager syndrome is a classic and so too is phenytoin overdose; a typical example is of a recurrently ataxic child with an epileptic grandma – the damn kid has been eating her pills.

You can usually tell that a question is one of the 'classics' due to the specific symptoms described. Here, the history of severe headaches with nasal stuffiness and a unilateral runny eye should alert you to an odd diagnosis. Chronic paroxysmal hemicrania, also known as Sjaastad syndrome, usually presents with several small attacks at any time during the day, with one of the diagnostic criteria being at least 50 attacks in a day. Trigeminal neuralgia has a specific distribution to the pain, precipitation factors, and also occurs at any time during the day. Migraine variants present with a host of symptoms such as an atypical sensory and motor aura, focal neurology, or even gastrointestinal manifestations. A normal CT scan rules out sinusitis. That leaves us with only one remaining option...

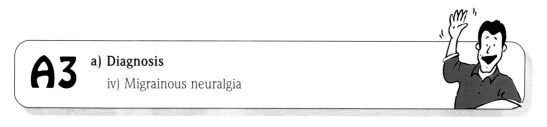

## A3  a) Diagnosis
 iv) Migrainous neuralgia

### ADDITIONAL BITS: THE BULLS**T BOX AND THE SURGICAL SIEVE

Some features in the history can give you clues. Traditionally, the examiners have been very keen to stereotype certain occupations with certain diseases, so below is a list of these.

### BULLS**T BOX

| PROFESSION | DISEASE |
|---|---|
| Health care professionals | Factitious illnesses (e.g. hypoglycaemia due to recurrent insulin administration) |
| Farmers | Farmer's lung |
| Scientists | Weil's disease or rat allergies |
| Bar staff/civil servants | Alcoholism |
| Travelling businessmen/bachelors | Sexually transmitted diseases |

We apologise to these professions, but it is honestly not our fault. In fact, some traditional stereotypes appear in the examinations, but are too defamatory to print in this book. Keep your eyes open and prepare your own list! And once you have it, keep it to yourself. For remember the two most important rules in life:

### 1) DON'T TELL EVERYONE EVERYTHING YOU KNOW

### 2)

Occasionally, your mind might go blank when faced with a question. You can spot the obvious pathology, but cannot remember the appropriate list. Under such circumstances, you need to make up your own list 'on the hoof'. We have a strategy for this, involving the mnemonic TIE HIM IN: trauma, infection, endocrine, haematological, iatrogenic, metabolic, idiopathic, neoplastic. For almost all of these, there is a subdivision:

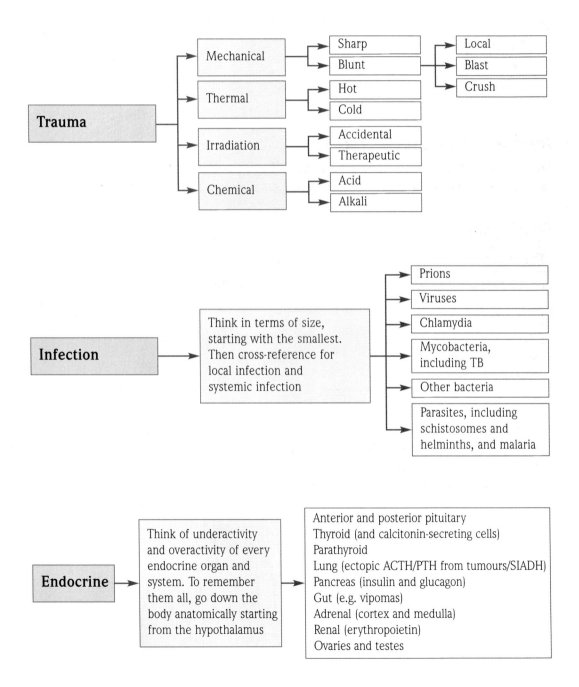

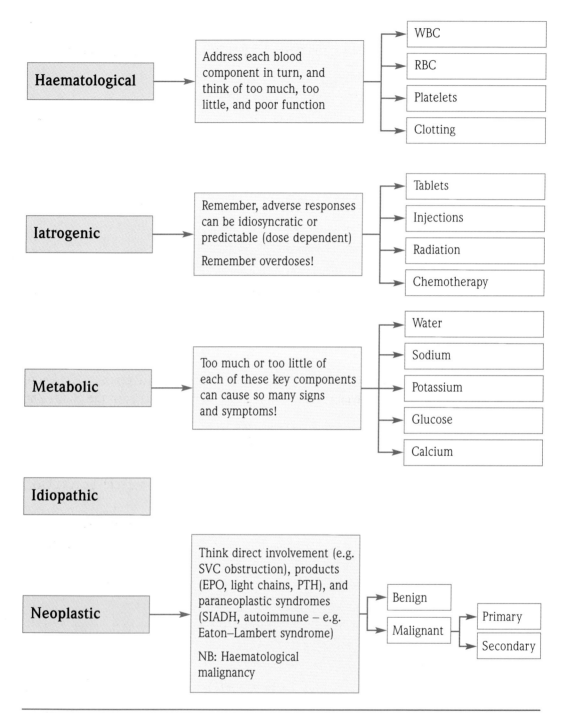

ACTH: adrenocorticotrophic hormone; EPO: erythropoietin; PTH: parathyroid hormone; RBC: red blood cell; SIADH: syndrome of inappropriate antidiuretic hormone secretion; SVC: superior vena cava; TB: tuberculosis; WBC: white blood cell.

## CROSS-CHECKS

Once you have gone through this sieve, run through a few final cross-checks. Have you checked:

- each system in turn: respiratory, central nervous system, etc.?
- occupational, tropical, and autoimmune diseases?
- those diseases peculiar to the young or old?
- the usual suspects (systemic lupus erythematosus, sarcoidosis, amyloidosis, tuberculosis)?

If nothing on your list seems to fit, then think:

- overdose? (Has the patient been eating grandma's phenytoin?)
- is this a 'syndrome' I should recognise?

**Always** remember intoxication and drugs – you can be sure that the patients and examiners will lay traps for you.

## SUMMARY

From these questions, you should be able to see how to tackle the MRCP examination. These are the same rules that we use when making a diagnosis on the wards or in the clinic. The plan is simple:

1) Ignore the 'white smoke' and write down all the findings that are *always abnormal*.
2) From these findings, select those for which there is a *limited list* of potential causes.
3) Write down the list of causes for each finding. Don't worry – we shall be teaching you these as we go along. You have already learnt two.
4) Look at the lists you have written down. The correct diagnosis must appear on all of the lists. If there is only one overlapping factor, then this is the diagnosis that you seek.
5) If there is more than one diagnosis that appears on all of your lists, then go through factors that might *exclude* some diagnoses.
6) Look at those you have left. From the information you have available, select the diagnosis that fits best, and run with this one.

If there seem to be no useful lists then it is likely that this is one of the 'you either recognise it or you don't' questions. There is not much of a strategy to adopt here. However, we will try to cover most of the 'classic cases' as we go along.

Rather than going through lists in a random order, we shall try to approach them in groupings by system or symptom. You will find that lists appear again and again; this is to help you learn by repetition. We have also tried to vary the way in which you can learn a list: some are alphabetical, some equations, some mnemonics, some acronyms, and some appear as pictures or verse. Please do not feel constrained by the way lists are presented – feel free to find your own way to remember them.

Good luck and enjoy. Remember, like other books in the 'Joy of...' series, you can work on this alone or, even better, with friends, anytime and anywhere!

# QUIZ SPOT!

### CRITERIA CONNECTIONS

Connect the Duckett Jones criteria to the right class: major criteria or minor criteria. Which ones are missing, and how many criteria are needed to make the diagnosis of rheumatic fever (answers on page 220)?

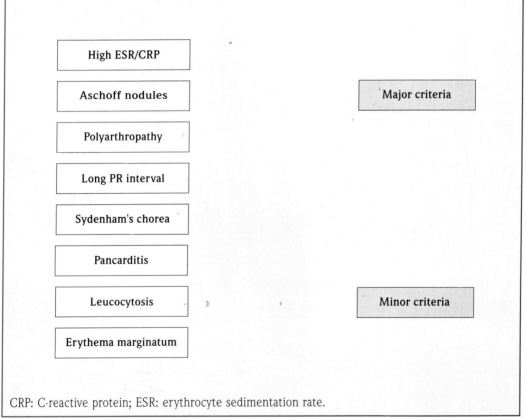

CRP: C-reactive protein; ESR: erythrocyte sedimentation rate.

# 2

# NERVOUS TICKS ON THE LIST

NEUROLOGICAL MRCP LISTS

## CAUSES OF INTRACRANIAL CALCIFICATION

| | |
|---|---|
| Tumours | Glioma (astrocytoma, oligodendroglioma), meningioma, craniopharyngioma (90% in children), ependymoma, pinealoma, teratoma, chordoma, dermoid, and cholesteatoma. Lipomas are usually midline and have typical curved bands of calcification |
| Vascular | Atheroma, aneurysm, angioma, subdural haematoma, and intracerebral haematoma |
| Infection and infestation (often multiple) | Tuberculosis (basal meninges), toxoplasmosis (paraventricular), cytomegalovirus, cysticercosis (usually supratentorial), pyogenic abscess, hydatid, and *Paragonimus westermani* |
| Miscellaneous | Phakomatosis: tuberous sclerosis, Sturge–Weber syndrome (characterised by tram lines), von Hippel–Lindau syndrome, neurofibromatosis types 1 and 2, and Gorlin's syndrome<br>Renal failure plus dialysis |
| Basal ganglia | Birth anoxia (idiopathic [most common] bilateral and symmetrical), radiation, mitochondrial diseases, Fahr's disease, hypoparathyroidism, pseudohypoparathyroidism, and infarction |

**Q4** A 72-year-old man presents complaining that he has had to give up smoking against his will. Painters have been redecorating his flat for some weeks. He has been effectively housebound and feels that he has been continually exposed to the fumes. His smoker's cough has worsened and precipitated his cigarette abstinence. His GP has prescribed erythromycin and amoxycillin for what appears to be an almost constant cough. He has taken arrowroot as a homeopathic remedy. He has found it increasingly difficult to handle his cigarettes and matches during this period. He says that his hand is weak, as it was when he had Guillain–Barré syndrome 10 years ago.

## On examination

- Coarse skin
- Rattling chest
- Beefy, red tongue
- Downgoing left plantar; right plantar is equivocal
- Guttering between the metacarpals of both hands
- Wax blocking left ear
- Right pupil = 3 mm diameter; left pupil = 4 mm diameter. Both react well to light.
- Forehead furrowed
- Eyebrows raised

### a) What is the diagnosis?

    i)    lead poisoning

    ii)   Pancoast tumour

    iii)  hypothyroidism

    iv)  Guillain–Barré syndrome

    v)   syringomyelia

OK. This is easy enough for some. As always, there is much evidence given to try to confuse. The paint story is to make you think about toxic solvents. The past Guillain–Barré syndrome is a red herring. The inclusion of dry skin is probably an effort to make you think of myxoedema. Wax in the ear – ignore it. Here the trick is to tease out what we really know to be the abnormalities, and they have been deliberately obscured. We know that a hand is weak, and that there is 'guttering'. This tells us that he has wasting of the intrinsic muscles of the hands, which are supplied by T1. Could this be a T1 lesion in a smoker? Yes. This is a classic case of Pancoast tumour. What about the eye? One pupil is definitely smaller than the other. The eyebrows are raised, which suggests compensation for a ptosis. Ptosis plus a small pupil suggests classic Horner's syndrome.

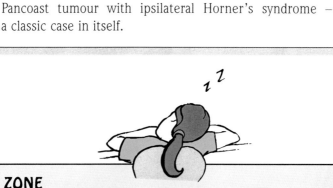

**A4** a) **Diagnosis**
ii) So, we have a slight variation. You have had to spot two classic cases and put them together. The patient has a Pancoast tumour with ipsilateral Horner's syndrome – a classic case in itself.

**REVISION ZONE**
These classics rely upon a knowledge of the typical pupillary syndromes, of which there are four: Horner's syndrome, third nerve palsy, Argyll Robertson pupil, and Holmes–Adie syndrome. So let's have a look at these.

### HORNER'S CORNER, TRAMPS, LADIES OF THE NIGHT, AND HERMITS

*(Little Jack) Horner's syndrome*

How would you feel if you had just stuck in your thumb and pulled out a plum? Just like Miss Muffet sitting on her tuffet, this might generate some form of sympathetic response. Facially, you might be expected to go wide-eyed, sweaty, and for your eyes to pop out like organ stops. Loss of sympathetic activity (causing Horner's syndrome) produces the exact opposite – a sunken eye (enophthalmos) with a small pupil, partial ptosis, and ipsilateral loss of sweating. The course of the sympathetic supply may be interrupted at one of two main points:

- its origin: stroke, syrinx, tumour, encephalitis, multiple sclerosis (MS) plaque, or anything else in the surgical sieve that might hit the brainstem
- the neck: carotid aneurysm, Pancoast tumour, or trauma

Alternatively, the features and causes can be remembered another way:

*Little Jack Horner, 'e SSATT\* in the corner*
*There with his sunken eye*
*His small pupil hid*
*'Neath his poor drooping lid*
*With the side of his face crisp and dry!*

\*Encephalitis, Stroke, Syrinx, Aneurysm of the carotid, Tumour (including Pancoast), Trauma

Congenital Horner's syndrome is benign and often associated with heterochromia (one iris differs in colour from the other).

*Tramps*

Why is a third nerve palsy known as the tramps' palsy? Because of the complete ptosis or the dilated pupil? No; it is because the eye is found to be looking 'down and out'!

Third nerve palsy complicates the diagnosis of raised intracranial pressure, as the third nerve stretches under the uncus and palsy produces a false lateralising sign. Equally, in the presence of a headache (painful third nerve palsy), the diagnosis is of a rapidly expanding posterior communicating artery aneurysm until proven otherwise; this is a reason for immediate admission and a computed tomography (CT) or magnetic resonance imaging (MRI) scan. The pupil is frequently involved because the parasympathetic fibres from the Edinger–Westphal nucleus to the pupil lie on the outside of the third nerve, where they are vulnerable to an expanding mass. Diabetes mellitus can cause a palsy that is usually painless. Diabetes can also cause inflammation or thrombosis of the vasa nervorum to the third nerve, which predominantly affects the central nerve fibres of the third nerve, hence resulting in pupillary sparing.

Examinations often refer to Weber's syndrome (third nerve palsy with contralateral hemiplegia), which is due to a basilar artery event causing infarction of a cerebral peduncle.

*Put another way,* **the causes** *of a third nerve palsy* are those that damage the origin of the nerve in the midbrain (e.g. midbrain amyloid, MS, Weber's syndrome), those that damage the nerve vasculature (e.g. diabetes, vasculitis due to systemic lupus erythematosus, rheumatoid arthritis, polyarteritis nodosa), and nerve compression and stretch (e.g. posterior cerebral artery aneurysms, tumours). Transient and repetitive paroxysmal third nerve palsies can occur with migraines.

*Ladies of the night*

The Argyll Robertson pupil was classically said to be due to syphilis and, in a weak pun, earned the name of the 'prostitute's pupil', as it does not like the light much, but is very accommodating; it is characterised by small, irregular pupils that do not react to light, but do accommodate. This is a little unfair, now that the most common cause is diabetes mellitus. Other aetiologies include: long-standing Adie's syndrome, encephalitis, amyloidosis, midbrain tumours (e.g. pinealoma), sarcoidosis, Lyme disease, and the presence of chronic iritis.

*Hermits*

Holmes–Adie pupil usually occurs in women, and is mostly unilateral. It is characterised by a myotonic pupil – a dilated pupil that responds sluggishly to light. Unlike the Argyll Robertson pupil, the hermit's Holmes–Adie pupil does not like the light much (if at all) and is not very accommodating, although it can be persuaded to accommodate slowly. Knee and ankle jerks may be absent.

## CAUSES OF A DILATED PUPIL (MYDRIASIS)

- Topical mydriatic drugs (e.g. atropine, homatropine, tropicamide, cyclopentolate)
- Sympathomimetic drugs (e.g. amphetamines)
- Anticholinergic drugs (e.g. tricyclic antidepressants)
- Third nerve lesion (note that some lesions may be pupillary sparing)
- Holmes–Adie syndrome
- Phaeochromocytoma
- Retrobulbar neuritis/optic atrophy
- Iridectomy
- Congenital

## CAUSES OF A CONSTRICTED PUPIL (MIOSIS)

- Drugs: opiates (reversed by naloxone), parasympathomimetics (e.g. pilocarpine), organophosphate toxicity, cholinesterase inhibitors, phenothiazines
- Pontine haemorrhage (obtunded patient with Cheyne–Stokes respiration and focal neurological signs)
- Encephalitis
- Horner's syndrome
- Iritis and keratitis
- Argyll Robertson pupil
- Sleep and sedatives
- Congenital

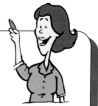

# Q5

You are asked to examine a 23-year-old woman with recurrent headaches on one of the medical wards. She has had the headaches for about 1 year, and they have occurred at all times of the day. She denies any paraesthesia, but complains of an occasional episode of blurred vision. No episodes of loss of consciousness have occurred. According to her medical history, she had mild asthma as a child, suffered from a prolonged attack of measles at the age of 4 years, and suffered whiplash in a road traffic accident 5 years ago. Her father and paternal grandfather suffered from migraine. Her only medication at the moment is the oral contraceptive pill, which she has been taking for 7 years. Apart from the occasional muscle ache after exercise, she admits to no other symptoms. She has two jobs – one working in a cake shop by day and one on a petrol forecourt in the evenings – which she finds very stressful.

On examination, she is 5 ft tall and weighs 120 kg. Her blood pressure is 132/72 mmHg and she has a pulse of 91 beats/min. Examination of the respiratory and cardiovascular systems shows nothing remarkable. Her reflexes are normal and her plantar response is downgoing. Apart from some slight difficulty with past-pointing, she has no other cerebellar signs. Fundoscopy shows that both disc margins are blurred, but she has no signs of other retinopathy. Her gastrointestinal examination is normal.

| INVESTIGATIONS | RESULTS |
| --- | --- |
| Urea and electrolytes | Normal |
| Full blood count | Normal |
| Serum calcium/phosphate levels | Normal |
| Arterial blood gas analysis | Normal |
| Chest X-ray | Normal |
| CT scan of the head | Unremarkable |
| MRI scan of the brain | Normal |
| Lumbar puncture | No oligoclonal bands |

## a) What is the most likely diagnosis?

   i)    subacute sclerosing panencephalitis

   ii)   migraine

   iii)  benign intracranial hypertension

   iv)  central retinal vein thrombosis

   v)   MS

**b) What is the most important step in her management?**

   i)    repeated lumbar puncture

   ii)   start acetazolamide

   iii)  daily ophthalmic survey

   iv)  lose weight

   v)   stop the oral contraceptive pill

There are a myriad of red herrings here – stress, past head injury, and a family history of migraine, to name but a few. There is only *one* finding that is always pathological, and for which there is a limited list of causes, and this is papilloedema. Write down your list now. *Don't look down – no cheating!*

_____

_____

_____

_____

_____

Once you have established that the patient is not hypertensive and has no respiratory problems, and excluded the possibility of mass lesions and MS through investigations, then the diagnosis should be easy. She is of entirely normal weight – *for someone 7 ft tall!* To anyone else, she is at best 'vertically and nutritionally challenged'. In addition, she takes the oral contraceptive pill. Together, these facts should swing you towards a diagnosis of benign intracranial hypertension. The only problem left to you now is to know the management. Being the MRCP examination, it is tempting to think of the most bizarre forms of treatment. In reality, the examiners would like you to be sensible. Do not be too clever.

**A: Papilloedema**

- benign intracranial pressure
- malignant hypertension
- mass lesions
- hypercapnia
- central retinal vein or cavernous sinus thrombosis
- hydrocephalus
- vitamin A toxicity
- lead poisoning and optic neuritis

The only serious and permanent complication of benign intracranial hypertension is loss of vision. Although the treatment involves acetazolamide, in certain situations the very first lumbar puncture may resolve the symptoms, obviating its need. In other cases, repeated lumbar punctures will only transiently drop the pressures. The ophthalmic survey should include visual acuity testing and visual field testing (perhaps the most sensitive indicator). Deteriorating vision is an indication for urgent surgery to relieve papilloedema.

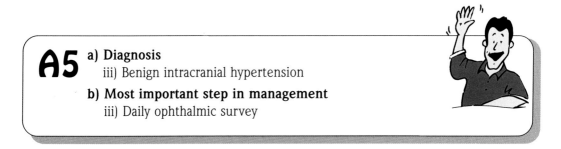

**A5** a) **Diagnosis**
   iii) Benign intracranial hypertension
   b) **Most important step in management**
   iii) Daily ophthalmic survey

## FOR THE RECORD

Benign intracranial hypertension is also known as pseudotumour cerebri. It occurs most frequently in women aged 15–44 years. There are many presumptive risk factors, most notably a high body mass index (obesity), pregnancy, and use of the oral contraceptive pill. Other associations used in MRCP examinations include the use of tetracyclines (e.g. patients treated for acne), corticosteroids, or lithium.

## Q6

A 23-year-old woman presents to her GP with headache, nausea, and vomiting. She works as a cleaner in a local supermarket. She is married with three children. She had an appendectomy at the age of 6 years and has complained of dysmenorrhoea since her periods started at the age of 14 years. She is otherwise relatively fit and well. Examination reveals bilateral blurring of the optic discs. She has a mild degree of past-pointing bilaterally on testing, and a broad-based gait. Otherwise, examination of the nervous system is unremarkable. Her blood pressure is 120/90 mmHg and she has a pulse rate of 90 beats/min. Clinical examination, including gynaecological examination, is otherwise entirely normal.

| INVESTIGATIONS | RESULTS |
| --- | --- |
| Plasma sodium | 132 mmol/l |
| Plasma potassium | 3.9 mmol/l |
| Plasma bicarbonate | 24 mmol/l |
| Plasma urea | 4.3 mmol/l |
| Plasma glucose | 3.6 mmol/l |
| Haemoglobin | 20.2 g/dl |
| White cell count | $3.6 \times 10^9/l$ |
| Platelets | $189 \times 10^9/l$ |
| Erythrocyte sedimentation rate | 1 mm in first hour |
| Kidneys | Normal |
| Liver | Normal |
| Spleen | Normal |
| Ovaries and uterus | Appear normal |

## a) Which test would you order next?

i) total red cell volume or red cell mass

ii) urine or blood erythropoietin level

iii) CT or MRI scan of the brain

iv) visual field testing by static or kinetic perimetry

v) bone marrow biopsy

**b) Why is the erythrocyte sedimentation rate (ESR) only 1?**

_____

_____

**c) What is the most likely diagnosis?**

    i)     polycythaemia rubra vera

    ii)    cerebellar haemangioblastoma

    iii)   Gaisböck's syndrome

    iv)   medulloblastoma

    v)    MS

_Cover the page below, and read line by line._

Here we go again!

First, what are the key findings that are _always_ abnormal and for which there are defined lists of causes? Write them down.

Now, which diagnosis appears on all of the lists?

_Don't turn over until you have finished your lists and come up with your answer._

Your list here...

_____

_____

_____

_____

_____

_____

_____

_____

_____

_____

This question requires you to notice that this patient has a grossly abnormal elevated haemoglobin level and papilloedema.

## PAPILLOEDEMA

Papilloedema may be benign (benign intracranial pressure, which of course isn't benign) or malignant (malignant hypertension or tumour). Other causes include:

- mass lesions in (abscess or benign tumour) or around (e.g. chronic subdural) the brain
- too much blood getting in: hypercapnia causes loss of cerebral autoregulation
- too little blood getting out: central retinal vein, sagittal sinus, or cavernous sinus thrombosis
- too little cerebrospinal fluid (CSF) getting out: hydrocephalus, including post-subarachnoid haemorrhage
- lead poisoning, optic neuritis, vitamin A toxicity

## POLYCYTHAEMIA

*Relative*

- dehydration
- Gaisböck's syndrome (stress)

*Primary*

- polycythaemia rubra vera
  (splenomegaly, raised platelets)

*Secondary*

- hypoxia
- chronic obstructive pulmonary disease
- altitude
- abnormal haemoglobins
- sleep apnoea

*Excess erythropoietin*

- cerebellar haemangioma
- hepatoma
- phaeochromocytoma
- hypernephroma
- polycystic/transplant kidneys
- uterine leiomyoma/fibroma

## WORKING IT OUT

This is a tricky question, and takes our thoughts to a slightly higher and 'more devious' level. Clearly, any 'true' polycythaemia causes hyperviscosity and can lead to cerebral vessel thrombosis, whether cavernous sinus, sagittal sinus, or central vein. These can all cause papilloedema, and so all causes of true polycythaemia suddenly become candidates. However, there can only be one correct answer. There is usually a 'list overlap' or a clue, and in this case you have both.

Something is going on in the cerebellum (the clues being the past-pointing and balance problem). You will know all the signs of cerebellar disease – they were first comprehensively described by Gordon Holmes (Professor of Neurology at the National Hospital for Neurology, Queen Square, London, UK) based on his meticulous observations of soldiers with cerebellar bullet wounds in the First World War. These signs include atonia (low tone), ataxia, overshoot, asynergy and dysdiadochokinesis, past-pointing, and intention tremor, along with a broad-based gait, impaired eye movements including nystagmus (towards the lesion), and scanning speech. Remember that these signs are predominantly from the cerebellar hemispheres, not the vermis. Midline (or vermis) lesions often have none of these signs, but such patients are troubled by truncal ataxia or the inability to maintain posture, along with marked nausea, vomiting, and vertigo.

*Those who have strokes at the back of the brain*
*Will vomit and say they can't walk straight again*
*Ataxic, nystagmic, past-point finger-nose*
*Intent on a tremor, they scan with their prose*
*If hit in the vermis they all comb their hair*
*Instead they can't walk or sit down on a chair*

So, are there any cerebellar problems on the 'polycythaemic' list? Yes! Cerebellar haemangioblastomas are seen in von Hippel–Lindau syndrome.

Does this fit with the list of causes of papilloedema? Yes – a vascular tumour. Of course, you could have reached the same conclusion by using your list of causes of cerebellar syndromes. Write one down now. We shall be telling you what the list is in a moment.

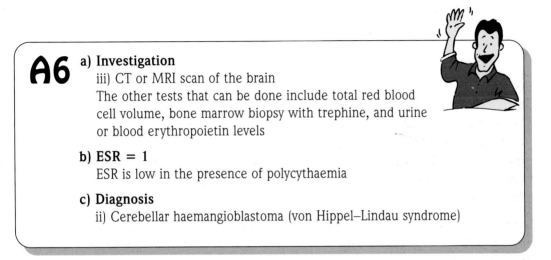

**A6**

**a) Investigation**
   iii) CT or MRI scan of the brain
   The other tests that can be done include total red blood cell volume, bone marrow biopsy with trephine, and urine or blood erythropoietin levels

**b) ESR = 1**
   ESR is low in the presence of polycythaemia

**c) Diagnosis**
   ii) Cerebellar haemangioblastoma (von Hippel–Lindau syndrome)

# QUIZ SPOT!

**Q:** What are the causes of a very low ESR?

**A:** Polycythaemia
Afbrinogenaemia and hypofibrinogenaemia
Remember, as a simple rule the ESR should be age ÷ 2 (and in females, add 10 to the result)

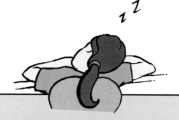

**REVISION ZONE**

**The eyes have it!**

We have had a nice (common) case of papilloedema. You now need to remind yourself of the other common problems at the back of the eye.

## OPTIC ATROPHY (THE PALLID DISC)

Write down your list of causes in the space below. Then check it against ours (which follows).

Your list here...

## OUR LIST

In the presence of pallor posterior to the pupil, proceed to peruse paediatrics (Friedreich's ataxia, Leber's optic atrophy, and Wolfram's syndrome [DIDMOAD – diabetes insipidus, diabetes mellitus, optic atrophy, and deafness] are the main congenital ones to remember), papilloedema (longstanding), pressure (e.g. compression by tumour or glaucoma), poisons (quinine overdose, tobacco amblyopia, wood alcohol), Paget's disease, pernicious anaemia and poor diet (vitamin B$_{12}$ deficiency), pulselessness (retinal artery ischaemia), psyphilis, and pmultiple sclerosis (it is a little known fact that these last two have a silent 'p').

Now list the causes of papilloedema (already learnt; see page 29)...

-----------------------------------------------------------------------------------------------
-----------------------------------------------------------------------------------------------
-----------------------------------------------------------------------------------------------
-----------------------------------------------------------------------------------------------
-----------------------------------------------------------------------------------------------
-----------------------------------------------------------------------------------------------
-----------------------------------------------------------------------------------------------
-----------------------------------------------------------------------------------------------
-----------------------------------------------------------------------------------------------
-----------------------------------------------------------------------------------------------
-----------------------------------------------------------------------------------------------
-----------------------------------------------------------------------------------------------
-----------------------------------------------------------------------------------------------
-----------------------------------------------------------------------------------------------

*Angioid retinal streaks*

These are seen as visible thickening and calcification of the elastic layer of Bruch's membrane. The causes may be remembered as the female who is doing a streak.

"...**perhaps** she **shall bicycle across** the road with **her elastic** loose"

or

"...**Paget's** she **thal bisickle acro** the road with **Ehlers elasticum** loose"

Paget's disease, thalassaemia, sickle cell anaemia, acromegaly, Ehlers–Danlos syndrome, pseudoxanthoma elasticum.

*Pseudoxanthoma elasticum*

- recessive or dominant inheritance of a defect in a cholesterol transporter gene

- the recipe for 'chicken skin' lesions? Saggy skin with buttery papules and plaques (seen in the face, neck, axilla, antecubital fossa, popliteal fossa, and groin)

- cardiovascular complications include premature vascular disease with claudication or myocardial infarction

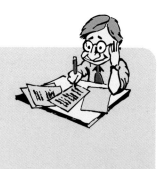

**CHOROIDORETINITIS**

Repeat after me:

*Choroid makes it hard to see*
*When hit with all the nasty three*
*But sarcoid, syphilis, TB*
*With tox may go, and CMV!*

CMV: cytomegalovirus; sarcoid: sarcoidosis; TB: tuberculosis; tox: toxoplasmosis and toxocariasis.

*Retinitis pigmentosa*

Remember that retinitis pigmentosa usually affects the peripheral retina, sparing the macula and, therefore, resulting in tunnel vision.

Diseases associated with retinitis pigmentosa (corpuscular retinal pigmentation) are:

- hereditary ataxias such as Friedreich's ataxia, an autosomal recessive or sex-linked condition. Spinal cord atrophy occurs with degeneration of the spinocerebellar tracts (hence cerebellar signs), corticospinal tracts (hence long-tract signs), and dorsal columns. Peripheral neuropathies make this one of the causes of extensor plantars and absent ankle jerks. It also causes cardiomyopathy, scoliosis, and pes cavus
- Refsum's disease: an autosomal recessive neuropathy causing anosmia, deafness, and sensory neuropathy, with cerebellar ataxia and a high CSF protein concentration
- Laurence–Moon–Biedl syndrome: an autosomal recessive disorder characterised by obesity, polydactyly, intellectual retardation, hypogonadism, renal dysgenesis, diabetes mellitus, and endocrinopathies
- Alport's syndrome: hereditary nephritis
- Kearns–Sayre syndrome: a mitochondrial disease caused by deletions of mitochondrial DNA – note the link with mitochondria
- Usher's syndrome: causes sensorineural hearing impairment
- abetalipoproteinaemia and vitamin E deficiency

## A QUICK JOKE

A woman accompanied her husband to the doctor, on account of his failing vision. Afterwards, the doctor takes the wife aside. "Do all I say, or your husband will go blind. You must make him his favourite breakfast each morning, to set him up for the day. In the evening, let him relax while you prepare a sumptuous five-course spread. Don't let him do any household chores. Have sex with him as often as he likes, and fulfil his every whim and fancy – no matter how depraved!"

On the way home, the husband turns to his wife. "I saw the doctor take you aside. Is everything going to be OK?"

"No," she replied, "you're going to go blind."

## BEFORE WE MOVE ON...

Have a quick think. Can you remember:

- the causes of polyarthralgia?

------------------------------------------------
------------------------------------------------
------------------------------------------------
------------------------------------------------

- the revised Duckett Jones criteria?

------------------------------------------------
------------------------------------------------
------------------------------------------------
------------------------------------------------

- all about the three phases of Lyme disease?

------------------------------------------------
------------------------------------------------
------------------------------------------------
------------------------------------------------

Can you write down the surgical sieve?

------------------------------------------------
------------------------------------------------
------------------------------------------------
------------------------------------------------
------------------------------------------------
------------------------------------------------

Now check your answers against the lists: causes of polyarthralgia (page 5), the revised Duckett Jones criteria (page 7), the three phases of Lyme disease (page 10), and the surgical sieve (pages 13–14).

## BRAIN BITS AND CORD CHUNKS

*Cerebellar syndromes*

Remind yourself of the clinical features. In particular, is the nystagmus oscillation towards or away from the lesion? Remember that vermis lesions are different. Can you recite the verse you should have learnt (page 30)?

For the causes of cerebellar syndromes, go through the usual surgical sieve, but remember: they need a: **FAT CAT** Scan for **MS**.

Friedreich's ataxia
Alcohol*
Tumours:         primary:      cerebellar haemangioblastomas
                                      von Hippel–Lindau syndrome
                      secondary:  especially lung cancer as a paraneoplastic syndrome
Congenital:     ataxia telangiectasia and Arnold–Chiari malformations
Strokes
MS

Rarer causes of cerebellar syndromes include:

- metabolic causes (thiamine deficiency, hypothyroidism)
- drugs and toxins (phenytoin, barbiturates, alcoholism, lead poisoning)

Note that ataxia telangiectasia is associated with immunodeficiency, cancer susceptibility, radiosensitivity, and elevated serum α-fetoprotein levels.

*Alcohol abuse causes cerebellar degeneration. Strangely, this happens to us acutely and reversibly, with 10 pints of finest lager causing ataxia, slurred speech, nausea, and vertigo. This syndrome – known to experts as 'bed spin' – is poorly detailed in standard texts. You can try it out for yourselves on the night that you pass this damned examination. You'll find that we are right.

## Spastic paraparesis

Anatomically, there are few options for the site of the lesion. Being spastic, it has to be an upper motor neurone problem. The only site that will hit both legs (only) is across the spinal cord, or parasagittally with something (usually a parasagittal meningioma) pressing on the cortical motor strip. If there are no sensory signs at all, then the latter is the most likely diagnosis, especially if there are any other signs above the foramen magnum (such as raised intracranial pressure, epilepsy, or other focal neurology). If there is a sensory level deficit and no signs above the foramen magnum, a cord lesion is more likely. Use your sieve to produce a list of cord lesion causes:

## OK? FINISHED?

Well, barring all the usual causes of cord compression, the main ones (and those that people miss) are:

- transverse myelitis complicating a viral infection (such as HIV), MS, or a paraneoplastic syndrome
- sudden vascular occlusion: this can be due to compression by a tumour or extradural abscess, or secondary to a vasculitis. In the case of an abscess or tumour, there may not be loss of a complete sensory level (e.g. posterior columns may be spared)
- tropical spastic paraparesis: this is a complication of human T-cell lymphoma virus type I/III infection, the other complication of which is lymphoma. It is most commonly seen in those of Afro-Caribbean descent, and presents with a very slow (over decades) paralysis after initial backache and constipation

## ABSENT ANKLE JERKS, EXTENSOR PLANTARS

Work out your own way of remembering this list of causes. As to whether it is actually of any use is debatable; nobody we know remembers this ever turning up as a part II question. The main causes are:

- syringomyelia
- taboparesis (syphilis)
- Friedreich's ataxia
- cervical spondylosis and peripheral neuropathy
- motor neurone disease
- subacute combined degeneration of the cord

## Brain juice

Look out for the following changes:

*Lymphocytosis*

Think 'inflammation without ordinary bacteria'. Work your way through your surgical sieve, write a list, then compare it with ours.

Your list here...

## OUR LIST

The 'not ordinary bacteria' list includes all of the 'odd-ball' infections:

- viruses (including HIV)
- fungi
- syphilis
- *Rickettsia* (Lyme disease, caused by *Borrelia burgdorferi*)
- *Listeria*
- *Brucella*
- *Coxiella*
- *Mycoplasma*
- Whipple's disease

Abscess and tuberculous meningitis/encephalitis are the ones most commonly found in the MRCP examination.

The 'not infections at all' list includes:

- tumours
- MS
- systemic lupus erythematosus
- sarcoidosis
- Behçet's syndrome

Remember, there are some catches. Cerebral lymphoproliferative disease can produce CSF full of 'lymphocytes'. A woman treated with steroids for $>1$ year for flares of cerebral sarcoidosis (the MRI scan had suggested cerebral sarcoidosis and the CSF was full of lymphocytes) complained of gum bleeding when brushing her teeth. A blood film showed her to have acute lymphoblastic leukaemia. The cells in the CSF were not lymphocytes, but mature lymphoblasts. She had responded well to steroids, which are very good at killing lymphoblasts.

Another catch? Partially treated bacterial meningitis may present with a CSF lymphocytosis.

## Raised protein, normal CSF cells

Note that Guillain–Barré syndrome is a motor neuropathy that occurs after an infection (often viral). It can be recurrent. The catches? Well, they can sell it to you as respiratory failure, and with sensory symptoms (although *signs* are usually absent). Beware, also, that the presence of a raised CSF cell count (especially lymphocytosis) is *not* compatible with Guillan–Barré syndrome, although a raised CSF protein level is compatible. The other causes of a raised CSF protein level with normal cell count are lead poisoning, cord compression, spinal block (Froin's syndrome), cord malignant deposits, syphilis, and subacute sclerosing panencephalitis.

## Is part II getting on your nerves yet?

## Peripheral polyneuropathy

Here is one way of remembering the list.

| | |
|---|---|
| Born unlucky: | Friedreich's ataxia, Refsum's disease, Charcot–Marie–Tooth disease |
| Three dejected: | • alcoholics due to the effects of alcohol |
| | • vitamin $B_1$, $B_6$, and $B_{12}$ deficiencies |
| | • isoniazid used to treat tuberculosis – which is why people receiving tuberculosis treatment must receive pyridoxine supplements |
| Two infected: | • leprosy |
| | • Guillain–Barré syndrome* |
| Two injected: | • paraneoplasia* in cancer patients, or the effects of its treatments such as vincristine and isoniazid |
| | • diabetes mellitus |
| One connected: | connective tissue disease, such as rheumatoid arthritis/systemic lupus erythematosus/polyarteritis nodosa |
| Granuloma suspected: | sarcoidosis, Churg–Strauss syndrome |
| Hypothyroid: | which just refuses to rhyme |

Sometimes, there is a motor neuropathy alone. This may be due to the duo starred* causes above, diabetic amyotrophy and diphtheria, porphyria (acute intermittent), polymyositis, or lead poisoning.

Another way of classifying neuropathies is as follows:

| AXONAL | DEMYELINATING | MONONEURITIS MULTIPLEX |
|---|---|---|
| • HSMN type I | • HSMN type II | • Diabetes mellitus |
| • Diabetes mellitus | • Diabetes mellitus | • Leprosy |
| • Vitamin $B_{12}$ deficiency | • Vitamin $B_{12}$ deficiency | • Connective tissue diseases |
| • Folate deficiency | • Paraprotein neuropathy | (e.g. PAN, SLE, RA, GCA) |
| • Renal failure | • Inflammation: | • Sarcoidosis |
| • Carcinomatous neuropathy | Guillain–Barré syndrome | • Malignancy |
| • Porphyria | and chronic inflammatory | • Amyloidosis |
| • Amyloidosis | demyelinating neuropathy | • Neurofibromatosis |
| • Toxins (e.g. phenytoin, | | • HIV infection/AIDS |
| isoniazid, nitrofurantoin, | | • Churg–Strauss syndrome |
| dapsone, organophosphate, | | |
| vincristine, alcohol, | | |
| heavy metals) | | |
| • HIV infection | | |
| • Critical care neuropathy | | |

GCA: giant cell arteritis; HSMN: hereditary sensory and motor neuropathy; PAN: polyarteritis nodosa; RA: rheumatoid arthritis; SLE: systemic lupus erythematosus.

You can make up your own ways of remembering these, if you want!

## CARPAL TUNNEL SYNDROME

The causes 'have got to be PRAM' (have **g**out **TB P²RA²M**).

**G**out, tuberculosis (**TB**), **p**regnancy/**p**ill, **r**heumatoid arthritis, **a**cromegaly, **a**myloidosis, and **m**yxoedema. Renal disease is said to be another 'r', and diabetes mellitus may be associated through amyloidosis.

# Q7

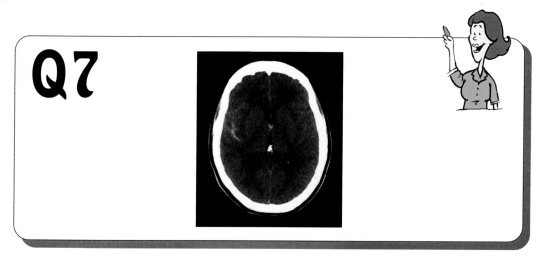

## a) What does this unenhanced CT scan show?

i)    acute extradural haematoma

ii)   acute subdural haematoma

iii)  nothing, it's normal

iv)   haemorrhagic infarct

v)    subarachnoid haemorrhage

### LET'S LOOK AT EACH OPTION IN TURN...

*Acute extradural haematoma*

High attenuation (white) on a scan indicates acute bleeding. It occurs in the periphery with a convex inner margin (see diagram, below left, shaped like an 'E' for extradural).

*Acute subdural haematoma*

This is a high attenuation lesion in the periphery. It has a crescent shape with an inner concave margin as blood accumulates between the dura and arachnoid mater (see diagram, below right, shaped like an 'S' for subdural). Look out for mass effect with subdural haematoma.

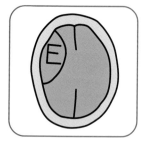
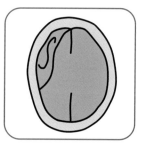

*Haemorrhagic infarct*

Haemorrhagic infarct appears white on the CT scan, whereas thromboembolic infarct appears black (low attenuation). The abnormality follows the distribution of the vascular supply of the brain.

*Subarachnoid haemorrhage*

Subarachnoid blood (white) replaces CSF in the basal cisterns, Sylvian fissures, sulci, and ventricles, as shown in the CT scan.

**b) Which of the following conditions is not associated with subarachnoid haemorrhage?**

   i)    fibromuscular dysplasia

   ii)   arteriovenous malformation

   iii)  polycystic kidney disease

   iv)  glioblastoma multiforme

   v)   coarctation of the aorta

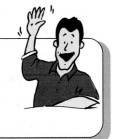

**A7**   **a) The CT scan shows**
            v) Subarachnoid haemorrhage
         **b) Not associated with subarachnoid haemorrhage**
            iv) Glioblastoma multiforme

The main cause of subarachnoid haemorrhage is a ruptured saccular aneurysm. Other causes include arteriovenous malformation, coagulopathy, and head injury. There are multiple risk factors, including hypertension (coarctation of the aorta causes hypertension), polycystic kidney disease, and connective tissue disease (fibromuscular dysplasia).

**DID YOU KNOW...**

...5% of subarachnoid haemorrhages are not evident on a CT scan (especially those with small bleeds).

...if the CT head scan is normal and clinical suspicion remains high, lumbar puncture should be carried out at least 12 hours after the onset of headache to look for xanthochromia. Its key pigment is bilirubin, resulting from the breakdown of red blood cells in the cerebrospinal fluid.

...xanthochromia can be detected 2–3 weeks after the onset of subarachnoid haemorrhage.

# Quiz Spot!

**Q:** Abdominal pain and peripheral neuropathy ought to flag up two classic MRCP examination thoughts. What are they?

A: Lead poisoning and acute intermittent porphyria

## Phew! Time for a drink and a break

When you start again, make sure that you have all of these lists completely sorted before you move on. This should be your habit on working through the book. Whenever you start again, run through **all** of the lists that you have learnt up to that point, and make sure that you still have them off pat.

## But before we finish, another quick joke...

As the businessman aged, he suffered increasingly frequent and severe headaches. He sought specialist help. The neurologist examined him thoroughly. "You have a one-in-a-million condition in which your testicles are pressed against the base of your spine. I can cure your headaches," he said, "but this will require castration. The way to relieve the pressure – and hence the headache – is to remove the testicles." Recognising the seriousness of the condition, the businessman felt that he had no choice.

With a clear mind (no headache and a considerably lighter undercarriage) the man left hospital after the operation. To cheer himself up, he decided to buy a suit. The salesman looked at him and, without blinking, said "Size 42 long." "Correct! How did you know?" The suit fitted perfectly. "It's my job. New shirt?" asked the salesman, "34 sleeve and $15\frac{1}{2}$ collar?" "Yes, and correct!" said the man. "How did you know?" "It's my job. Shoes? Size 10?" "Yes! Amazing! Perfect fit! How did you know?" "It's my job." "How about new underwear? Size 36?" "No," said the man, "I always wear size 34!" "Oh, no! No! No!" the salesman said. "You can't do that! It will push your testicles against the base of your spine and give you one hell of a headache."

## NEUROLOGY CLASSICS

Finally, there are some 'classic cases' that you ought to recognise. Here they are!

### Friedreich's ataxia

This is characterised by absent ankle jerks/extensor plantars, cerebellar ataxia, pyramidal tract disease, dorsal column/spinocerebellar sensory neuropathy, pes cavus, and optic atrophy.

It is associated with hypertrophic cardiomyopathy in up to 90% of patients and diabetes mellitus in 10%–20%. Various other features include sensorineural deafness, marfanoid features (kyphoscoliosis and high-arched palate), low IQ, and retinitis pigmentosa. Patients usually present early in their teens with debilitating neurology and die in their fourth decade of cardiac failure. They may appear as a case of 'absent ankle jerks and upgoing plantars' or dementia.

### Guillain–Barré syndrome

This is characterised by viral/coryzal illness, demyelinating neuropathy (sensory or motor), and bulbar weakness. The Miller–Fisher variant of Guillain–Barré syndrome is characterised by viral/coryzal illness, external ophthalmoplegia, descending motor neuropathy, and sensory ataxia.

Both patients with Guillain–Barré syndrome and those with Miller–Fisher syndrome have a very high CSF protein level. Other causes of a demyelinating neuropathy include diabetes mellitus, vitamin $B_{12}$ deficiency, diphtheria, and Charcot–Marie–Tooth disease.

### Hartnup disease

This is characterised by convulsions, cerebellar signs, mental retardation, diarrhoea, and photosensitivity.

### Huntington's disease

This is characterised by chorea, akinesia, rigidity, dementia, and genetic anticipation.

### Laurence–Moon–Biedl syndrome

This is characterised by retinitis pigmentosa, mental retardation, obesity, hypogonadism, and polydactyly. It is also associated with dwarfism and renal defects.

*Refsum's disease*

This is characterised by sensorimotor neuropathy, cerebellar ataxia, retinitis pigmentosa, and deafness. It is also associated with cataracts and ichthyosis (scaly skin). Like Friedreich's ataxia, it is also associated with cardiomyopathy and optic atrophy. Unlike Friedreich's ataxia, however, the symptoms of Refsum's are reversible with a diet low in phytanic acid.

*Shy–Drager syndrome*

This is characterised by parkinsonism (tremor, rigidity, and bradykinesia) and primary autonomic failure (e.g. postural hypotension).

Note that this is now part of the multi-system atrophy syndrome.

*Steele–Richardson–Olszewski syndrome*

This is characterised by parkinsonism (with marked axial rigidity), progressive supranuclear palsy, frontal lobe features, and dementia.

*Wilson's disease*

This is characterised by parkinsonism/dementia in younger patients, jaundice/cirrhosis, and proximal renal tubular acidosis.

Note that it is an autosomal recessive disease that causes failure of copper secretion into bile, hence causing acute liver failure, chronic hepatitis, or cirrhosis. The diagnosis is based upon decreased serum caeruloplasmin, increased urinary copper, haemolytic anaemia, slit lamp investigations that reveal Kayser–Fleischer rings, and liver biopsy. Treatment is copper chelation with penicillamine.

*Sturge–Weber syndrome*

This is characterised by port-wine stain, epilepsy, optic atrophy, choroid angioma, and squint.

*Wallenberg's syndrome*

This is characterised by ipsilateral Horner's syndrome/cerebellar signs/dysphagia/dysarthria/ trigeminal pain, contralateral spinothalamic sensory loss/mild hemiparesis, and hiccups. It is also known as lateral medullary syndrome or posterior inferior cerebellar artery syndrome. It usually presents with acute vertigo and vomiting.

*Wernicke's encephalopathy*

This is characterised by cerebellar ataxia, ophthalmoplegia with nystagmus, peripheral sensory neuropathy, and, of course, heavy alcohol use. It is largely due to thiamine/vitamin $B_1$ deficiency. A confirmatory test is an assay of red cell transketolase, which is reduced when thiamine is deficient. Some laboratories can now perform direct red cell thiamine assays.

*Acute intermittent porphyria*

This is characterised by peripheral motor neuropathy, papilloedema, abdominal pain, and syndrome of inappropriate antidiuretic hormone secretion. It is also associated with epilepsy in 20% of patients, fever, sinus tachycardia, hypertension, hypercholesterolaemia, psychosis, and, not surprisingly, depression!

*Chronic lead poisoning*

This is characterised by peripheral motor neuropathy, papilloedema/optic atrophy, abdominal pain, convulsions, aseptic meningitis, sideroblastic anaemia, chronic interstitial nephritis, and a blue line on the gums.

Note that high lead levels result in raised porphyrin levels due to an interruption of porphyrin metabolism. So, if the information given does not seem to fit with any of the porphyrias, think lead! Don't forget that lead poisoning also produces basophilic stippling on the blood film. In the MRCP examination, it occurs in plumbers, painters, or children with a pica for paint! It is treated with intravenous penicillamine, which acts as a chelating agent.

*Langerhans' cell histiocytosis (histiocytosis X)*

This is characterised by cranial diabetes insipidus, otitis externa, exophthalmos, rash, and lytic lesions on skull X-ray.

*Tuberous sclerosis*

This is characterised by epilepsy, mental retardation, adenoma sebaceum, subungual fibromata, café-au-lait spots, ash-leaf macules, and shagreen patches. It is associated with a higher than normal incidence of malignancy – in particular, retinal phakomas, renal and pulmonary hamartomas, and rhabdomyosarcomas.

*Syringomyelia*

This is characterised by lower-limb spastic paraparesis, upper-limb lower motor neurone weakness/wasting, Horner's syndrome, nystagmus, and 'balaclava' sensory loss.

Note that sneezing and coughing both increase intracerebral pressure and therefore exacerbate the symptoms in syringomyelia. It can also be associated with neural tube defects (e.g. myelomeningocele), a tethered spinal cord, and Chiari malformation of the skull and brainstem.

*Phenylketonuria*

This is characterised by epilepsy, mental retardation, and hypopigmentation. Phenylketonuria is routinely screened for in the UK on day 5 following birth using the Guthrie test. If positive, the treatment is a low-alanine diet in the first few months of life.

*von Hippel–Lindau syndrome*

This is characterised by retinal angiomas, cerebellar signs due to cerebellar haemangioblastomas, and polycythaemia due to excess erythropoietin production. It is an autosomal dominant disease.

*Mollaret's meningitis*

This is characterised by recurrent episodes of aseptic meningitis associated with recurrent herpetic infection, raised CSF pressure, and CSF lymphocytosis.

# 3

# PANTS

RESPIRATORY MRCP LISTS

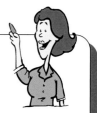

**Q8** A 63-year-old man presents to the outpatient department with a history of recurrent dyspnoea over the past 6 months. He finds that he gets breathless on moderate exertion, but has not had any sputum production. Before this he had no respiratory illnesses and was fit and well, but returned from voluntary work in an orphanage in Tasmania 8 months ago. He is not sure whether he had a BCG vaccination in the past. He has never smoked and drinks "about 8 pints on a Saturday". He is married with two grown-up children. He previously worked in the aerospace industry and had a brief spell of no more than 2 years in the atomic industry. Before he retired he had also worked in a local newsagent's shop. He denies any asbestos contact, fever, weight loss, haemoptysis, skin rashes, or arthralgia. He has no history of epilepsy. He has never had any renal tract problems, although he admits to symptoms of prostatism. On examination, he appears well and has no evidence of lymphadenopathy. He has a blood pressure of 130/80 mmHg and a pulse of 72 beats/min. He has no neurological signs and the abdominal examination is unremarkable. Fine crepitations can be heard at both lung bases.

| INVESTIGATIONS | RESULTS |
| --- | --- |
| Full blood count | Normal |
| Liver function tests | Aspartate aminotransferase 32 IU/l (normal: 5–15 IU/l) |
| | Alanine aminotransferase 23 IU/l (normal: 5–15 IU/l) |
| | Bilirubin 6 μmol/l |
| | Alkaline phosphatase 95 IU/l |
| Serum calcium | 2.32 mmol/l |
| Serum ACE | Normal |
| Echocardiography | Good LV function, valves appear normal |
| Chest X-ray | Bilateral hilar lymphadenopathy, with midzone reticulonodular shadowing. No evidence of cavitation |
| Lung function tests | KCO 72% |
| | FEV$_1$ 1.8 l |
| | FVC 2.1 l |
| | DLCO 70% predicted |
| Urinalysis and electrolytes | Normal |
| Abdominal ultrasound | Normal |
| Liver biopsy | No evidence of malignancy, possible granuloma seen |

ACE: angiotensin-converting enzyme; DLCO: carbon monoxide diffusion in the lung; FEV$_1$: forced expiratory volume in 1 second; FVC: forced vital capacity; KCO: transfer coefficient of carbon monoxide; LV: left ventricular.

## a) What is the most likely diagnosis?

    i)     tuberculosis (TB)

    ii)    sarcoidosis

    iii)   lymphoma

    iv)   histiocytosis X

    v)    hypersensitivity pneumonitis

## b) Which investigation would you use to confirm the diagnosis?

    i)     routine CT scan of the chest

    ii)    high-resolution CT scan of the chest

    iii)   mediastinoscopy and lymph node biopsy

    iv)   Kveim test

    v)    Mantoux test

Although there is a lot of information in this question, the two most obvious problems are the presence of bilateral hilar lymphadenopathy and restrictive lung function with other features of fibrosis. If we revise the causes of these two problems then the diagnosis should become apparent.

First of all – as usual – jot down the lists of causes as best you can in the space below:

Your lists here...

**Bilateral hilar lymphadenopathy**                    **Lung fibrosis**

## CAUSES OF BILATERAL HILAR LYMPHADENOPATHY

Fortunately, this is a short list of causes. Remember it with **Two pairs** are C²HEAP²: there are two pairs of obvious causes and six less obvious causes. Obvious causes (two pairs) are sarcoidosis and TB, and lymphoma and cancers. The six less obvious causes (C²HEAP²) are cystic fibrosis, Churg–Strauss syndrome, HIV infection, extrinsic allergic alveolitis (hypersensitivity pneumonitis), phenytoin treatment, and pneumoconioses (especially berylliosis). Remember that Churg–Strauss syndrome may encompass glomerulonephritis, gut involvement causing ulcers and diarrhoea, skin involvement, and mononeuritis multiplex.

## CAUSES OF LUNG FIBROSIS

Any chronic diffuse lung inflammation will, in general, cause fibrosis. Any toxic agent may directly cause damage. Otherwise, the main causes are shown below.

Main causes of lung fibrosis:

- TB
- drugs: e.g. amiodarone, bleomycin, busulphan
- pneumoconioses: silicosis, asbestosis
- acute rheumatic disease (e.g. rheumatoid arthritis, systemic lupus erythematosus)
- radiation
- sarcoidosis
- hypersensitivity pneumonitis (e.g. pigeon breeder's lung)
- paraquat
- pulmonary haemosiderosis
- histiocytosis X

Remember: Pigeon **CRA²PS:** cryptogenic fibrosing alveolitis\*, radiation, amiodarone, (extrinsic) allergic alveolitis, pigeon breeder's lung, sarcoidosis

\*Remember that cryptogenic fibrosing alveolitis is associated with other autoimmune diseases, especially rheumatoid arthritis, ankylosing spondylitis, Sjögren's syndrome, chronic active hepatitis, Hashimoto's disease, and inflammatory bowel disease, and also with renal tubular acidosis. In essence, this is the same list as that for the associations of chronic active hepatitis (covered in the 'Gastrointestinal Tracts' chapter), so learn it only once! It is associated with clubbing and (like chronic active hepatitis) with positive anti-nuclear antibodies and anti-mitochondrial antibodies.

Also sneaking in there as other causes of a cellular lung infiltrate and fibrosis are the histiocytosis X files:

- eosinophilic granuloma
- Hand–Schüller–Christian disease
- Letterer–Siwe disease: hepatosplenomegaly, anaemia, diabetes insipidus, Rhesus factor positive, pulmonary hypertension

In this case, a possible granuloma seen on the liver biopsy suggests a granulomatous disease. This would indicate that the probable answer is sarcoidosis, TB, or berylliosis (which mimics sarcoidosis). Berylliosis should come to mind considering the patient's previous employment in the aerospace and atomic industries. Other relevant occupational exposures include the early manufacture of fluorescent lightbulbs or golf-club heads. TB can cause both granuloma and fibrosis, but is unlikely as the patient is otherwise well and afebrile. The patient's age and the fact that he is male should not let you be put off from the diagnosis. The second part of the question is easy if you have got the first part right. *Do not* leave any questions out: the examination is not negatively marked.

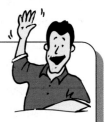

**A8** **a) Diagnosis**
    ii) Sarcoidosis
  **b) Investigations**
    iii) Mediastinoscopy and lymph node biopsy

A high-resolution CT scan of the chest would be useful to differentiate between acute sarcoidosis and chronic fibrosis. The Kveim test is not used very often, and the only test that will yield a presumptive diagnosis is a biopsy.

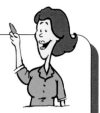

**Q9** A 23-year-old woman presents to the respiratory outpatient department with wheeze, nocturnal cough, and shortness of breath over the last 6 months. She has also had two episodes of haemoptysis within the last 3 weeks. On both occasions she attended the emergency department, was told that she had a chest infection, and was discharged with antibiotics. As a child, she had severe atopic eczema until the age of 5 years. She had the usual childhood vaccinations against measles, mumps, rubella, and whooping cough. Apart from the recent chest infections, she has otherwise been extremely well. There is a family history of atopy and her brother is a severe asthmatic. She smokes 10 cigarettes per day and works as a legal secretary in the city. She is also a keen sportswoman and until 6 months previously was in the university 100 m running team, but she now gets breathless even on mild exertion. She has only travelled to France in recent years, where she was pleased to see the French team beaten at rugby. (In this respect, then, quite normal.) A chest X-ray taken from her emergency admission shows a shadow in the right mid-zone. A repeat chest X-ray in the clinic shows clearing of the first shadow, but with a suspicion of another shadow in the left lower zone. Examination shows few physical signs, except for some expiratory wheeze.

| Investigations | Results |
| --- | --- |
| Lung function tests | FEV$_1$ 1.6 l |
| | FVC 3.0 l |
| | PEFR 200 l/min |
| CT scan of the chest | Proximal bronchiectasis |
| Full blood count | Haemoglobin 10.6 g/dl |
| | White cell count 6.2 × 10$^9$/l (75% neutrophils and 10% lymphocytes) |
| | Platelets 154 × 10$^9$/l |
| Urinalysis and electrolytes | Normal |
| Stool culture | Negative |
| Ca$^{2+}$ | Normal |
| ACE | Normal |
| Immunoglobulin G | 10 g/dl (normal: 10–15 g/dl) |
| Sputum culture | Negative |

ACE: angiotensin-converting enzyme; FEV$_1$: forced expiratory volume in 1 second; FVC: forced vital capacity; PEFR: peak expiratory flow rate.

## a) What is the most likely diagnosis?

i)     sarcoidosis

ii)    TB

iii)   Churg–Strauss syndrome

iv)   $\alpha_1$-antitrypsin deficiency

v)    allergic bronchopulmonary aspergillosis

## b) What test would you do next?

i)     Mantoux test

ii)    transbronchial biopsy

iii)   skin-prick test for *Aspergillus*

iv)   serum $\alpha_1$-antitrypsin levels

v)    perinuclear anti-neutrophilic cytoplasmic antibodies

## c) What would be the most appropriate treatment?

i)     anti-TB drug therapy

ii)    prednisolone

iii)   $\alpha_1$-antitrypsin protease inhibitor

iv)   intravenous amphotericin

v)    immunosuppressive therapy

Again this should be a straightforward question if you have followed the principles given in the text so far. Do not look at the lists on the next page but, on your own, try to decide which are the key findings that are always pathological and for which there are a limited list of causes. Write a list of these causes. Which diagnosis appears on both lists? This is likely to be the answer.

*Don't turn over! (Cheat!)*

Your list here...

_____

_____

_____

_____

_____

The two lists you should have produced are for the causes of eosinophilia and proximal bronchiectasis. Here are the lists you ought to remember:

## CAUSES OF EOS⁴I³N³OP⁶HI⁵LIA

| | |
|---|---|
| Skin: | rheumatoid arthritis with cutaneous manifestations |
| | dermatitis herpetiformis |
| | scabies |
| | atopic eczema |
| Immune: | asthma |
| | atopy |
| | any drug reactions |
| Neoplastic: | Hodgkin's lymphomas |
| | acute lymphoblastic lymphoma |
| | all solid malignancies |
| Pulmonary: | increases in sputum and peripheral blood eosinophil counts are caused by: |

- allergic bronchopulmonary aspergillosis (asthma, cough, sputum plugs, proximal bronchiectasis)
- Löffler's syndrome (cough, fever, yellow sputum, malaise, fluffy X-ray infiltrates)
- tropical eosinophilia (microfilaraemia, ascariasis, ankylostomiasis, toxocariasis, strongyloidiasis)
- drug reactions (cotrimoxazole, busulphan, methotrexate, nitrofurantoin, or anything at all!)
- Churg–Strauss syndrome* (small/medium-vessel vasculitis, asthma, eosinophilia)
- adult asthma

| | |
|---|---|
| Infective: | nematodes – roundworms (e.g. *Toxocara*, *Ascaris lumbricoides*) |
| | cestodes – tapeworms (e.g. *Echinococcus*) |
| | hookworms |
| | trematodes – flukes |
| | *Schistosoma* and other parasites |
| | Whipple's disease |

*Remember that Churg–Strauss syndrome often has gut involvement, with diarrhoea and gut ulceration. In addition, there is often skin involvement, glomerulonephritis, and mononeuritis multiplex.

## CAUSES OF BRONCHIECTASIS (TACKY HI²P)

- Post-TB
- Aspergillosis
- Cystic fibrosis/bronchial compression
- Kartagener's syndrome (dysmotile cilia with situs inversus and infertility)
- Yellow nail syndrome
- Hypogammaglobulinaemia
- Idiopathic
- Inhalation of foreign body
- Post-childhood infection (whooping cough/pertussis, measles)

Note:

- Examiners seem to love Kartagener's syndrome: if there is the slightest hint of sinusitis, quiet heart sounds (dextrocardia), or infertility, it should be considered.
- $\alpha_1$-anti-trypsin deficiency can cause bronchiectasis, but is better recognised for emphysema, chronic liver disease, or hepatocellular carcinoma. Diagnosis is made by serum electrophoresis.

The combination of eosinophilia and bronchiectasis has therefore led you immediately to the diagnosis. It couldn't be easier, could it? In terms of the tests to confirm your diagnoses, you will learn these answers from our book and others.

**A9**

a) **Diagnosis**
v) Allergic bronchopulmonary aspergillosis (allergic asthma)

b) **Investigations**
iii) Skin-prick testing for *Aspergillus*

c) **Treatment**
ii) These patients should be given prednisolone at an initial dose of 30 mg daily, which readily reduces the pulmonary infiltrate. Frequent episodes of this disease can be prevented by steroid treatment, but unfortunately high doses are required (10–15 mg/day).

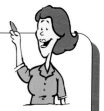

# Q10

Your house officer is concerned that a patient in the emergency department, a 25-year-old student, has 'apical shadowing' on his chest X-ray. The patient comes from India and has never had a BCG vaccination. He has been studying in the UK for the last 3 years and returned from his summer holidays in India 2 months ago. He denies any systemic symptoms, but admits to having had a dry cough since returning to the UK, which he attributes to the weather.

### a) What would you advise your house officer to do?

i)   admit, isolate, and start treatment for TB

ii)  Mantoux test

iii) give a BCG vaccination

iv)  arrange for bronchoscopy and lavage

v)   morning urine test

### b) The patient has confirmed pulmonary TB. Which of the following anti-TB drugs most commonly causes peripheral neuropathy?

i)   rifampicin

ii)  streptomycin

iii) isoniazid

iv)  pyrazinamide

v)   ethambutol

### c) On contact tracing, the patient is found to live with two housemates from university. They do not have any respiratory or systemic symptoms. Both housemates had BCG vaccinations during childhood. How would you manage them?

i)   admit and start treatment for TB

ii)  Mantoux test

iii) interferon-γ test

iv)  chest X-ray

v)   no investigation required

The NICE guidelines recommend that patients with suspected active pulmonary TB should have at least three sputum samples sent for culture and microscopy for acid-fast bacilli prior to treatment, and one of these should be an early-morning sample. As this patient does not have a productive cough, his diagnostic tests should include either induced sputum for culture or bronchoscopy and lavage.

## TB DRUGS AND THEIR SIDE EFFECTS

High-dose isoniazid causes peripheral neuropathy, hence patients on TB treatment also receive pyridoxine prophylaxis. Ethambutol can also cause peripheral neuropathy, but less commonly than isoniazid.

## CONTACT TRACING

Contacts infected with TB can be asymptomatic – but latent TB can develop into active TB, particularly in children or young adults, or reactivate many years later.

The patient's housemates, who are both aged <35 years old and have had BCG vaccinations, should have a Mantoux test. A positive skin test (≥15 mm) should prompt further investigations with an interferon-γ test. A positive interferon-γ test should then be investigated with a chest X-ray. Those with a normal chest X-ray following positive Mantoux and interferon-γ tests should be treated for latent TB infection, requiring rifampicin and/or isoniazid, depending on whether the index case has isoniazid-resistant TB. Abnormal chest X-rays should be investigated for active TB.

Contacts >35 years old should have a chest X-ray as their initial investigation for latent TB. Those who have not received a BCG vaccination will need a Mantoux test.

# QUIZ SPOT!

Match the following anti-TB drugs to their side effects. Some drugs can cause more than one side effect:

| | |
|---|---|
| Rifampicin | Orange–red colour |
| Pyrazinamide | Abnormal liver function tests |
| Isoniazid | Optic neuritis |
| Ethambutol | Gout |

A: Rifampicin: orange–red colour/abnormal liver function tests; pyrazinamide: abnormal liver function tests/gout; isoniazid: abnormal liver function tests; ethambutol: optic neuritis.

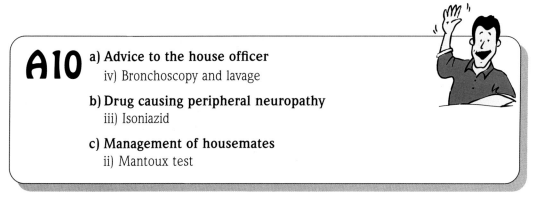

**A10** a) **Advice to the house officer**
iv) Bronchoscopy and lavage

b) **Drug causing peripheral neuropathy**
iii) Isoniazid

c) **Management of housemates**
ii) Mantoux test

## DID YOU KNOW...

...Studies have shown encouraging results with interferon-γ as a diagnostic or screening test for TB exposure. It is thought to be more specific in diagnosing exposure to TB than tuberculin skin tests. Interferon-γ tests use *Mycobacterium tuberculosis* antigens to assess host response. These antigens are not found in BCG vaccines and are only present in a few other mycobacteria, which reduces the false-positive rate of tuberculin skin tests. Further studies will determine its effectiveness as a diagnostic and screening tool for TB exposure – watch this space!

## NON-PULMONARY TB

- Can occur in meninges, spinal cord, pericardium, lymph nodes, bone, and joints.
- Requires culture from biopsied tissue and needle aspiration to confirm TB and check for multidrug resistance.
- Can coexist with pulmonary TB. Check for this in all patients with extrapulmonary TB.

## SOME PRACTICAL POINTS FROM THE INFECTION-CONTROL POLICE

### ACTIVE PULMONARY TB

| | |
|---|---|
| Symptoms | Cough, haemoptysis, weight loss, fever, dyspnoea, or night sweats |
| Chest X-ray | Abnormalities include patchy or nodular shadowing, loss of volume, fibrotic changes, or cavitation in the upper zones |

**Infection risk to others and isolation**

| | |
|---|---|
| Sputum-smear-positive, non-MDR TB | • Single side room if the ward does not have immunocompromised patients<br>• If there are immunocompromised patients, the patient should be admitted to a negative-pressure side room<br>• The patient should wear a surgical mask whenever they leave the room<br>• The patient is usually considered noninfectious after 2 weeks of treatment with good compliance and clinical improvement |
| Sputum-smear-negative TB | If the ward does not have immunocompromised patients, the index case can be managed on the ward |
| Sputum-smear-positive, MDR TB | Admit the patient to a negative-pressure side room |
| Treatment for pulmonary, non-MDR TB | 2 months of isoniazid, rifampicin, pyrazinamide, and ethambutol, then isoniazid and rifampicin for another 4 months |

MDR: multidrug-resistant; TB: tuberculosis.

### LATENT TB

| | |
|---|---|
| Symptoms | Asymptomatic |
| Chest X-ray | Normal |
| Infection risk to others and isolation | Not infectious to others |
| Treatment | See contacting tracing question |

TB: tuberculosis.

# Q11

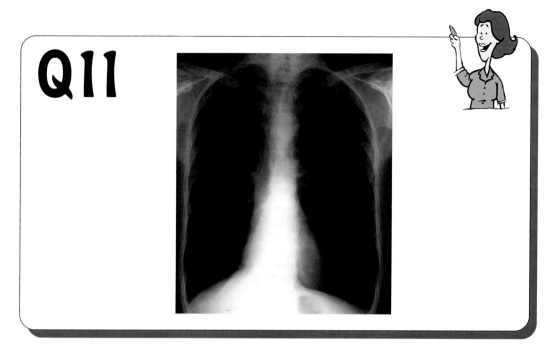

## a) What does this chest X-ray show?

i) right lower lobe consolidation

ii) hiatus hernia

iii) right pleural effusion

iv) nothing – it's normal

v) right lower lobe collapse

This chest X-ray shows the features of right lower lobe collapse:

- loss of clarity over the medial border of the right hemidiaphragm
- a triangular density behind the right heart border
- the right heart border remains visible as it is anterior to the lower lobe

Collapse of a lobe is caused by proximal obstruction of a bronchus – think about malignancy or mucus plugging (allergic bronchopulmonary aspergillosis). In children, mind the swallowed peanut!

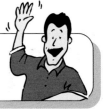

**A11** a) **Shown in chest X-ray**
   v) Right lower lobe collapse

## Additional bits: Aspergillus

Much confusion underlies *Aspergillus*. The organism:

- can colonise a lung cavity as an aspergilloma (causing cough, haemoptysis, and fever, as with any lung infection)
- may invade through the lung interstitium and then disseminate around the body
- may asymptomatically colonise the lung, or establish an allergic response causing asthma, cough, and the production of plugs of yellow eosinophilic sputum

The prick test or radioallergosorbent test are positive in the case of an allergic response, but not in the case of the other causes. Here is a short summary:

| Problem | Features | Prick test | Precipitins/culture |
|---|---|---|---|
| Colonisation | Frequently asymptomatic | – | + |
| Aspergilloma | Cough, haemoptysis, fever | – | + |
| Invasive | Solely in immunosuppressed patients, often spreads around the body | +/– | +/– |
| Asthma | May be occupational | + | + |
| ABPA | Asthma, cough, sputum plugging. Patchy infiltrates on chest X-ray, may show bronchiectasis | + | + <br> Raised IgE |

ABPA: allergic broncho-pulmonary aspergillosis; Ig: immunoglobulin.

## Another quick joke

A doctor arrives in the clinic with a rectal thermometer behind his ear. One of the nurses points this out. "Damn!" he says, "Who the hell has got my pen?"

## ADDITIONAL BITS: PLEURAL EFFUSIONS

Can you remember a list of causes of pleural effusions? The causes should be clear if you construct your usual 'surgical sieve'. You should always have your own sieve. Remember – our favourite is 'TIE HIM IN', to which we add a few 'can-do-anything' checks (syphilis, hypothyroidism and hyperthyroidism, sarcoidosis, and amyloidosis) and a system review (think of anything that can affect, for example, the respiratory, central nervous, or gastrointestinal systems). Ensure that you remember this sieve. If you cannot, revise it now (pages 13–14).

Use the sieve, and apply it to transudates and exudates in turn:

Trauma

Infection

Endocrine

Haematology

Iatrogenic

Metabolic

Idiopathic

Neoplastic

TB

Syphilis

Amyloidosis

Sarcoidosis

Autoimmune

Systems review

The ones people often miss are:

*Transudates*

- congestive heart failure
- nephrosis
- cirrhosis
- protein-losing enteropathy
- peritoneal dialysis
- renal failure
- hypoalbuminaemia

*Exudates*

- infection (pneumonia, TB)
- mesothelioma, local malignancy
- pulmonary embolus
- uraemia
- hypothyroidism
- subphrenic abscess
- yellow nail syndrome (NB: bronchiectasis)
- Dressler's syndrome
- pancreatitis
- local trauma
- vasculitic diseases
- lymphoma
- Meigs' syndrome (+ benign ovarian fibroma or thecoma +/− ascites)
- connective tissue diseases (systemic lupus erythematosus, rheumatoid arthritis)

Note: classically a protein concentration of <3 g/dl (<30 g/l) has been used to distinguish a transudate from an exudate. However, better still, the effusion is an exudate if it meets one or more of Light's criteria: ratio of pleural to serum protein levels of >0.5; ratio of pleural to serum lactate dehydrogenase (LDH) levels of >0.6; or a pleural fluid LDH level of less than two-thirds the upper limit for serum LDH levels. Alternatively, a serum/pleural albumin concentration of <1.2 g/dl indicates exudation.

Assessment of a pleural effusion thus requires:

- cell count with differential, total protein level, glucose level, LDH level, amylase level, and pH (provides important prognostic information in tumours)
- cytological analysis
- Gram staining, auramine/Ziehl–Neelson/acid-fast bacilli staining, fungal staining (India ink/cryptococcal antigen), culture, and sensitivity testing for aerobic and anaerobic organisms and fungi
- determination of simultaneous serum total protein, albumin, glucose, LDH, and amylase levels

# Q12

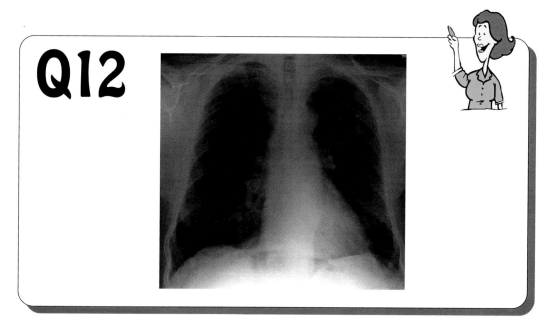

## a) Which of these conditions does not cause this chest X-ray appearance?

- i) TB
- ii) Wegener's granulomatosis
- iii) pulmonary embolus
- iv) pleural plaque
- v) rheumatoid nodule

The chest X-ray shows a cavitating lesion. See the rhyme on page 69 for the causes.

'Pleural plaque' is therefore our odd man out. Pleural plaques are white, and are usually multiple and bilateral on the diaphragm or posterolateral aspect. They are caused by at least 10–20 years of asbestos exposure. The patient is usually asymptomatic, and is not entitled to industrial compensation on the basis of pleural plaques alone under current UK legislation.

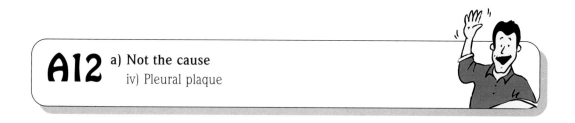

# A12
a) Not the cause
iv) Pleural plaque

Two last lists now.

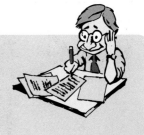

### Cavitating lesions in the lung

*Cancers\* cause cavities, so can TB*
*Wegener's, rheumatoid\*\*, also PE*
*Think of the 'oses' of which there are three*
*Also of abscesses\*\*\*, klebsielli*

\*Squamous cell cancer; \*\*progressive massive fibrosis/rheumatoid nodules associated with rheumatoid arthritis; \*\*\*think staphylococcal, *Klebsiella*, amoebic, aspiration; 'oses': histoplasmosis, coccidioidomycosis, and aspergillosis; PE: pulmonary embolism; TB: tuberculosis; Wegener's: Wegener's granulomatosis.

### Mass lesions in the lung

Work out your own way of remembering these lists.

*Single well-rounded large opacities* are due to:

Neoplasms:     primary malignant or metastatic (may have spiculation or cavitation)
               hamartomas (may have popcorn calcification)

Infections:    bacterial – abscesses
               tuberculoma (may have calcification or satellite shadowing)
               fungal – mycetoma
               parasitic – hydatid cyst

Vascularities: arteriovenous malformations
               haematoma (post-traumatic)

*Multiple well-rounded large opacities* are due, in particular, to:

* sarcoidosis
* metastases
* hydatid cyst
* abscesses or septic emboli

*Multiple small (<5 mm) opacities* are usually suggestive of:

- miliary TB
- sarcoidosis
- pneumoconioses
- interstitial fibrosis/alveolitis

*Localised radiolucencies* are due to:

- cavitation in an abscess/carcinoma/TB
- bullae
- pneumatoceles (think of cystic fibrosis)
- cystic bronchiectasis

Sarcoidosis seems to arise frequently in the MRCP examination, and especially in respiratory cases. Remember that it can cause lymphadenopathy and hepatosplenomegaly (and thus can mimic lymphoma). It may produce a rise in γ-globulins, β-cells, total lymphocyte count, and serum ACE levels.

The space below is left blank for you to work out your own 'memory trick' for the list.

*Your memory trick*

## BEFORE MOVING ON TO THE NEXT CHAPTER...

- What are the features of Horner's syndrome and its causes?

- What are the causes of papilloedema? Polycythaemia? Optic atrophy?

- What are the causes of choroidoretinitis? Retinitis pigmentosa?

- Write down the bilateral hilar lymphadenopathy list

# 4

# METABOLLOCKS

THE METABOLIC MRCP LISTS

Abnormal biochemical findings feature heavily in the MRCP examination. Sometimes, the finding is solitary, such as hypercalcaemia. At other times, you might be expected to recognise a pattern, such as hypokalaemic alkalosis. Of all the abnormal biochemical findings seen, the most common relate to calcium levels and, in particular, high calcium.

## In a nutshell

Remember that the calcium pool in the blood comes from gut absorption, renal calcium reabsorption, and bone resorption. Control of calcium levels requires normal renal, bone, and gut function, and three normally functioning hormone systems:

| | |
|---|---|
| 1) parathyroid hormone (PTH) | **increases plasma calcium**<br>increases renal tubular resorption<br>increases osteoclast activity (bone resorption)<br>increases renal conversion of 25-hydroxy-vitamin D to 1,25-dihydroxy-vitamin D |
| | **decreases plasma phosphate**<br>decreases renal phosphate reabsorption<br>increases osteoclast activity with release of phosphate from bone |
| 2) vitamin D | **increases plasma calcium**<br>increases renal tubular reabsorption<br>increases gut reabsorption<br>increases osteoclast activity |
| | **increases plasma phosphate**<br>increases renal phosphate reabsorption |

3) **hormones that broadly affect 'growth' also raise blood calcium:**
   e.g. growth hormone excess, oestrogen excess, thyrotoxicosis, excess steroids

## Causes of hypercalcaemia

*Abnormal control*

- excess PTH:
  - primary and tertiary hyperparathyroidism
  - multiple endocrine neoplasia types I and II
  - ectopic PTH/PTH-related protein (PTHrP) (e.g. from oat cell carcinoma of the lung)

- vitamin D toxicity
- high hormone levels (**COAT**):
  - Cushing's disease/Addison's disease
  - oestrogen excess
  - acromegaly
  - thyrotoxicosis

*Bone destruction/resorption*

- metastatic malignancy: the tumours that most commonly metastasise to bone are 'the 5 bs': bronchus, breast, byroid, brostate, and bidney
- multiple myeloma and lymphoma

*Five are MIIIST from the lists*

- milk-alkali syndrome
- iatrogenic (lithium, thiazides), idiopathic infantile (supravalvular aortic stenosis, elfin facies)
- sarcoid* (phosphate often normal)
- tuberculosis (TB)* (and leprosy)

*Granulomas in general may raise calcium levels. Thus, other causes include histoplasmosis, coccidioidomycosis, and Wegener's granulomatosis.

## HYPOCALCAEMIA...

...has a more limited list of causes:

- hypoparathyroidism and parathyroid gland excision: pseudohypoparathyroidism
- low vitamin D levels: think low-fat diet or malabsorption. The four fat-soluble vitamins are A, D, E, and K
- malabsorption syndromes
- chronic renal failure: tubules are resistant to hormone action, resulting in low calcium and high phosphate levels. Compensatory high calcium production can lead to metastatic soft-tissue calcification
- acute pancreatitis: calcium is sequestered as 'soaps'
- rhabdomyolysis

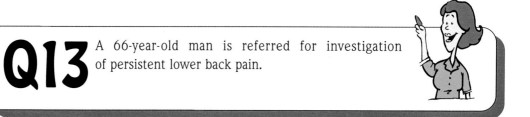

**Q13** A 66-year-old man is referred for investigation of persistent lower back pain.

| Investigations | Results | Investigations | Results |
|---|---|---|---|
| DEXA T score spine | −2.5 | Corrected calcium | 3.28 mmol/l |
| Bone scan | Normal | Serum total protein | 84 g/l |
| Haemoglobin | 97 g/l | Serum albumin | 40 g/l |
| Mean corpuscular volume | 84 fl | IgG | 38 g/l |
| White cell count | 2.1 × 10⁹/l | IgA | <0.2 g/l |
| Platelets | 105 × 10⁹/l | IgM | <0.2 g/l |
| Plasma urea | 5.9 mmol/l | Serum protein electrophoresis | Presence of a paraprotein band |
| Plasma creatinine | 87 μmol/l | Urine electrophoresis | Negative |
| Urine dipstick | Negative | | |

DEXA: dual energy X-ray absorptiometry; IgA: immunoglobulin A; IgG: immunoglobulin G; IgM: immunoglobulin M.

## a) What is the most likely diagnosis?

   i)     multiple myeloma

   ii)    osteoperosis

   iii)   metastatic carcinoma

   iv)   MGUS

   v)    Waldenström's macroglobulinaemia

Great, a 66-year-old man with back pain! But look, he also has pancytopenia, hypercalcaemia, immune paresis, high levels of serum protein and IgG paraprotein – but no urinal paraprotein. His DEXA score is consistent with osteoporosis, and he has a normal bone scan. So the answer is…

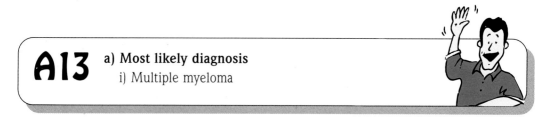

**A13** a) Most likely diagnosis
   i) Multiple myeloma

Multiple myeloma (clonal plasma cell proliferation) can manifest itself in many ways. Don't forget it. Essential diagnostic criteria, based on the International Myeloma Working Group Classification 2003:

- >10% plasma cells on biopsy from bone or other tissue (plasmacytoma) AND
- Monoclonal protein (serum and/or urine) AND
- Evidence of end organ damage: one or more of CRAB (hypercalcaemia, renal impairment, anaemia, bone disease)

## More on multiple myeloma:

- Patients typically over 65 years old
- Males more commonly affected
- Most common symptoms are fatigue, weight loss, bone pain (classically not tender on palpation) and recurrent infections. It may be asymptomatic, picked up on routine blood tests
- Other presenting complaints/complications include fractures, spinal cord compression, bleeding, hypercalcaemia, hyperviscosity, neurological manifestations, renal impairment, and PUO
- ~30% are Bence Jones protein negative
- Most common paraprotein is IgG, then IgA, and IgM
- Median survival is 3 years

## Other important facts:

- Bone scans are not helpful in identifying the lytic lesions of multiple myeloma. Bone metastases of solid tumours characteristically show as 'hot-spots'
- A DEXA scan is also not helpful. Patients are typically treated with regular bisphosphonates; therefore, confirmation of osteoporosis (associated with multiple myeloma) would not alter their management
- X-rays typically show 'punched out' lesions (the pepper-pot skull). Remember, multiple myeloma tends to affect the axial skeleton and long bones
- Treatment with thalidomide is associated with peripheral neuropathy and an increased risk of thromboembolic events. Beware the question: A patient with multiple myeloma who has recently started treatment presents with shortness of breath… pulmonary embolism!
- Long-term treatment with bisphosphonates is linked to osteonecrosis of the jaw

- Causes of renal impairment in multiple myeloma. The list is long, but worth remembering...hypercalcaemia; nephrocalcinosis and urate nephropathy; light chain/Bence Jones protein damage (kappa chains are worst at this: 'kappa kills kidneys'); dehydration; infection due to immunoparesis; plasma cell infiltration of the kidney; nonsteroidal anti-inflammatory drug damage (taken for the back pain); amyloidosis

*Before you proceed, would you expect his PTH to be high/low/normal?*

- Low – because of his high calcium level. However, remember in renal failure – frequently associated with multiple myeloma – this response may be suppressed, leaving him with a normal PTH. Now, what can you remember about hypo- and hyperparathyroidism?

## The other options...

Monoclonal gammopathy of uncertain significance (MGUS) is a monoclonal gammopathy with no clinical manifestations and <10% plasma cells in the bone marrow, and a serum paraprotein concentration <3 g/dl. It is premalignant and it has a 1% annual risk of transforming to multiple myeloma, so these patients should be routinely followed up. This man had bony involvement and hypercalcaemia; therefore, MGUS is not the answer. Just a reminder... Osteoporosis is defined as a BMD 2.5 SD below peak bone mass, (T score −2.5 and below). Osteopenia is defined as a T score between −1.0 and −2.5.

### Finally, Waldenström's macroglobulinaemia in a nutshell:

- Lymphoproliferative disease, patients typically over 65 years old, males more commonly affected, key feature is IgM paraprotein
- Other laboratory features: anaemia (both the direct and indirect antiglobulin test can be positive so watch out), raised LDH and erythrocyte sedimentation rate (ESR), and increased serum viscosity. Of interest it can cause false positive RhF
- Clinical features: fatigue, weight loss, bleeding, Raynaud's phenomenon, peripheral neuropathy, visual disturbances, lymphadenopathy, and hepatosplenomegaly (rare in multiple myeloma). Bone pain is rare.

Both Waldenström's macroglobulinaemia and multiple myeloma may cause cryoglobulinaemia. Of note, $\beta_2$-microglobulin is of prognostic value in both Waldenström's and myeloma.

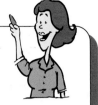

# Q14

A 73-year-old man presents with a 3-month history of weight loss and the recent onset of confusion. He thinks that he might have had one episode of haemoptysis 2 days before his clinic visit. He denies other symptoms, but his wife says that he has been complaining of intermittent headaches, has appeared 'distant' over the same period of time, and has lost interest in his main pastime of gardening. (We view this hobby as evidence of a *long-standing* impairment of mental function!) He gave up smoking 5 years earlier, after a 60 pack-year history. He was previously diagnosed as having mild chronic bronchitis and uses salbutamol and beclomethasone inhalers for this. On further questioning he says that he has lost his appetite. He denies any associated fevers. There is no history of recent foreign travel, although he did serve in the army during the war and was stationed in North Africa where he suffered from one episode of malaria. He denies any gastrointestinal symptoms and has never suffered with cardiac disease. He does admit to coughing up sputum most mornings and this has been worse recently.

On examination, he appears cachectic with proximal muscle wasting. He has evidence of a peripheral neuropathy, more pronounced in the arms than the legs. Fundoscopy is normal and there is no evidence of long tract, parietal, or cerebellar signs. He is in atrial fibrillation with a pulse rate of 100 beats/min. His blood pressure is 123/72 mmHg. There are no signs in the respiratory tract. Abdominal examination is unremarkable.

| Investigations | Results |
| --- | --- |
| Serum sodium | 135 mmol/l |
| Serum potassium | 3.6 mmol/l |
| Serum urea | 10.8 mmol/l |
| Plasma creatinine | 98 µmol/l |
| Creatinine phosphokinase | 100 IU/l |
| Serum alkaline phosphatase | 100 IU/l |
| Serum aspartate aminotransferase | 8 IU/l |
| Serum alanine aminotransferase | 6 IU/l |
| Serum calcium | 2.65 mmol/l |
| Serum albumin | 30 g/l |
| Parathyroid hormone | Normal |
| Sputum acid-fast bacilli | Negative × 3 |
| Serum electrophoresis | No monoclonal bands seen |
| Chest X-ray | Cavitating lesion in the right midzone |

### a) What is the most likely diagnosis?

    i)     squamous cell carcinoma of the bronchus

    ii)    TB

    iii)   Wegener's granulomatosis

    iv)   sarcoidosis

    v)    polyarteritis nodosa

### b) Give two reasons for his confusion.

### c) What investigation would you perform next?

    i)     CT scan of the chest

    ii)    cytoplasmic anti-neutrophilic cytoplasm antibodies

    iii)   serum ACE level

    iv)   CT scan of the head

    v)    nerve conduction tests

Even if you spotted the answer straight away, work your way through the method and learn the lists. What are the findings that are always abnormal and for which there are limited lists of causes? Decide, and then write down the relevant lists. Which diagnosis appears on all of the lists? This is the correct answer. Again, *don't look down!*

The definitively abnormal findings are hypercalcaemia, peripheral neuropathy, and a cavitating lesion in the lung. You already have a list for the causes of peripheral neuropathy. You now need lists for the causes of hypercalcaemia and lung cavitation.

Let's first deal with the hypercalcaemia. You should have this off to a tee by now.

You have already learned the causes of peripheral neuropathy. Fill in the list below to refresh your memory...

## PERIPHERAL NEUROPATHY

Congenital (born unlucky): _____

Three dejected: _____

Two infected: _____

Two injected: _____

One connected: _____

_____ suspected and _____ , which just refuses to rhyme.

And here are the causes of lung cavitation... Do you remember the rhyme (Pants, page 69)?

### CAVITATING LESIONS IN THE LUNG

- Cancers (squamous cell carcinoma)
- TB
- Wegener's granulomatosis
- Rheumatoid arthritis
- Pulmonary embolism
- Three 'oses': histoplasmosis, coccidioidomycosis, and aspergillosis
- Abscesses: staphylococcal, *Klebsiella*, amoebiasis, and aspiration

Untreated, TB is not commonly a cause of peripheral neuropathy. If the patient is receiving treatment with isoniazid, however, then this is a potential diagnosis.

Vasculitis can also be associated with peripheral neuropathy, and a Wegener's-like granulomatosis might be considered, except for the hypercalcaemia. Sarcoidosis, too, might be considered as a cause of neuropathy and hypercalcaemia, but is not a cause of lung *cavitation*.

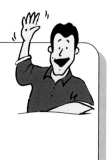

**A14**

a) **Diagnosis**
   i) Squamous cell carcinoma of the bronchus

b) **Reasons for confusion**
   Hypercalcaemia
   Cerebral metastases

c) **Investigations**
   i) CT scan of the chest

**Q15** A 45-year-old woman presents to her GP with polyuria and polydipsia. She is not diabetic and her blood sugar is normal. On further questioning she admits to having had intermittent abdominal pain for several months, accompanied by vomiting and constipation. She is very worried because her father died last year from oesophageal carcinoma and she herself has smoked 20–30 cigarettes per day since she was 16 years old. There is nothing to find on examination. Her GP arranges to see her in 1 month, and meanwhile organises a plain abdominal film and some screening blood tests.

| INVESTIGATIONS | RESULTS |
| --- | --- |
| Abdominal X-ray | Evidence of bilateral nephrocalcinosis |
| White cell count | $8.4 \times 10^9$/l |
| Haemoglobin | 11.7 g/dl |
| Platelets | $376 \times 10^9$/l |
| Plasma urea | 8.1 mmol/l |
| Plasma creatinine | 165 μmol/l |
| Plasma sodium | 140 mmol/l |
| Plasma potassium | 4.3 mmol/l |
| Serum calcium | 2.80 mmol/l |
| Serum phosphate | 0.70 mmol/l |

### a) Which is the most likely diagnosis?

i)   paraneoplastic hypercalcaemia of malignancy

ii)  primary hyperparathyroidism

iii) familial hypocalciuric hypercalcaemia

### b) Which would be the most helpful investigation?

i)   PTH assay

ii)  urinary cyclic adenosine monophosphate (cAMP)

iii) hydrocortisone suppression test

iv)  24-hour urinary calcium excretion

v)   PTHrP radioimmunoassay

**A15** a) **Diagnosis**

ii) The obvious abnormal feature here is hypercalcaemia. You really ought, by now, to have the table of causes 'off pat'. Of the choices given, nephrocalcinosis only occurs in primary hyperparathyroidism, so this must be the diagnosis. You might not have known this before, but you do now!

b) **Test**

iii) The most helpful test is the one that excludes the other diagnoses. In this instance, it is the hydrocortisone suppression test; hydrocortisone suppresses calcium levels in other causes of hypercalcaemia, but not in primary hyperparathyroidism.

## CHOROIDORETINITIS CAUSES

Find the right start square, then follow to adjacent boxes (only vertically or horizontally) to find some causes of choroidoretinitis. There are a few other words in there which are not causes. What are they? Once you have finished, look at the answers (page 116) and revise the causes (page 34).

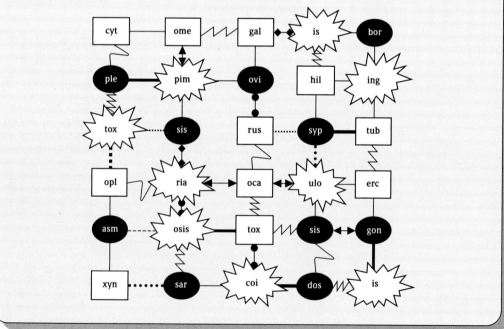

# REVIEW OF POSSIBLE DIAGNOSES

Here is a quick summary of the main features of the three possible diagnoses.

| PRIMARY HYPERPARATHYROIDISM | HYPERCALCAEMIA OF MALIGNANCY | FAMILIAL HYPOCALCIURIC HYPERCALCAEMIA |
| --- | --- | --- |
| 80% single adenoma 10% gland hyperplasia 2% parathyroid carcinoma | Squamous cell carcinoma (lung, oesophagus) renal/breast/ovary/ pancreas/bladder/lymph | Autosomal dominant Abnormal calcium receptors |
| Very high PTH | High PTHrP | High/normal PTH |
| High calcium, low phosphate | High calcium, low phosphate | Very high calcium – stays high post parathyroidectomy |
| High urinary cAMP | High urinary cAMP | High/normal urinary cAMP |
| High 24-hour urine calcium | High 24-hour urine calcium | Low 24-hour urine calcium |
| Polyuria/polydipsia | Polyuria/polydipsia | Benign/asymptomatic |
| Nephrocalcinosis | No nephrocalcinosis | No nephrocalcinosis |
| Subperiosteal erosions | Bony erosions | No bony abnormalities |
| Less acute onset | More acute onset | Usually found by chance |
| Bones, moans, stones, and abdominal groans | Symptoms and signs of primary cancer | |
| Associated with a hyperchloraemic metabolic acidosis | May have hypochloraemic metabolic alkalosis if much vomiting/polyuria | |
| Hydrocortisone suppression test doesn't suppress calcium in primary hyperparathyroidism, but does in other causes of hypercalcaemia | PTH radioimmunoassay readily differentiates between PTH and PTHrP | Familial hypocalciuric hypercalcaemia = CaCl/CrCl <0.01 Primary hyperparathyroidism >0.01 |

CaCl: calcium clearance; cAMP: cyclic AMP; CrCl: creatine clearance; PTH: parathyroid hormone; PTHrP: parathyroid hormone-related protein.

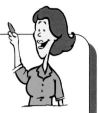

# Q16

A young girl is seen in the endocrine clinic after referral from her GP who found her to be hypocalcaemic. She has a fairly long-standing history of intermittent diarrhoea, which has never been investigated. She was achieving well at school until last year. She confides in you that some of the bigger girls in her year have been bullying her. She has no significant medical history other than mild asthma, which is well-controlled. She has never been hospitalised. On examination, she is a pretty girl, with a round face. You notice that on her right hand she has shortened ring and little fingers. Examination is otherwise unremarkable.

| INVESTIGATIONS | RESULTS |
| --- | --- |
| Serum calcium | 1.95 mmol/l (corrected) |
| Serum phosphate | 1.7 mmol/l |
| Plasma urea | 4.3 mmol/l |
| Plasma creatinine | 121 μmol/l |
| Plasma sodium | 137 mmol/l |
| Plasma potassium | 3.9 mmol/l |
| Serum albumin | 39 g/l |
| Iron studies | Normal |
| Clotting | Normal |
| Haemoglobin | 12.6 g/dl |
| White cell count | $5.8 \times 10^9$/l |
| Platelets | $234 \times 10^9$/l |

## a) What is the diagnosis?

i)   type I pseudohypoparathyroidism

ii)  type II pseudohypoparathyroidism

iii) Turner's syndrome

iv)  pseudopseudohypoparathyroidism

v)   malabsorption syndrome

## b) Which is the most discriminating test?

i)   PTH estimation

ii)  response to PTH infusion

iii) serum magnesium level

iv)  buccal smear

v)   anti-endomysial immunoglobulin A antibodies

The key abnormal finding that has a limited list of causes is hypocalcaemia. List the causes now in the space below. When you have done this, they are given below to refresh your memory.

_____

_____

_____

## Causes of hypocalcaemia

- Hypoparathyroidism and parathyroid gland excision: pseudohypoparathyroidism
- Low vitamin D levels (remember low-fat diet/limited sunlight/low absorption)
- Malabsorption syndromes
- Chronic renal failure
- Acute pancreatitis (calcium sequestered as 'soaps')
- Rhabdomyolysis

In this case, the patient clearly does not have acute pancreatitis/rhabdomyolysis. Chronic renal failure is excluded by the normal urea and creatinine levels. By telling you that the albumin and iron studies are normal, the examiners are trying to tell you that there is no significant malabsorption. In particular, the normal international normalised ratio, which has been given in the investigations, suggests normal vitamin K levels, and hence a low likelihood of abnormal absorption of fat-soluble vitamins: with normal sunlight exposure, this makes vitamin D levels likely to be normal. She might thus be thought to have pseudohypoparathyroidism (type I). The causes are listed in the summary table on the next page. Learn it now. You now ought to be able to figure out that she actually has 'pseudopseudohypoparathyroidism', or Albright's hereditary osteodystrophy, and the most helpful investigation is the PTH infusion test. This involves taking baseline, 30-, 60-, and 90-minute urine samples for phosphate and cyclic AMP, while giving 200 units of PTH intravenously over 10 minutes between collections; this is usually performed in a metabolic unit!

At this point, it is worth reviewing the familial hypocalcaemic/hypophosphataemic syndromes. In examinations, a patient will be presented with familial hypocalcaemia and hypophosphataemia; they will be symptomatic, with signs and symptoms of hypocalcaemia and rickets. Although these cases are almost always presented badly the answer is invariably simple.

Low calcium and low phosphate levels (as well as rickets) must mean a defect in vitamin D metabolism. Once this is appreciated, quickly think back to vitamin D metabolism. Vitamin D is either ingested or converted from cholesterol by sunlight in the skin and further metabolised in the liver to 25-hydroxy-cholecalciferol, and finally in the kidneys to active 1,25-dihydroxy-vitamin D. It then acts upon its intracellular receptor.

Thus, low calcium/phosphate levels are either due to poor diet or vitamin D absorption, poor sun exposure, or failure of liver/kidney metabolism or receptor function. Familial type I rickets is a failure of kidney metabolism with low 1,25-dihydroxy-vitamin D, and is easily treated with 1,25-dihydroxy-vitamin D supplementation. Familial type II rickets is a receptor defect, and is characterised by end-organ resistance. In such cases, 1,25-dihydroxy-vitamin D levels are high, and the condition is treated (though less effectively) with high doses of vitamin D and phosphate. Untreated, both of these conditions cause raised PTH levels.

Do not confuse these with the X-linked hypophosphataemic rickets (X-linked dominant), which is associated with normal calcium and PTH levels, low phosphate levels, and rickets.

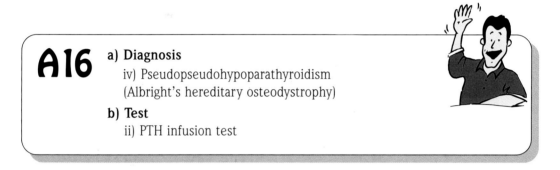

**A16**  a) **Diagnosis**
iv) Pseudopseudohypoparathyroidism
(Albright's hereditary osteodystrophy)
b) **Test**
ii) PTH infusion test

### REVIEW OF POSSIBLE DIAGNOSES

Here is a quick summary of the main features of the four possible diagnoses.

|  | TYPE I PSEUDO-HYPOPARATHYROIDISM | TYPE II PSEUDO-HYPOPARATHYRODISM | PSEUDOPSEUDO-HYPOPARATHYROIDISM | TURNER'S SYNDROME |
|---|---|---|---|---|
| Nature | G-protein disorder with end-organ resistance to PTH | Failure of renal response to cAMP | No abnormal pathology | XO genotype |
| PTH | Appropriately high | Appropriately high | Normal | Normal or slightly high |
| Calcium | Low | Low | Normal | Normal |
| Phosphate | High | High | Normal | Normal |
| Phenotype | Unusual, with round face and short fourth and fifth metacarpals | Normal | Unusual, as for AHO | Can be associated with short fourth and fifth metacarpals |
| Urine | Low urine phosphate and cAMP response to PTH infusion | Normal urine cAMP but low urine phosphate in response to PTH infusion | Normal urine cAMP and phosphate in response to PTH infusion | Normal urine cAMP and phosphate in response to PTH infusion |

AHO: Albright's hereditary osteodystrophy; cAMP: cyclic AMP; PTH: parathyroid hormone.

*Turner's syndrome*

Patients with Turner's syndrome (XO) have short stature, a wide carrying angle, webbed neck, widely spaced nipples, shield chest, and ovarian failure, which causes osteoporosis. They may also suffer autoimmune hypothyroidism/diabetes mellitus, renal dysgenesis, aortic coarctation/dissection, lymphoedema, and gonadoblastoma. X-linked recessive disorders that usually affect men include haemophilia.

Time for a quick **WORDSEARCH** over a cuppa. Find the 11 syndromes or tests bearing the discoverer's name in the grid below. They can occur diagonally, vertically, and horizontally, either backwards or forwards. Write down three lines on each as you find them. These syndromes will be covered throughout the book.

| A | L | B | R | I | G | H | T | S | H | J | G | Q | S | T | A | R | D | D | A |
|---|---|---|---|---|---|---|---|---|---|---|---|---|---|---|---|---|---|---|---|
| W | A | S | D | F | G | Y | T | L | L | L | E | D | T | B | N | J | K | L | R |
| A | S | D | K | R | D | E | F | G | H | S | S | G | Q | U | I | H | C | L | M |
| I | O | P | E | E | C | F | E | O | L | L | D | E | W | C | V | N | H | K | L |
| O | R | F | S | H | S | D | G | N | C | M | W | E | I | L | S | M | R | M | M |
| W | J | K | E | E | D | S | E | C | M | S | W | F | F | F | D | W | I | I | U |
| H | L | B | L | L | W | W | R | F | G | W | E | K | L | J | K | R | S | X | M |
| A | S | W | A | A | S | Y | U | E | O | P | H | O | D | S | U | I | T | N | E |
| M | W | E | S | D | D | D | C | X | I | S | W | G | O | W | L | P | M | M | D |
| S | S | D | E | E | S | N | M | R | R | R | D | W | V | M | K | D | A | P | S |
| T | W | J | F | R | H | K | L | X | F | R | A | R | K | F | D | S | S | G | E |
| E | E | V | N | H | D | S | W | W | B | M | N | D | E | O | F | U | L | P | I |
| S | S | W | E | S | G | K | R | E | E | E | H | K | M | N | E | X | K | D | I |
| T | E | S | E | I | G | D | N | S | G | T | L | J | N | A | F | I | G | D | H |
| W | A | I | D | F | V | B | D | E | S | D | H | I | W | S | H | L | E | D | R |
| W | P | K | P | P | F | J | Q | A | V | M | Z | S | W | J | K | W | L | Y | E |
| F | V | A | V | V | R | E | I | L | U | O | S | D | R | A | N | R | E | B | G |
| F | A | S | C | G | U | H | W | I | L | J | A | K | L | G | S | D | Q | T | A |
| X | C | A | S | U | J | L | F | W | E | E | G | E | W | S | D | J | F | E | R |
| W | O | W | P | J | W | A | S | S | S | R | A | F | R | E | S | A | J | K | D |
| W | P | A | B | D | H | L | S | A | W | E | H | W | A | F | A | N | H | U | Y |
| D | L | K | G | S | J | J | R | S | E | V | C | S | H | L | H | E | Q | U | H |
| C | N | G | D | S | G | H | P | S | S | Q | D | G | K | E | K | E | A | C | S |
| F | I | K | F | S | E | J | Q | P | G | S | H | C | Z | M | J | G | F | E | E |
| Y | L | F | A | N | C | O | N | I | S | R | G | E | O | H | P | O | L | E | S |

**Answers:** Albright's, Behçet's, Bernard–Soulier, Chagas', Christmas, Darier's, Fanconi's, Ham's test, Kawasaki's, Shy–Drager, Weil's

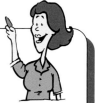

**Q17** A 29-year-old man presents to his GP with polydipsia and polyuria. He drinks 8–10 pints of water daily and wakes several times in the night to pass water and because of thirst. He is afebrile and has lost no body mass. His mother, who is of Antiguan origin, has poorly controlled diabetes but does not yet take insulin. His father is hypertensive and there is no other relevant family history. The patient works in the music industry and has no medical history of note. Clinical examination is unremarkable.

| GP PRELIMINARY INVESTIGATIONS | RESULTS |
| --- | --- |
| BM (blood sugar) | 4.2 mmol/l |
| Urine dipstick | No glucose, protein, or blood |
| | Specific gravity low |

| ENDOCRINE CLINIC INVESTIGATIONS | RESULTS |
| --- | --- |
| Plasma sodium | 141 mmol/l |
| Plasma potassium | 3.7 mmol/l |
| Plasma urea | 8.0 mmol/l |
| Serum albumin | 40 g/l |
| Serum calcium | 2.3 mmol/l |
| Plasma glucose | 4.5 mmol/l |
| Plasma osmolality | 293 mOsmol/l |
| Urine osmolality | 80 mOsmol/l |
| Water deprivation test | Posm at 6 hours = 308 mOsmol/l |
| | Uosm at 6 hours = 100 mOsmol/l |
| | Posm after DDAVP = 290 mOsmol/l |
| | Uosm after DDAVP = 900 mOsmol/l |
| Chest X-ray | Bilateral hilar lymphadenopathy, mild |
| | reticular shadowing in apical lung fields |

DDAVP: 1-deamino-8-D-arginine vasopressin; Posm: plasma osmolality; Uosm: urine osmolality.

## a) What is the cause of this man's symptoms?

i) diabetes mellitus

ii) nephrogenic diabetes insipidus

iii) cranial diabetes insipidus

iv) water intoxication

v) none of the above

b) **What would you expect to find on transbronchial biopsy?**

 i)   eosinophilic granuloma

 ii)  normal biopsy

 iii) abnormal lymphocytes

 iv)  caseating granuloma

 v)   noncaseating granuloma

c) **What is the underlying diagnosis?**

 i)   sarcoidosis

 ii)  histiocytosis X

 iii) psychogenic polydipsia

 iv)  TB

 v)   lymphoma

The key abnormal findings here are:

 • cranial diabetes insipidus

 • bilateral hilar lymphadenopathy

We have already been through the causes of bilateral hilar lymphadenopathy. Jot them down here.

Now check that you got them all:

- sarcoidosis and TB
- lymphoma and cancers
- Churg–Strauss syndrome, phenytoin treatment, extrinsic allergic alveolitis, pneumoconioses (especially berylliosis), cystic fibrosis, and HIV infection

The patient has nothing at all to suggest Churg–Strauss syndrome or HIV infection, has not been exposed to beryllium, and is not receiving phenytoin treatment. The absence of systemic features or findings is against TB, lymphoma, or another malignancy. Thus, the most likely diagnosis is sarcoidosis.

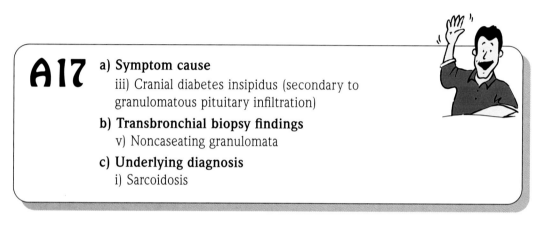

**A17**
a) **Symptom cause**
iii) Cranial diabetes insipidus (secondary to granulomatous pituitary infiltration)
b) **Transbronchial biopsy findings**
v) Noncaseating granulomata
c) **Underlying diagnosis**
i) Sarcoidosis

## TREATMENT

The treatment of choice for cranial diabetes insipidus is administration of synthetic vasopressin. The most convenient route of administration is intranasally, usually 2–3 times daily.

## WATER, WATER EVERYWHERE...

The last few questions might have alarmed you by reminding you about diabetes mellitus, diabetes insipidus, and the causes of polyuria and polydipsia. Fear not! Here is all you need to know about water.

Firstly, water is the most important molecule on the planet, being the primary constituent of beer. Any other facts are superfluous.

Water overload causes dilution. Low levels of urea, sodium, and potassium together should alert you to the diagnosis. Causes are divided into the 'too much in' and 'too little out' categories.

*Too much in*

Causes include: psychogenic polydipsia, hypothalamic tumour (leading to excess thirst), iatrogenic (drip), and water retained in excess of salt, such as in states of oedema – congestive heart failure, cirrhosis, nephrotic oedema, and myxoedema.

*Too little out*

In the syndrome of inappropriate antidiuretic hormone secretion (SIADH), plasma osmolality is low, but urine osmolality is higher than that of plasma. Urinary sodium excretion may also be raised. Sorry (in advance) for the bad pun, but the causes of SIADH are **CCCP**, as *there ain't no water 'Russian' out!*

| | |
|---|---|
| Chest: | infections (abscess, effusions, pneumonia, TB), tumours (small cell carcinoma especially) |
| Cerebral: | infections (abscess, meningitis, TB), tumours (cerebral) |
| Cancers: | lungs and other sites rarely, such as the pancreas |
| Ps: | pleural effusions, pancreatitis, porphyria, and pills **CCCAN** (carbamazepine, chlorpropamide, clofibrate, antipsychotics, nonsteroidal anti-inflammatory drugs) |

Pure salt depletion is unusual as a cause of hyponatraemia, but can occur with diarrhoea/vomiting if adequate water intake is sustained. Beware pseudohyponatraemia, when cholesterol and fat levels in the blood take up space in the sample volume and lead to erroneous assessment of serum sodium. This occurs in nephrotic syndrome and ketoacidosis.

### ...AND NOT A DROP TO DRINK

*Diabetes insipidus*

This is due to a lack of antidiuretic hormone action, which may be due to:

- low production: anything destroying posterior pituitary function: hypothalamic damage, craniopharyngioma, pituitary stalk damage (e.g. Sheehan's syndrome of pituitary stalk infarction complicating post-partum haemorrhagic shock), pituitary tumours, basal meningitis (particularly tuberculous meningitis), sarcoidosis (work your way through your surgical sieve)
- resistance to action
    - drugs: such as lithium, or amphotericin therapy

- – electrolytes: prolonged hypercalcaemia, hypokalaemia or hyponatraemia, or distal tubular disease

- – inherited: nephrogenic diabetes insipidus (X-linked)

Note: hypoadrenalism also prevents the normal concentration of urine.

Answers to the causes of erythema nodosum (page 182): sarcoidosis, TB, the pill, sulphonamides, bromides, iodides, streptococci, IBD, histoplasmosis, blastomycosis (and horse and mules).

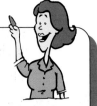

**Q18** A 25-year-old man is admitted to the emergency department following a road traffic accident, during which he briefly lost consciousness. He had lost control of the vehicle and tells you that he had taken Ecstasy and drank two beers that night. He is found to have a closed fracture of his left tibia and fibula. Despite the fact that the orthopaedic senior house officer is keen to discharge the patient with a Tubigrip, he is admitted for surgical treatment under general anaesthesia. Afterwards, he complains of a slight headache and coryza with a runny nose. He was treated for non-Hodgkin's lymphoma at the age of 18 years, and smokes 15 cigarettes per day. He occasionally takes cocaine on Saturday nights. Some 36 hours post-operatively, he appears to have developed an acute confusional state. The nurses report that he has oliguria. His blood tests from that morning are as follows.

| INVESTIGATIONS | RESULTS |
| --- | --- |
| Plasma sodium | 120 mmol/l |
| Plasma urea | 2.8 mmol/l |
| Plasma potassium | 3.2 mmol/l |
| Plasma creatinine | 45 μmol/l |
| Plasma glucose | 5.2 mmol/l |

a) **What is the most probable cause of the above results?**

   i)    Ecstasy overdose

   ii)   SIADH

   iii)  fluid overload

   iv)   pseudohyponatraemia

   v)    psychogenic polydipsia

b) **What is the immediate management of this patient?**

   i)    admit to intensive care

   ii)   CT scan of the head

   iii)  fluid restriction

   iv)   hypertonic (3%) saline

   v)    arginine vasopressin antagonists

This poor fellow has severe hyponatraemia following surgery. The temptation is immediately to blame the orthopaedic consultant for his fluid management. *In general, this is a good idea and is to be encouraged. Please speak slowly, however, so that they can keep up. Wave a £20 note intermittently to keep their attention.*

However, you must remember that the patient has also had a closed head injury. The fact that he is oliguric suggests that he might be suffering from SIADH.

Finally, Ecstasy overdose can lead to a variety of metabolic abnormalities, as can excessive drinking of fluids whilst taking it. However, probably too much time has lapsed for these effects to be responsible for the patient's symptoms.

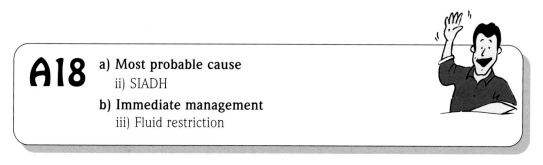

**A18**　a) **Most probable cause**
　　　　ii) SIADH
　　　b) **Immediate management**
　　　　iii) Fluid restriction

Another favourite scenario in the examination is that under different circumstances trauma may lead to central diabetes insipidus due to damage to the posterior pituitary.

### HYPONATRAEMIA

It is useful to think of hyponatraemia in terms of a patient's fluid balance, as below.

| OEDEMATOUS | NORMAL FLUID BALANCE | DEHYDRATED |
|---|---|---|
| Excess body water > excess sodium | Excess body water + normal body sodium | Sodium loss > water loss |
| Examples: | Examples: | Examples: |
| • CHF | • SIADH (all causes) | • adrenal insufficiency |
| • cirrhosis | • pseudohyponatraemia (hyperglycaemia, hyperlipidaemia multiple myeloma) | • GI losses (diarrhoea and vomiting, fistula) |
| • nephrotic syndrome | | • renal losses (diuretics, osmotic diuresis, renal tubular disease) |
| • myxoedema | • psychogenic polydipsia | |

CHF: congestive heart failure; GI: gastrointestinal; SIADH: syndrome of inappropriate antidiuretic hormone secretion.

Remember, too, that:

$$\text{Calculated plasma osmolality} = 2(Na + K) + urea + glucose$$

You can use this trick in the emergency department. Calculate the osmolality, then ask the laboratory to measure it. They are usually happier to do this than to measure a blood alcohol level. Work out the difference between the calculated and real measurements. This difference must be ascribed to some metabolically active agent in the blood. If the patient has been drinking, you can assume that this substance is alcohol. As 1 mmol of alcohol is responsible for 1 mOsmol, you can now calculate the mmol/l of alcohol. Knowing the relative molecular mass of alcohol (from its formula $C_2H_5OH$) you can calculate the number of mg/dl!

## Potassium

### Potassium and pH

Hydrogen and potassium ions can be considered to compete for cellular handling. Thus, as potassium levels rise, fewer hydrogen ions can enter into cells, and plasma hydrogen levels rise. At the renal tubule, excess potassium also limits hydrogen excretion. Thus, primary hyperkalaemia is associated with acidosis (hyperkalaemic acidosis) and primary potassium depletion with alkalosis (hypokalaemic alkalosis). The same association of potassium and hydrogen is seen in primary metabolic acidosis and alkalosis. Thus, hypokalaemic alkalosis is seen in situations of excess potassium loss. Hypokalaemic acidosis, on the other hand, needs a loss of both bicarbonate and potassium. Draw up a list of causes of hypokalaemic alkalosis and hypokalaemic acidosis; then check it against the list below.

*and remember...*

...glucocorticoids and mineralocorticoids are sodium sparing and potassium wasting.

| Hypokalaemic alkalosis | Hypokalaemic acidosis |
| --- | --- |
| 'STEROID hormones GIVe VILe Diuresis' | 'PARADE' |
| **Steroid:** Conn's syndrome, Cushing's disease, corticosteroid treatment, phaeochromocytoma, liquorice and carbenoxolone | Partially treated diabetic ketoacidosis (already acid: insulin drives potassium into cells) |
| | Acetazolamide |
| **GI:** Vomiting | Renal tubular Acidosis (type I = distal, type II = proximal) |
| VIllous adenoma, Laxative | Diarrhoea and hypovolaemic shock |
| Diuretics (e.g. thiazides) | Enteric (ureterosigmoidostomy or biliary/pancreatic fistula leading to bicarbonate loss: vipoma with MEN type I) |

GI: gastrointestinal; MEN: multiple endocrine neoplasia.

*Remember the inherited tubulopathies*

Defects in the loop of Henle channels, which actively reabsorb sodium from the distal convoluted tubule, lead to excessive distal convoluted tubule salt loading and eventually salt loss (e.g. in Bartter's or Gitelman's syndromes). The result is biochemically similar to blockade from loop diuretics: polyuria, hypokalaemic alkalosis, hypocalcaemia, and high salt secretion are seen. For various reasons (led by high angiotensin II levels), patients also exhibit growth inhibition and intellectual retardation. They may be dysmorphic or have sensorineural hearing loss. *Thus, you might* **say** *that the patient with Bartter's syndrome is strangely 'short' on IQ, potassium, sodium, and calcium, but he might not hear you!*

Treatment includes sodium, potassium, calcium, and magnesium supplementation, use of spironolactone (an aldosterone antagonist), amiloride, and ACE inhibitors. Growth hormone is used to treat short stature.

In addition, prolonged hypokalaemia is a cause of polyuria and polydipsia. Other causes to bear in mind are:

- prolonged hypercalcaemia
- diabetes mellitus and diabetes insipidus
- recovery phase of acute tubular necrosis, or after release of obstruction
- psychogenic polydipsia
- chronic renal impairment

*Now three quick questions to keep you going...*

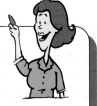

**Q19** A 55-year-old man presents to the emergency department with lethargy, polyuria, and polydipsia. He finds this distressing as he is unable to go ballroom dancing, which he usually does at the weekends. He has been widowed for the last 18 months and takes no regular medication. His clinical examination is unremarkable other than his blood pressure, which is 175/105 mmHg. His blood test results are shown below.

| INVESTIGATIONS | RESULT |
| --- | --- |
| Plasma sodium | 148 mmol/l |
| Plasma bicarbonate | 37 mmol/l |
| Serum calcium | 2.3 mmol/l |
| Plasma potassium | 2.5 mmol/l |
| Plasma chloride | 98 mmol/l |
| Serum albumin | 38 g/l |
| Plasma creatinine | 100 μmol/l |
| Plasma glucose | 5.2 mmol/l |

a) **What is the underlying diagnosis?**

   i)    Conn's syndrome

   ii)   diabetes insipidus

   iii)  type I renal tubular acidosis

   iv)  Bartter's syndrome

   v)   Gitelman's syndrome

b) **Which two biochemical tests would you use next to confirm the diagnosis?**

   i)    plasma aldosterone and plasma renin

   ii)   serum aldosterone and 24-hour urinary aldosterone

   iii)  urine potassium and urine aldosterone

   iv)  serum magnesium and 24-hour urinary calcium

   v)   anion gap and urine pH

c) **Which two radiological tests would you use to further confirm the diagnosis?**

   i)    CT scan of the brain and adrenal veins

   ii)   X-ray and ultrasound scan of the abdomen

   iii)  CT scan of the abdomen and bilateral adrenal vein sampling

   iv)   MRI scan of the brain and adrenal veins

   v)    MRI scan of the adrenal veins and bilateral adrenal vein sampling

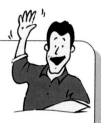

**A19**

a) **Diagnosis**

i) The patient has a hypokalaemic alkalosis. He is also hypertensive. Thus, the diagnosis is Conn's syndrome.

b) **Biochemical tests**

ii) The plasma aldosterone to plasma renin activity ratio is a useful screening test for Conn's syndrome. A ratio of >25 has 95% sensitivity and 75% specificity. However, it is only useful as a screening tool and a more definitive test would be serum and 24-hour urine aldosterone (this is the most useful test), which would be confirmatory.

c) **Radiological tests**

i) CT scan of the abdomen and bilateral adrenal vein sampling (differentiates a unilateral aldosterone-producing adenoma from bilateral adrenal hyperplasia).

Generally, an MRI scan of the adrenals is no more useful than a high-resolution CT scan.

Note: if there is hypokalaemic/hypochloraemic alkalosis, think vomiting/gastric outlet obstruction.

## CONN'S SYNDROME

This results from a primary excess of mineralocorticoids, causing sodium retention and potassium loss. However, the sodium retention causes hyperosmolality, and thus increased antidiuretic hormone secretion and volume expansion. There is hypokalaemic alkalosis with low bicarbonate levels, low/normal or only slightly elevated sodium levels, and hypertension.

## Polyuria and polydipsia

The patient also complained of polyuria and polydipsia. In this case, the biochemical tests showed the patient to be hypokalaemic. However, in the absence of any other data, the causes of polyuria and polydipsia are useful to know. Revise them now, then check your answers against the list on page 98.

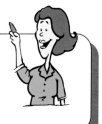

**Q20** A 45-year-old woman presents to surgeons with abdominal pain, weight loss, and malaise. Apart from mild hypothyroidism she has otherwise been well. On examination, she appears to be somewhat dehydrated.

| INVESTIGATIONS | RESULT |
| --- | --- |
| Pulse | 110 beats/min |
| Blood pressure | 90/45 mmHg |
| Temperature | 36.6°C |
| Abdominal examination | Generalised abdominal tenderness |
| Urinalysis | Normal |
| Plasma sodium | 125 mmol/l |
| Plasma potassium | 6.9 mmol/l |
| Plasma urea | 16 mmol/l |
| Plasma bicarbonate | 15 mmol/l |

### a) What is the diagnosis?

i) renal tubular acidosis type 4

ii) Addison's disease

iii) gastrointestinal malignancy

iv) drug-induced thyrotoxicosis

v) acute renal failure secondary to haemorrhage

### b) How could this be confirmed quickly?

i) 24-hour urine potassium levels

ii) short tetracosactrin test

iii) CT scan of the abdomen

iv) thyroid function tests

v) ultrasound of the abdomen

**A20** a) **Diagnosis**
ii) The obvious feature here is a hyperkalaemic acidosis. The patient also has abdominal pain and hypotension. Thus, the diagnosis is Addison's disease.

b) **Quick test**
ii) The test is a short tetracosactrin (ACTH: adrenocorticotrophic hormone) test followed by a therapeutic trial of steroids.

## ADDISON'S DISEASE

This is caused by adrenal failure. Patients may be tanned, with scar/palmar crease/buccal pigmentation. Acute cortisol deficiency causes nausea and vomiting, general malaise, and weight loss. This compounds the renal sodium loss due to adrenal hormone deficiency, and hyponatraemia, hypotension, uraemia, and hyperkalaemic acidosis are seen. A normal cortisol level at any time of the day excludes the diagnosis, as does a normal short tetracosactrin test (tetracosactrin 250 µg i.m. raises cortisol levels by >200 nmol/l to >550 nmol/l), a 5-hour test (tetracosactrin 1 mg intramuscular [i.m.]: cortisol levels are 600–1300 nmol/l at 1 hour and 1000–1800 nmol/l at 5 hours), or a 3-day test (tetracosactrin 1 mg daily: check levels daily at 5 hours; a rising response over 3 days suggests a chronic lack of adrenocorticotrophic hormone).

*Causes of Addison's disease*
You should know these. Construct a quick list here from your surgical sieve:

*Our list*

Remember:

**Congenital**: rare – congenital adrenal hyperplasia is the most common cause

**Acquired**:

T: –

I: TB, fungi (including *Cryptococcus*, coccidioidomycosis, histoplasmosis), *Neisseria meningitidis* (Waterhouse–Friderichsen syndrome)

E, H, I, M: –

I: drugs such as rifampicin, phenytoin, carbamazepine

N: metastases

...and autoimmune adrenal failure

Note: patients must be warned to increase their dose of maintenance steroids during intercurrent infection and during treatment with enzyme inducers, such as rifampicin; in examinations, beware of a patient with Addison's disease who is being treated for TB.

# QUIZ SPOT!

**Q:** Polycythaemia rubra vera, myelofibrosis, and myeloproliferative disorders cause a raised leucocyte alkaline phosphatase level. What else does?

A: Hodgkin's lymphoma

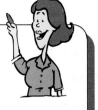

# Q21

An 11-year-old girl is admitted with a history of abdominal pain, vomiting, and malaise. She has no previous history of any illnesses. Clinical examination reveals only mild abdominal tenderness.

| INVESTIGATIONS | RESULTS |
| --- | --- |
| Pulse | 110 beats/min |
| Blood pressure | 95/65 mmHg |
| Temperature | 36.8°C |
| Plasma sodium | 128 mmol/l |
| Plasma potassium | 6.8 mmol/l |
| Plasma urea | 12 mmol/l |
| Plasma bicarbonate | 7 mmol/l |

a) **What is the diagnosis?**

   i)    Addison's disease

   ii)   Henoch–Schönlein purpura

   iii)  acute intermittent porphyria

   iv)  diabetic ketoacidosis

   v)   phaeochromocytoma

b) **What is your immediate management, after confirmation of your suspicions?**

**A21**

a) Diagnosis

iv) This is a classic MRCP examination case of diabetic ketoacidosis. Often, the sodium will be presented as much lower, due to pseudohyponatraemia from high blood lipid/cholesterol levels.

b) **Immediate management**

After confirming the diagnosis with a blood glucose level and urinalysis, aggressive normal saline rehydration is the key. Only when the patient has intravenous fluids being infused should a sliding scale of insulin be started and the cause of this complication be addressed.

## MORE ABOUT ADDISON'S DISEASE

Why is the diagnosis in this case not Addison's disease? Addison's disease rarely causes such a severe metabolic acidosis as diabetic ketoacidosis. The bicarbonate level in Addison's disease rarely falls below 15 mmol/l.

However, it is worth remembering that Addison's disease can present in a patient with diabetes. This association is known as Schmidt's syndrome.

## DID YOU KNOW...

...that phaeochromocytomas cause hyperkalaemia and can be identified on ultrasound/MRI/CT scan, or using MIBG (meta-iodobenzylguanidine) scanning?

...that both Conn's syndrome and hyperosmolar nonketotic hyperglycaemia cause low potassium and high sodium levels?

## ACID HOUSE PARTY

*In a nutshell...*

...remember the following equations:

1)  $H^+ + HCO_3^- \leftrightharpoons H_2CO_3 \leftrightharpoons H_2O + CO_2$

2)  $pH \propto \dfrac{\log[HCO_3^-]}{pCO_2}$

*Metabolic acidosis*

Metabolic acidosis adds hydrogen ions, which lower the bicarbonate concentration and pH. Compensation is achieved by increased respiratory drive, blowing off carbon dioxide, and normalising pH (equation 2).

*Metabolic alkalosis*

Metabolic alkalosis loses hydrogen ions. The first equation therefore moves from right to left, and the bicarbonate concentration and pH rise (equation 2). Compensation is achieved by retaining carbon dioxide (equation 2).

Think of acid loss (potassium loss, chloride depletion, pyloric stenosis, hyperaldosteronism) or alkali gain (forced alkaline diuresis, excess alkali in chronic renal failure).

*Respiratory acidosis*

Respiratory acidosis gains carbon dioxide, causing the bicarbonate and hydrogen concentrations to rise, and the pH to fall. Compensation is achieved by retaining bicarbonate (equation 2).

Think:

- respiratory depression (raised intracranial pressure, drugs such as opioids and barbiturates, and overdoses)
- neuromuscular disease (neuropathy such as Guillain–Barré syndrome, motor neurone disease), myopathy
- skeletal disease (thoracic cage abnormalities: kyphoscoliosis and ankylosing spondylitis)
- severe asthma, chronic obstructive pulmonary disease

*Respiratory alkalosis*

Respiratory alkalosis loses carbon dioxide, equation 1 moves from left to right, and hydrogen and bicarbonate concentrations and pH fall. Compensation is achieved by losing bicarbonate (equation 2).

Remember that hypoxia should normally drive a respiratory alkalosis (except in 'blue bloaters'). Think of pulmonary oedema and lung fibrosis – both may be associated with unremarkable chest X-rays. An inappropriately increased respiratory drive (amphetamines, panic attack, early salicylate poisoning) is another catch.

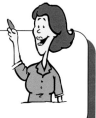

**Q22** A 16-year-old boy has been receiving chemotherapy for a teratoma. He presents to the emergency department 3 days after his latest course in a confused state with hyperventilation.

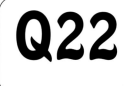

| INVESTIGATIONS | RESULTS |
| --- | --- |
| Arterial blood $pO_2$ (or $PaO_2$) | 17.5 kPa |
| Arterial blood $pCO_2$ (or $PaCO_2$) | 2.9 kPa |
| Plasma bicarbonate | 12 mmol/l |
| Plasma sodium | 135 mmol/l |
| Plasma potassium | 7.2 mmol/l |
| Plasma chloride | 98 mmol/l |
| Plasma urea | 45 mmol/l |
| Plasma creatinine | 280 μmol/l |
| Plasma glucose | 3.8 mmol/l |

a) **What is the patient's anion gap?**

b) **What is the most likely diagnosis?**

  i)    diabetic ketoacidosis
  ii)   sepsis secondary to immunosuppression
  iii)  salicylate poisoning
  iv)   acute anxiety attack
  v)    tumour lysis syndrome

c) **What is the acute management?**

  i)    intravenous fluids and insulin infusion
  ii)   intravenous broad-spectrum antibiotic
  iii)  intravenous calcium chloride and dextrose–insulin infusion
  iv)   β-blockers and benzodiazepines
  v)    activated charcoal, intravenous fluids, and urinary alkalinisation

Aha! The bl**dy anion gap! Always a pain. Actually, however, it is not so difficult.

## Mind the gap

To maintain electrical neutrality in the blood, the concentration of cations and anions in the blood must be equal. However, the concentrations of routinely measured cations (sodium and potassium) and routinely measured anions (chloride and bicarbonate) never match; there are many anions that are not measured. This concentration of unmeasured anions is called the 'anion gap'. In other words:

$$([Na^+] + [K^+]) - ([HCO_3^-] + [Cl^-]) = \text{the anion gap}$$

The anion gap is normally 15–20 mmol/l.

Thus, the presence of excess unmeasured acids will soak up buffering bicarbonate ions and the anion gap will increase. Coming up is a list of these situations. Cover it up now, write down your own list, and then check it against the table below.

### Causes of metabolic acidosis with a high anion gap

| Condition | Causes |
|---|---|
| Ketoacidosis | Diabetic ketoacidosis |
| Lactic acidosis: | |
| Type A (tissue hypoxia) | Circulatory shock (sepsis, cardiogenic shock, left ventricular failure, bleeds, severe anaemia) |
| Type B (no tissue hypoxia) | Acute hepatic failure |
| | Renal failure (acute and chronic) |
| | Leukaemias |
| | Biguanides (metformin, phenformin) |
| Poisoning with acids | Salicylates |
| | Methanol and ethanol |

If the bicarbonate loss is matched by loss of cations then the anion gap will be normal. Thus, when you see an acidosis with normal anion gap, think of conditions where bicarbonate and sodium/potassium are lost together. Write yourself a checklist of such causes, and then compare it with the following list.

### Causes of metabolic acidosis with a normal anion gap

- Renal tubular acidosis
- Severe diarrhoea (remember villous adenomata, where potassium can be lost in quantity!)
- Carbonic anhydrase inhibitors (cause potassium and bicarbonate loss)

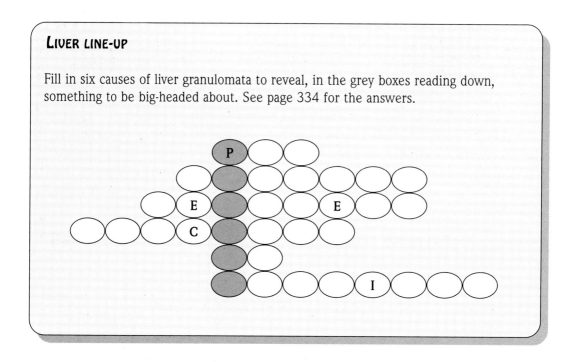

### LIVER LINE-UP

Fill in six causes of liver granulomata to reveal, in the grey boxes reading down, something to be big-headed about. See page 334 for the answers.

Here you are actually given the answer in the question. The patient is clearly in renal failure and you only have to make the obvious assumption that the cause of his renal failure is secondary to hyperuricaemia as a consequence of his chemotherapy. Such cases are quite rare these days, as patients are routinely predosed with allopurinol and preloaded with fluids. But that doesn't stop the examiners thinking that this is a good question.

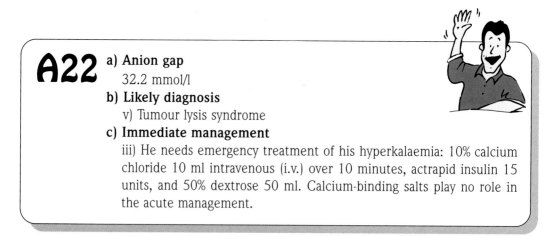

**A22** a) **Anion gap**
32.2 mmol/l
b) **Likely diagnosis**
v) Tumour lysis syndrome
c) **Immediate management**
iii) He needs emergency treatment of his hyperkalaemia: 10% calcium chloride 10 ml intravenous (i.v.) over 10 minutes, actrapid insulin 15 units, and 50% dextrose 50 ml. Calcium-binding salts play no role in the acute management.

# Q23

A 60-year-old woman presents to the emergency department with breathlessness. She has been increasingly short of breath over the last week. She is an ex-smoker of 10 pack years, but her husband continues to smoke 10–15 cigarettes per day. On direct questioning, she denies a cough productive of sputum, haemoptysis, or chest pain. She does voluntary work for her local church arranging flowers for weddings, and keeps a parrot. She returned from New Mexico 1 month ago, where she had been on holiday. She is diabetic and until recently was diet-controlled. However, she has recently put on 3 stone in weight ("but I hardly eat anything") and started oral hypoglycaemic agents 2 weeks ago.

## ON EXAMINATION

- Body mass index = 32 kg/m$^2$
- Respiratory rate = 34 breaths/min
- Early cataract in right eye

## INVESTIGATIONS

- Haemoglobin = 12 g/dl
- Plasma sodium = 138 mmol/l
- Plasma glucose = 7.2 mmol/l
- White cell count = 7.1 × 10$^9$/l
- Plasma potassium = 4.6 mmol/l
- Plasma bicarbonate = 14 mmol/l
- Platelets = 382 × 10$^9$/l
- Plasma urea = 8.1 mmol/l
- Plasma chloride = 93 mmol/l
- Plasma creatinine = 112 μmol/l
- SaO$_2$ = 97%

SaO$_2$: oxygen saturation in arterial blood.

## a) What is the cause of her current presentation?

i) silent myocardial infarction

ii) extrinsic allergic alveolitis

iii) coccidioidomycosis

iv) metformin toxicity

v) acute exacerbation of chronic obstructive lung disease

Hmmm. Not so straightforward at first glance. The history is full of red herrings, and most of the biochemistry, at first glance, looks pretty unremarkable. You know, by now, that there must be an abnormal finding with a limited list of causes. Either that, or this is a 'classic case' that you just need to recognise.

Remember that breathlessness may be due to hypoxia, central drive abnormalities, or metabolic acidosis. Hypoxia is excluded by the normal $SaO_2$, and there is nothing to suggest a neurological component centrally. Thus, there is likely to be a metabolic acidosis.

The anion gap is high (35.6 mmol/l).

What are the causes of high anion gap metabolic acidosis? They were given earlier, but refresh your memory by filling in the table.

| CONDITION | CAUSES |
| --- | --- |
| Ketoacidosis | |
| Lactic acidosis: | |
| Type A (tissue hypoxia) | |
| | |
| Type B (no tissue hypoxia) | |
| | |
| | |
| | |
| Poisoning with acids | |

We have no evidence of tissue hypoxia or ketoacidosis and she is unlikely to have been poisoned with methanol or salicylates.

Non-insulin-dependent diabetes mellitus, overweight, new drug, thus suggests...

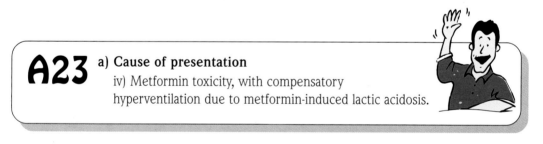

**A23** a) **Cause of presentation**
iv) Metformin toxicity, with compensatory hyperventilation due to metformin-induced lactic acidosis.

## LESSONS TO LEARN FROM THIS QUESTION

- If a new medication has recently been started, this should be suspected as the cause of or a contributor to the pathology.
- If the test results include chloride and bicarbonate, you're probably meant to use them!

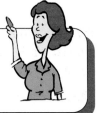

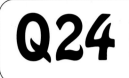

**Q24** A 14-year-old girl presents to the emergency department with confusion. She is usually fit and well, apart from occasional headache.

| INVESTIGATIONS | RESULTS |
|---|---|
| Arterial blood $pO_2$ (or $PaO_2$) | 17.3 kPa |
| Arterial blood $pCO_2$ (or $PaCO_2$) | 2.2 kPa |
| Plasma bicarbonate | 9 mmol/l |
| Plasma sodium | 139 mmol/l |
| Plasma potassium | 3.2 mmol/l |
| Plasma chloride | 102 mmol/l |
| Plasma urea | 6.3 mmol/l |
| Plasma creatinine | 65 μmol/l |
| Plasma glucose | 3.8 mmol/l |

## a) What investigation would you now order?

i) serum alcohol level

ii) salicylate level

iii) serum osmolality

iv) urine ketone levels

v) bone marrow biopsy

This is a severe metabolic acidosis with a high anion gap (31.2 mmol/l). The fact that the patient has intermittent headaches allows us to make the diagnosis of accidental salicylate overdose as being most likely. Salicylates may cause a primary respiratory alkalosis, a metabolic acidosis, tinnitus, deafness, visual obscurement, pulmonary oedema, renal failure, and hypoglycaemia.

A similar severe metabolic acidosis occurs in alcoholics who accidentally drink methanol. In the MRCP examination, the typical patient is a tramp, who is brought to the emergency department in a collapsed state from the local park, with severe metabolic acidosis. In that case, the patient is meant to have drunk methylated spirits. Even if your studies for the MRCP examination are not going well, we strongly advise you not to take this course of action. Like other activities said to be associated with solitary boredom, it can make you go blind.

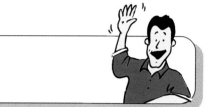

**A24**    **a) Investigation**
             ii) Salicylate level

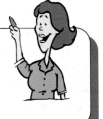

## Q25

A 23-year-old woman presents to the emergency department on Christmas Day with breathlessness. The emergency department senior house officer asks you to take a look at her blood gas results.

| INVESTIGATIONS | RESULTS |
| --- | --- |
| Arterial blood pH | 7.65 |
| Arterial blood $pO_2$ ($PaO_2$) | 9.8 kPa |
| Arterial blood $pCO_2$ ($PaCO_2$) | 7.8 kPa |
| Plasma bicarbonate | 12 mmol/l |
| Base excess | −5 |
| Plasma sodium | 141 mmol/l |
| Plasma potassium | 4.2 mmol/l |
| Plasma chloride | 106 mmol/l |
| Plasma urea | 3.3 mmol/l |
| Plasma glucose | 4.1 mmol/l |

## a) What would you do next?

   i)    ask the senior house officer to contact the intensive care unit immediately
   ii)   order an immediate chest X-ray and go to see the patient
   iii)  suggest nebulised salbutamol and intravenous aminophylline
   iv)   repeat the blood gases and look at the patient
   v)    ask the senior house officer to set up BiPAP (biphasic positive airway pressure) on the patient

This is a typical MRCP examination question that has come up on a number of occasions. Calculation shows that the patient has a high anion gap (27.2 mmol/l). Furthermore, respiratory compensation for this would be to hyperventilate to blow off carbon dioxide, but this is also high. This suggests that she has combined metabolic and respiratory acidosis, but in fact the pH shows that she is alkalotic. Thus, the results are impossible and would need to be repeated. (A quick look at the patient should inform the experienced clinician that this is a load of nonsense.)

The clue in the question is that this occurred on Christmas Day, and we can only conclude that either the emergency department senior house officer or the laboratory technician overindulged in the Christmas spirit. But fortunately, you as the medical registrar will save the day. Hurrah!

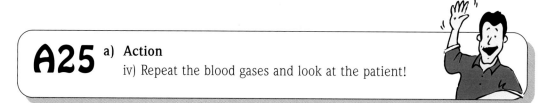

**A25** a) **Action**
iv) Repeat the blood gases and look at the patient!

Remember that, in the MRCP examination, trick questions such as this are loved by the examiners. They feel that they are a good discriminator between candidates, although, with all the MRCP books and courses available, people fall for these less often.

*Nonetheless, if a test does not appear to fit with the clinical situation then make sure that it is not a laboratory error.*

Answers to chorioidoretinitis causes (page 84): cytomegalovirus, syphilis, (boring), tuberculosis, toxocariasis, (pimple), toxoplasmosis, sarcoidosis.

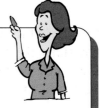

**Q26** A 63-year-old man who is otherwise well presents to the emergency department 3 days after experiencing his first epileptic seizure. This was witnessed by his wife, who described a classic tonic–clonic grand mal seizure. He was seen by his GP, who found no residual abnormality and arranged for an outpatient neurology referral. Since that time he has felt lethargic and slightly nauseous. He denies the consumption of excess alcohol or other drugs. It is noted in the emergency department that he is hyperventilating.

| INVESTIGATIONS | RESULTS |
| --- | --- |
| Arterial blood $pO_2$ (PaO$_2$) | 16.8 kPa |
| Arterial blood $pCO_2$ (PaCO$_2$) | 3.8 kPa |
| Plasma bicarbonate | 12 mmol/l |
| Arterial blood base excess | −7 |
| Plasma sodium | 141 mmol/l |
| Plasma potassium | 4.2 mmol/l |
| Plasma chloride | 106 mmol/l |
| Plasma urea | 33.3 mmol/l |
| Plasma creatinine | 290 µmol/l |
| Plasma glucose | 4.1 mmol/l |
| Salicylates | Negative |
| CT scan of the head | No abnormality detected |

### a) What would be a useful diagnostic test?

i) ultrasound of the kidneys

ii) creatinine kinase levels

iii) oral benzodiazepines

iv) serum prolactin levels

v) 24-hour urine collection

### b) What is the most likely diagnosis?

i) abdominal malignancy with cerebral metastasis

ii) acute renal failure secondary to rhabdomyolysis

iii) pseudoseizures

iv) acute on chronic renal failure

v) alcohol withdrawal

## b) What is the most likely diagnosis?

    i)      abdominal malignancy with cerebral metastasis

    ii)     acute renal failure secondary to rhabdomyolysis

    iii)    pseudoseizures

    iv)    acute on chronic renal failure

    v)     alcohol withdrawal

Again the clue to the question is the high anion gap metabolic acidosis. The cause of this is likely to be acute renal failure and, given that the patient has had a grand mal seizure, the likely diagnosis is rhabdomyolysis as a consequence of this.

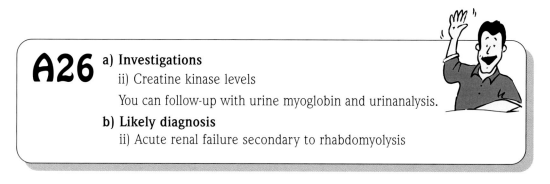

**A26**  **a) Investigations**
      ii) Creatine kinase levels
      You can follow-up with urine myoglobin and urinanalysis.
  **b) Likely diagnosis**
      ii) Acute renal failure secondary to rhabdomyolysis

Rhabdomyolysis crops up in the MRCP examination on a regular basis. It can occur as a consequence of a number of medical problems.

### CAUSES OF RHABDOMYOLYSIS

We have **TEASED** out the answers for you:

- trauma – ischaemic muscle damage (compartment syndrome), bullet wounds, road traffic accidents
- exertion, if severe – paratroopers, prolonged epileptic seizures
- alcoholics – via seizures, prolonged immobility, hypophosphataemia
- snake bites! (Unusual, it has to be said, in the UK)
- excessive temperature – malignant hyperthermia or environmental
- drug intoxication – cocaine or Ecstasy, or prolonged immobility from any other cause

There is a range of congenital causes, but these are rare and seldom turn up in examinations. Feel free to look up McArdle's disease and mitochondrial diseases.

## TREATMENT OF RHABDOMYOLYSIS

- Hydration – vigorous fluid replacement with central venous pressure measurements
- Alkalinisation of the urine (keep urine pH >7.6)
- Dialysis if necessary

## USEFUL INFORMATION

One last problem that is unique to rhabdomyolysis-induced acute renal failure is the development of hypercalcaemia during the recovery phase in about one-third of patients. This complication can be prevented to some degree by avoiding calcium therapy of hyperkalaemia during the acute stage.

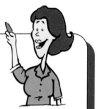

# Q27

A young man is brought to the emergency department by his fiancée. She is worried that he is unable to walk without assistance. When he tries to demonstrate his gait, he is extremely unsteady and has a tendency to veer to one side. In addition to this, she has noticed that his speech has become more slurred in the last day or so. Initially she thought he had been secretly drinking, but his symptoms did not improve even after she poured all of the alcohol away (except the Baileys!). On examination, he is icteric with early clubbing of the nails. He is not pallid. He has 3 cm hepatomegaly and mild ascites. There is a resting tremor. He has no cerebellar signs or specific nerve palsies.

| INVESTIGATIONS | RESULTS |
|---|---|
| Plasma sodium | 140 mmol/l |
| Plasma bicarbonate | 16 mmol/l |
| Plasma potassium | 3.1 mmol/l |
| Plasma chloride | 111 mmol/l |
| Plasma creatinine | 102 µmol/l |
| Plasma glucose | 5.6 mmol/l |
| Serum bilirubin | 38 µmol/l |
| Serum alanine aminotransferase | 80 IU/l |
| Serum alkaline phosphatase | 130 IU/l |
| Arterial blood pH | 7.29 |

### a) What is the cause of this man's symptoms?

- i) alcohol abuse with Wernicke's encephalopathy
- ii) Verner–Morrison syndrome
- iii) basal ganglia degeneration due to excess copper deposition
- iv) lead poisoning
- v) Friedrich's ataxia

### b) What would explain his biochemistry results?

- i) type I renal tubular acidosis
- ii) type II renal tubular acidosis
- iii) type III renal tubular acidosis
- iv) type IV renal tubular acidosis
- v) none of the above

**c) What one investigation will confirm the diagnosis?**

   i)     vitamin $B_{12}$ levels

   ii)    nerve conduction studies

   iii)   CT scan of the abdomen

   iv)   genetic tests for the frataxin gene

   v)    serum caeruloplasmin levels

**d) What treatment should be started?**

   i)     D-penicillinamine

   ii)    chlordiazepoxide and alcohol counselling

   iii)   diagnostic and therapeutic laparoscopic surgery

   iv)   physiotherapy

   v)    dimercaprol

This man evidently has liver disease – presumably with portal hypertension producing the ascites. He also has some neurological signs. But what is the *key abnormal finding* for which there is *a limited list of diagnoses?*

As has been mentioned before, if bicarbonate and chloride levels are given, then use them! In this case, the anion gap is normal. You therefore need to go to the list of hypokalaemic acidosis with normal anion gap that was covered earlier.

---

*Hypokalaemic acidosis with normal anion gap*

'PARADE'

Partially-treated diabetic ketoacidosis (already acid: insulin drives potassium into cells)

Acetazolamide

Renal tubular Acidosis (type I = distal, type II = proximal)

Diarrhoea + hypovolaemic shock

Enteric (ureterosigmoidostomy or biliary/pancreatic fistula leading to bicarbonate loss: vipoma with multiple endocrine neoplasia type I)

---

Severe diarrhoea causes loss of sodium bicarbonate in stools followed by renal sodium chloride retention. Ureterosigmoidostomy causes chloride uptake in the bowel; this operation is becoming obsolete due to the fact that it causes a hyperchloraemic metabolic acidosis with increased blood ammonium and total-body potassium depletion. It is also associated with a 500-fold increase in the incidence of bowel cancer.

## BILIARY OR PANCREATIC FISTULA

Vipoma with multiple endocrine neoplasia type I is also known as the Verner–Morrison syndrome.

By a process of elimination, we must be dealing with renal tubular acidosis. What are the causes of renal tubular acidosis, hepatocellular disease, and neurological signs? The answer is Wilson's disease.

You might approach this question in a number of ways. The 'list approach' narrows the diagnoses down, but eventually you need to 'just recognise the case'.

The heavy metal disorders are interesting and rare. Mercury is used in the treatment of vitiligo and homeopathic medicines, or is accidentally leaked from power plants, so watch out! Cadmium toxicity causes osteomalacia with tubular changes and lung emphysema.

| CAUSES OF RENAL TUBULAR ACIDOSIS | TYPE I | TYPE II |
|---|---|---|
| Idiopathic | — | — |
| Congenital | Autosomal dominant<br>Autosomal recessive | Wilson's disease<br>Cystinosis<br>Galactosaemia<br>Glycogen storage disease type I<br>Fanconi's syndrome |
| Secondary | Rheumatoid arthritis<br>Systemic lupus erythematosus<br>Sjögren's syndrome<br>Multiple myeloma<br>Cirrhosis<br>Sickle cell anaemia | Heavy metals (cadmium, lead, and mercury)<br>Amyloidosis<br>PNH |
| Drug-induced | Ifosfamide<br>Amphotericin<br>Lithium | Carbonic anhydrase inhibitors<br>Ifosfamide |

PNH: paroxysmal nocturnal haemoglobinuria.

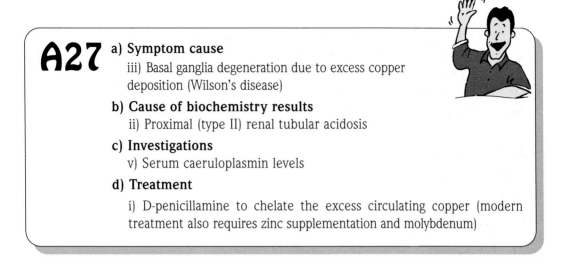

**A27**
**a) Symptom cause**
iii) Basal ganglia degeneration due to excess copper deposition (Wilson's disease)

**b) Cause of biochemistry results**
ii) Proximal (type II) renal tubular acidosis

**c) Investigations**
v) Serum caeruloplasmin levels

**d) Treatment**
i) D-penicillamine to chelate the excess circulating copper (modern treatment also requires zinc supplementation and molybdenum)

## A COMMON SCENARIO...

...is to sling in a question where the urea is disproportionately raised compared with the creatinine (e.g. urea 38 mmol/l and creatinine 160 µmol/l). To work it out, just think of creatinine as coming from muscle.

| | |
|---|---|
| Urea disproportionately raised compared with creatinine: | Huge high-protein meal (and this includes a big upper gastrointestinal bleed), dehydration*. |
| Increase in creatinine: | Trimethoprim and cimetidine interfere with creatinine secretion and falsely raise levels in excess of the glomerular filtration rate. |
| Decrease in both: | In chronic liver disease or malnutrition, urea production is reduced and creatinine also decreases as a result of reduced muscle mass. |

*Note: tetracycline prevents amino acid incorporation into protein. Amino acids are broken down to urea, raising the level inappropriately.

As you may remember, this question comes up more often in the Part 1 MRCP examination, but has also appeared a number of times in Part II. Due to only a limited number of causes, this question is easy to answer.

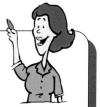

# Q28

A 21-year-old South African woman presents to the emergency department with a short history of abdominal pain and vomiting. She has been travelling around Europe with friends and has had no illnesses until now. Her current symptoms started suddenly after a brief visit to Brighton, but she cannot think of anything specific she could have eaten to cause this. She denies any diarrhoea or other symptoms. On direct questioning she admits to smoking occasionally, but denies illicit drug use and also claims that she does not drink alcohol, as it gives her a rash. Her only medication is the oral contraceptive pill, which she started recently.

## ON EXAMINATION

- Temperature = 37.5°C
- Pulse = 110 beats/min regular
- Blood pressure = 170/110 mmHg
- Cardiovascular system = normal
- Respiratory system = normal
- Abdomen tender in epigastric region, bowel sounds active
- Marked blistering rash on face, hands, forearms, and shins

## INVESTIGATIONS

- Haemoglobin = 13.5 g/dl
- Plasma sodium = 129 mmol/l
- Plasma potassium = 4.0 mmol/l
- Plasma urea = 8 mmol/l
- Plasma creatinine = 132 µmol/l
- White cell count = $11 \times 10^9$/l
- Neutrophils = 85%
- Platelets = $200 \times 10^9$/l
- Amylase = normal
- Abdominal X-ray = NAD

NAD: no abnormality detected.

## a) What is the diagnosis?

i)   acute intermittent porphyria

ii)  variegate porphyria

iii) porphyria cutanea tarda

iv)  systemic lupus erythematosus

v)   hereditary coproporphyria

**b) What one investigation would you do to confirm this?**

   i)    skin biopsy

   ii)   anti-nuclear antibodies

   iii)  anti-double-stranded DNA

   iv)  urine protoporphyrinogen

   v)   genetic study

This is one of those questions where you either recognise the answer or you don't. It is not really a 'list' question. In fact, in real life, the cause of her abdominal pain could have been a dodgy curry (the infamous vindaloo revenge). But this is the MRCP examination!

The abnormal features are as follows:

- blistering photosensitive rash (distributed in exposed areas)
- abdominal pain/tenderness
- tachycardia/hypertension/fever
- leucocytosis/SIADH
- rash with alcohol in a person of South African ethnicity
- newly commenced oral contraceptive pill

**A28** **a) Diagnosis**

ii) The diagnosis to consider is variegate porphyria. This is not porphyria cutanea tarda, which is nonacute and doesn't cause abdominal pain, hypertension, or SIADH. Equally, this cannot be acute intermittent porphyria, as this is not associated with photosensitive skin changes. Having features of both clinches the diagnosis – if you knew that this condition is more common in South Africans then you would have known the answer before reading the whole question!

**b) Investigation**

iv) Urine protoporphyrinogen

## FEATURES THAT SHOULD MAKE YOU THINK OF THE PORPHYRIAS

### ACUTE PORPHYRIAS

Attacks are SADly (sulphonamides, alcohol, dieting) precipitated by the pill, pregnancy, 'phit' medicines (barbiturates, carbamazepine, phenytoin), and phevers (infection). There are two types: acute intermittent porphyria and variegate porphyria.

*Acute intermittent porphyria (autosomal dominant)*

| | |
|---|---|
| Gastrointestinal: | abdominal pain, vomiting, constipation |
| Neurological: | peripheral, symmetrical motor neuropathy<br>occasional sensory symptoms/central nervous system palsies<br>epilepsy (20%)<br>papilloedema |
| Psychiatric: | depression, hysteria, psychosis |
| General: | fever, tachycardia, hypertension, leucocytosis, myocarditis, and raised cholesterol |
| Investigations: | elevated urea, abnormal liver function tests<br>SIADH<br>elevated D-alanine and porphobilinogen in urine<br>lowered porphobilinogen-deaminase activity<br>DNA screening |
| Treatment: | high carbohydrate diet, intravenous haematin (haem arginate), pain control with narcotic analgesics, β-blockers for hypertension, phenothiazines for psychological symptoms, anxiety, nausea, and vomiting, benzodiazepines and chloral hydrate for sedation and seizures; do not use conventional anticonvulsants (except gabapentin) |

*Variegate porphyria (autosomal dominant)*
- more common in South Africans
- neurological, abdominal, and general symptoms as above
- photosensitive blistering rash
- investigations reveal elevated urine protoporphyrinogen

## NONACUTE PORPHYRIAS

*Porphyria cutanea tarda (autosomal dominant or acquired)*

Skin:                 fragility, photosensitive blistering rash
                      pruritus, milia, bullae, scars, hyperpigmentation
                      hirsutism

Metabolic:            hepatomegaly, abnormal liver function tests
                      elevated serum iron and transferrin
                      diabetes

Investigations:       D-alanine and porphobilinogen are *never* elevated
                      elevated urinary uroporphyrin in attack
                      main precipitant is alcohol

Treatment:            perform venesection (haemoglobin <12 g/dl), give chloroquine, and
                      remove offending agents

Erythropoietic protoporphyria and congenital erythropoietic porphyria are other nonacute porphyrias.

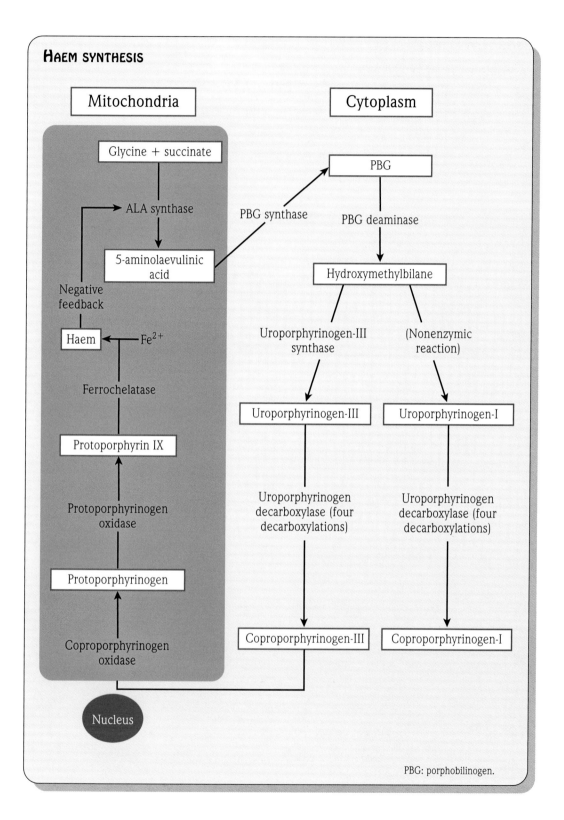

HAEM SYNTHESIS

## BEFORE MOVING ON...

Quickly jot down the causes of:

- hyperparathyroidism

_____

_____

_____

_____

_____

- bronchopulmonary eosinophilia

_____

_____

_____

_____

_____

- lung cavitation

_____

_____

_____

_____

_____

- hyponatraemia

_____

_____

_____

_____

_____

- renal tubular acidosis

- angioid retinal streaks

- lung fibrosis

- hypokalaemic alkalosis and acidosis

**Q29** A 54-year-old man presents with glycosuria. He is a little overweight. His mother had non-insulin-dependent diabetes mellitus. He works as a fish merchant and is an ex-petrol pump attendant. Two years ago he had a gastrectomy for a gastric carcinoma. He has been told that he should have regular vitamin injections, but has been lax about this. He is otherwise well. He undergoes a glucose tolerance test.

| Time (hours) | 0.0 | 0.5 | 1.0 | 1.5 | 2.0 |
|---|---|---|---|---|---|
| Serum glucose (mmol/l) | 4.8 | 4.2 | 8.9 | 3.4 | 3.6 |

## a) What is the result of the glucose tolerance test?

i)   diabetes mellitus

ii)  normal

iii) impaired glucose tolerance

iv)  lag storage curve

v)   impaired fasting glucose

## b) What is the likely cause in this man?

i)   type I diabetes

ii)  type II diabetes

iii) liver failure

iv)  post-gastrectomy

v)   vitamin deficiencies

Again, this is just one of the classic glucose tolerance test results that are shown in the MRCP examination. The causes of a lag storage curve are post-gastrectomy and liver failure. You have seen it now, so don't fall for it when it comes up in the data questions in the MRCP Part II examination.

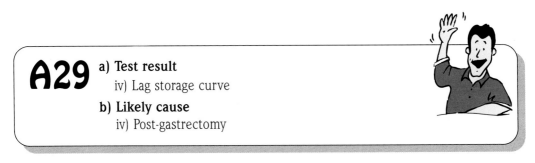

**A29** **a) Test result**
   iv) Lag storage curve

**b) Likely cause**
   iv) Post-gastrectomy

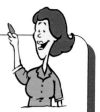

**Q30** A 28-year-old man presents to his GP with symptoms suggestive of a chest infection. Routine investigations find a random blood glucose level of 13 mmol/l, a total cholesterol level of 4 mmol/l, and a low-density lipoprotein cholesterol level of 1.4 mmol/l. He is 175 cm tall, weighs 70 kg, and has a blood pressure of 126/74 mmHg. His brother was diagnosed with type I diabetes at the age of 17 years, but has been fortunate to have persistently low insulin requirements. His sister, who is 34 years old, was diagnosed with type II diabetes 2 years ago; she is well controlled with dietary measures.

### a) What is the diagnosis?

    i)     maturity-onset diabetes of the young (MODY)

    ii)    type I diabetes

    iii)   type II diabetes

    iv)   Wolfram's syndrome

    v)    metabolic syndrome

### b) Lifestyle measures (exercise, dietary modification) fail. Which treatment should be commenced?

    i)     metformin

    ii)    acarbose

    iii)   glibenclamide

    iv)   rosiglitazone

    v)    troglitazone

## MATURITY-ONSET DIABETES OF THE YOUNG FOR THE MRCP...

*Points to remember*

- MODY is rare and is dominantly inherited.

- There are six subtypes, with variable penetrance.

- MODY may present with the classic signs and symptoms of diabetes. However, most patients are asymptomatic and are diagnosed on routine blood tests (especially during pregnancy) or screening of relatives.

- Normally, the diagnosis is initially assumed to be a more common form of diabetes. Many wonder who actually understood this disease before MRCP!

- The diagnosis is confirmed by identifying specific genetic mutations.

*So how and when would you suspect it?*

Look for:

- mild to moderate hyperglycaemia, especially if the patient is aged <25 years

- normal body–mass index, blood pressure, and lipid profile

- no evidence of other autoimmune disease in the patient or relatives (remember: a correlation exists between diabetes and autoimmune diseases)

- a strong family history of diabetes, to a similar degree and age of onset (easy to see why it gets misdiagnosed!)

*Treatment*

Sulphonylureas are the treatment of choice due to their mechanism of action. There are exceptions; insulin is more effective than oral hypoglycaemics in MODY types 1 and 3.

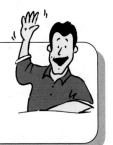

**A30** a) **Diagnosis**
　　　i) MODY
　　b) **Treatment**
　　　iii) Glibenclamide

# Q31

A 68-year-old man is brought to his GP by his wife. She complains that he's more tired than usual and is losing weight, despite home cooking. He has no medical history of note. He smokes 10–20 cigarettes per day. He is diagnosed with diabetes and given lifestyle advice. Despite this, his blood sugar control remains poor. His body–mass index is 30 kg/m², and his blood pressure is 154/88 mmHg. Urine dipstick shows + + + protein. He has confirmed microalbuminuria.

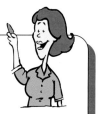

| INVESTIGATIONS | RESULTS |
| --- | --- |
| Haemoglobin | 13.4 g/dl |
| White cell count | 6.7 × 10⁹/l |
| Platelets | 340 × 10⁹/l |
| Plasma sodium | 138 mmol/l |
| Plasma potassium | 4.0 mmol/l |
| Plasma urea | 12.1 mmol/l |
| Plasma creatinine | 167 μmol/l |
| Bilirubin | 13 μmol/l |
| Serum alkaline phosphatase | 73 IU/l |
| Serum alanine aminotransferase | 20 IU/l |
| Plasma glucose | 13 mmol/l |
| Plasma calcium | 2.2 mmol/l |
| Plasma phosphate | 1.0 mmol/l |
| C-reactive protein | 34 mg/l |
| Total cholesterol | 9.0 mmol/l |
| High-density lipoprotein cholesterol | 1.3 mmol/l |
| Low-density lipoprotein cholesterol | 4.9 mmol/l |
| Triglycerides | 2.8 mmol/l |

## a) Which medications would you ensure he was on?

   i)    metformin, simvastatin, aspirin, ramipril

   ii)   metformin, simvastatin, aspirin, bendrofluazide

   iii)  glibenclamide, simvastatin, aspirin, ramipril

   iv)   metformin, gliclazide, simvastatin, aspirin, ramipril

   v)    metformin, aspirin, ramipril

We've made this easy for you! The patient has the full house and needs managing well or you'll be dealing with the complications on call. Although he has no cardiac history, he is trying his best to get one. He's obese, a smoker, hypertensive, and has dyslipidaemia. He's also just been told he's diabetic with end-organ damage (microalbuminuria).

## DIABETES!

You need to know the current guidelines:

- Lifestyle advice: weight loss, diet, exercise, and smoking cessation.

- Glucose control: glycosylated haemoglobin should be <6.5%. Check every 3–4 months (Diabetes Control and Complications Trial recommendation).

- Hypertension:

   - Does the patient have nephropathy? If yes, treat. ACE inhibitors are first-line in renal disease. If proteinuria, the target blood pressure is lower (<125/75 mmHg).

   - Is their blood pressure >160/100 mmHg? Treat!

   - A blood pressure between 160/100 and 140/80 mmHg is a little less specific. It should make you think about their 10-year coronary event risk. If high, treat. If low, monitor and treat as appropriate.

   - The optimal target is <130/80 mmHg.

- Statins: recommended in patients with hypertension or a 10-year coronary event risk of 15%.

- Antiplatelet treatment: NICE recommends 75 mg aspirin once daily if the patient has known cardiovascular disease or a high 10-year coronary event risk. Clopidogrel should not be used routinely.

- Long-term follow-up: remember the eyes, kidneys, and nerves.

Make sure you check the NICE website for up-to-date guidelines.

### Now for the oral hypoglycaemics...

- Metformin is first line if the patient is overweight (body–mass index >25.0 kg/m$^2$) and has poor glucose control despite lifestyle interventions. Metformin is contraindicated in renal impairment (creatinine >150 μmol/l).

- Sulphonylureas are the second-line agent in overweight patients with unsatisfactory glucose control. Consider them for first-line therapy when metformin is not tolerated/contraindicated or if the patient is not overweight.

- Thiazolidinediones are recommended as part of combination therapy with oral hypoglycaemics. They should not be co-prescribed with insulin. They may cause hypoglycaemia, liver dysfunction, and worsening of heart failure. They may improve the high-density lipoprotein cholesterol and triglyceride profile.

- Acarbose is an option if you are unable to use other oral hypoglycaemics. It has a high incidence of gastrointestinal side effects.

And, as you know, if glucose control remains unsatisfactory with optimised oral hypoglycaemics then insulin is the next step. That's more for the communication skills station of the PACES examination. Just remember that when you transfer a patient from oral combination therapy that includes metformin, continue the metformin.

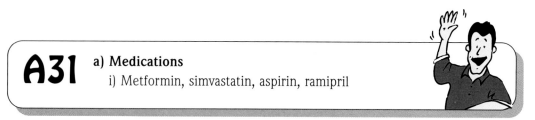

**A31**   a) Medications
       i) Metformin, simvastatin, aspirin, ramipril

## OTHER USEFUL POINTERS

- Proliferative retinopathy requires urgent referral.

- Maculopathy (more common in type II diabetes) and preproliferative retinopathy also require referral.

- Diabetic amyotrophy occurs in older men with poor glycaemic control. They complain of painful weakness and wasting of the thighs, and absent knee reflexes. Improve their glycaemic control and their symptoms should resolve. Can you remember the causes of absent knee reflexes? List them here:

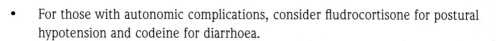

- For those with autonomic complications, consider fludrocortisone for postural hypotension and codeine for diarrhoea.

- We all know the diagnosis when a 'young, slim nurse' presents with hypoglycaemia, but can you remember how to confirm it?

  – Low glucose, high insulin, no ketones. If she's used insulin there will be no C-peptide. Try not to be too judgemental as she just may have an insulinoma!

  – A mnemonic for you: Light Girls Have Insulin Not Kake!

- As for the other causes of hypoglycaemia:

  – Low insulin, no ketones = nonpancreatic neoplasm.

  – Low insulin, high ketones = pituitary or adrenal failure, excessive alcohol intake... you after this examination!

# 5

# HAVE A HEART...

THE CARDIOLOGICAL MRCP LISTS

There aren't really any long cardiology lists. Indeed, the variety of cardiological cases that seem to appear in the MRCP examination is quite small. Favourites are bacterial endocarditis and atrial myxoma: both can appear with symptoms of general malaise, weight loss, fever, arthralgia, haematuria, and strange symptoms due to emboli, which may be, for example, neurological, dermatological, or mesenteric. In addition, both conditions can produce a variety of autoantibodies at low titre. The differential diagnosis of such symptoms lies between these two conditions, autoimmune diseases such as polyarteritis nodosa and systemic lupus erythematosus (SLE), HIV infection, and tuberculosis (TB).

## CAUSES OF FEVER, HAEMATURIA, MALAISE, AND POSSIBLE SPLENOMEGALY

- Polyarteritis nodosa
- SLE
- Bacterial endocarditis
- Left atrial myxoma
- Marantic endocarditis: found in those with malignancy, profound weight loss/cachexia
- Libman–Sacks endocarditis: an aseptic form of SLE endocarditis – previously thought to be benign, but can result in valve destruction and the need for surgery

The other pattern to recognise is that of cardiac failure and hepatomegaly. This is either due to hepatic engorgement from right heart failure, an infection that 'attacks' both the liver and heart, or an infiltrative/deposition process affecting both organs. The choice is wide, but the 'likely lads' are listed below.

## CAUSES OF CARDIAC FAILURE AND HEPATOMEGALY

- Congestive heart failure (with hepatic engorgement)
- Amyloidosis
- Lymphoma with cardiac involvement/tamponade
- Haemochromatosis
- Alcoholic cardiomyopathy
- Sarcoidosis

**Q32** A 60-year-old white man presents to his local emergency department with an episode of haemoptysis. On further questioning he admits to being a heavy smoker, particularly since his wife died 18 months ago. He also admits that he has been feeling somewhat low and tired in the last 8 months. He thinks he may have lost some weight, but on direct questioning denies more specific symptoms other than more recently having a productive cough and increased sweating at night-time.

## On examination

- Thin, cachectic with gingivitis
- Temperature = 38.5°C
- Pulse = 90 beats/min
- Blood pressure = 145/80 mmHg

*Cardiovascular*

- V waves visible in the JVP
- Heart sounds normal with a pansystolic murmur audible at the left sternal edge, louder on inspiration

*Respiratory*

- Coarse crepitations throughout both lung fields

*Abdomen*

- No tenderness/organomegaly
- Normal rectal examination

## Investigations

- Haemoglobin = 9.8 g/dl
- U&E = within normal limits
- White cell count = $15.3 \times 10^9/l$
- Platelets = $431 \times 10^9/l$

*Chest X-ray*

- Increased cardiothoracic ratio
- Multiple rounded opacities in both lung fields

JVP: jugular venous pressure; U&E: urinalysis and electrolytes; V: ventricular.

### a) What is the most likely diagnosis?

- i) TB
- ii) bacterial endocarditis with pulmonary emboli
- iii) adenocarcinoma of the lung
- iv) community-acquired pneumonia
- v) AIDS with *Pneumocystis jiroveci* infection

## b) What two investigations would be most helpful?

    i)     three samples of sputum for acid-fast bacilli and Mantoux testing

    ii)    CT scan of the chest and transbronchial biopsy

    iii)   sputum cultures and serial blood cultures

    iv)   serial blood cultures and echocardiography

    v)    HIV testing and bronchoalveolar lavage

This type of question can be difficult, as again there is so much 'social waffle'. Focusing on the purely pathological features should help to sort out the wood from the trees.

The 'always pathological' list is:

- cachexia
- fever
- tricuspid regurgitation
- bilateral multiple rounded opacities on chest X-ray

Of course, cachexia and fever are pretty nonspecific. Immediate thoughts are usually of cancer or infection – or even both. Lung tumours often present with chest infection in the affected territory due to bronchial obstruction. We are not much further forward. However, tricuspid regurgitation does have a limited list of causes, and so do rounded lung opacities.

Write out the list of causes of multiple rounded lung opacities now. You should remember them from the 'Pants' section. If not, revise pages 69–70.

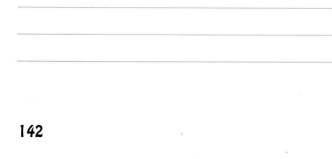

## Tricuspid regurgitation

Tricuspid incompetence may be due to primary problems with the valve or may be secondary to right heart dilatation or pressure overload.

*Valve problems*
- rheumatic heart disease
- bacterial endocarditis
- congenital heart disease (Ebstein's anomaly)
- carcinoid syndrome/slimming tablets
- myxomatous change

*Secondary to elevated pulmonary artery pressures*
- mitral valve disease
- cor pulmonale
- primary pulmonary hypertension

*Secondary to right ventricular dilatation*
- right ventricular infarction
- any dilated cardiomyopathy

Some of these conditions can immediately be discarded as there is nothing to suggest them in either the history or examination. Put a line through these now. Then select the cause that could most reasonably be expected to produce the chest X-ray appearance. As there is nothing in the history or examination to suggest a primary malignancy, and the patient has not complained of altered bowel habit and has no hepatomegaly or flushing, it is unlikely that either pulmonary metastatic disease or carcinoid syndrome is the diagnosis.

This ought to leave you with one likely diagnosis. Check it by cross-indexing your list of causes of tricuspid regurgitation with the causes of *multiple well-rounded large opacities*:
- sarcoidosis
- metastases
- hydatid cysts
- abscesses
- septic emboli

Right-sided bacterial endocarditis seems to be the cause. Septic emboli have showered gradually to both lungs, initially causing few symptoms, but progressing of late. Although right-sided bacterial endocarditis is classically associated with intravenous drug abuse, it can also be associated with general debility. The examiners have given a clue – gingivitis as a source of infection.

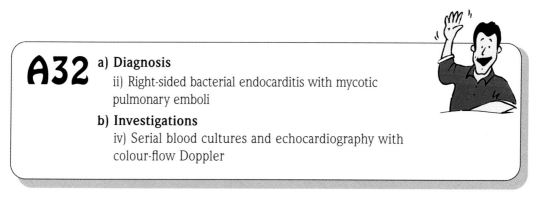

**A32**  a) **Diagnosis**
ii) Right-sided bacterial endocarditis with mycotic pulmonary emboli

b) **Investigations**
iv) Serial blood cultures and echocardiography with colour-flow Doppler

## EXTRA BITS: DOMINANT R-WAVES IN V1

Examiners always love electrocardiograms (ECGs) with a dominant R-wave in the right-side chest leads. This may be caused by:

- posterior myocardial infarction
- pulmonary embolus
- right ventricular hypertrophy (pulmonary hypertension/cor pulmonale/pulmonary stenosis, Noonan's syndrome, and Duchenne's muscular dystrophy)
- right bundle branch block
- Wolff–Parkinson–White syndrome type A
- dextrocardia

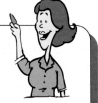

# Q33

A 45-year-old woman presents with a 3-week history of lethargy, malaise, and fever. One week before feeling unwell she had returned from a business trip in the Far East, but claims she had received all of the requisite immunisations beforehand and whilst there only drank bottled water. Two weeks ago she began having intermittent left-sided abdominal pain and also noticed that her urine seemed pink. For the last 5 days she has had severe night sweats. She presents today in a panic because she was transiently blind in her left eye for 2 hours this morning.

## ON EXAMINATION

- No rash, lymphadenopathy, or clubbing
- Temperature = 39°C
- Pulse = 110 beats/min regular
- Blood pressure = 145/60 mmHg

*Cardiology*
- Apex beat undisplaced
- Heart sounds normal, with pansystolic murmur heard at the apex
- Peripheral pulses all present and normal, with no bruits

*Respiratory system*
- Clear bilaterally

*Neurology*
- Normal central and peripheral nervous systems
- One small conjunctival haemorrhage noted

*Abdomen*
- Moderate tender splenomegaly
- No other organomegaly

## INVESTIGATIONS

- Haemoglobin = 9.8 g/dl
- Plasma sodium = 140 mmol/l
- Plasma potassium = 6.1 mmol/l
- Urinalysis: blood +++, protein +
- White cell count = 12.2 × 10⁹/l
- Neutrophils = 90%
- Platelets = 500 × 10⁹/l
- Erythrocyte sedimentation rate = 65 mm in first hour
- Rheumatoid factor positive at low titre
- Plasma urea = 45 mmol/l
- Plasma creatinine = 1035 μmol/l

*Ultrasound abdomen*
- Splenic enlargement with several high density peripheral wedge-shaped areas
- Kidneys normal size

a) **What is the most likely diagnosis?**

    i)     TB with renal involvement

    ii)    deep vein thrombosis with pulmonary and paradoxical emboli

    iii)   renal cell carcinoma

    iv)   bacterial endocarditis with mycotic emboli

    v)    pyelonephritis

b) **What two investigations would be most helpful?**

    i)     three sputum samples for acid-fast bacilli and Mantoux testing

    ii)    serial blood and urine cultures

    iii)   serial blood cultures and echocardiography

    iv)   Doppler scan of both legs and a CT pulmonary angiogram

    v)    CT scan of the abdomen and urine microscopy

The abnormal findings are:

- fever
- mitral incompetent murmur
- splenomegaly with evidence of splenic infarction
- conjunctival haemorrhage
- renal failure

In essence, this patient has systemic symptoms (lethargy, malaise, fever, night sweats) and evidence of infection (raised white cell count, fever, raised platelet count, raised erythrocyte sedimentation rate) accompanied by pathology of likely embolic origin, particularly transient blindness. We might also explain splenic infarction and conjunctival haemorrhage as being of embolic origin and renal failure as due to infection. The degree of renal failure might also suggest the development of rapidly progressive glomerulonephritis, of which bacterial endocarditis is one of the causes. However, without an echocardiogram it would be difficult to favour one of these diagnoses over the other, as a significant number of renal embolic lesions may produce a similar degree of failure.

A weak positive rheumatoid factor is common in subacute bacterial endocarditis. So too are many other autoantibody tests (including perinuclear anti-neutrophilic cytoplasmic antibody). Subacute bacterial endocarditis is also a cause of decreased complement levels.

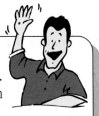

**A33**  **a) Diagnosis**

iv) Bacterial endocarditis with mycotic emboli (left sided). Another possibility would be a left atrial myxoma with systemic embolisation.

**b) Investigations**

iii) Serial blood cultures and echocardiography (transoesophageal would be better than transthoracic).

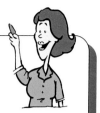

# Q34

A 60-year-old woman is admitted as an emergency with severe breathlessness. This has progressed steadily over the last 3 months, initially with exertional shortness of breath, but now with paroxysmal nocturnal dyspnoea, orthopnoea requiring four pillows, and breathlessness at rest. Over the last 10 days, she has also noticed progressive swelling of her legs and intermittent abdominal pains.

She has had rheumatoid arthritis for the last 15 years. Currently this is quiescent, although she has required methotrexate and other disease-modifying medications in the past, and 4 months ago she was hospitalised for acute pain management and a course of penicillamine. She currently takes low-dose prednisolone, together with nonsteroidal anti-inflammatory drugs as required. She has had asthma all her life, but tends to use her salbutamol inhaler only when it is cold. Otherwise, she has no other illnesses and has never before been hospitalised. She recently retired, having spent the last 25 years working in human resources. She has just moved into a newly built house (which she has been redecorating), and lives with her husband of 45 years. On direct questioning she says she keeps two budgerigars and a pet vole.

## On examination

- No cyanosis, lymphadenopathy, or clubbing
- Afebrile
- Pulse = 92 beats/min regular
- Blood pressure = 140/90 mmHg

*Cardiovascular*
- JVP elevated 8 cm with positive Kussmaul's sign
- Apex beat 6th intercostal space, anterior axillary line
- HS: S1, S2 + S3 gallop + S4
- Gross pitting oedema to mid-thigh

*Respiratory*
- Dull percussion note bibasally
- Reduced breath sounds bibasally, with inspiratory crepitations to mid-zone

*Abdomen*
- Abdomen soft, bowel sounds active, smooth hepatomegaly 4 cm, mild ascites

## Investigations

- Full blood count = normal
- Plasma sodium = 134 mmol/l
- Plasma potassium = 3.8 mmol/l
- Serum albumin = 23 g/l
- Bilirubin = 17 μmol/l
- Plasma urea = 8 mmol/l
- Plasma creatinine = 175 μmol/l
- Serum alanine aminotransferase = 20 IU/l
- Serum alkaline phosphatase = 125 IU/l

*Urinalysis*
- Protein + + +
- Blood trace
- 24-hour urine collection: 7 g protein/ 24 hours

*Electrocardiogram*
- Right bundle branch block

*Chest X-ray*
- Bilateral upper lobe blood diversion
- Bilateral pleural effusions
- Alveolar shadowing

HS: heart sounds; JVP: jugular venous pressure.

a) **What is the most likely diagnosis?**

    i)     cor pulmonale

    ii)    haemochromatosis

    iii)   amyloidosis

    iv)   lymphoma with cardiac involvement

    v)    ischaemic cardiomyopathy

b) **How would you confirm this?**

    i)     echocardiography

    ii)    genetic testing for the C282Y mutation

    iii)   CT scan of the chest and abdomen

    iv)   serum amyloid precursor (SAP) scan

    v)    kidney biopsy

Evidently, the patient has hepatomegaly and biventricular failure. You have already learned the causes for these. Write them down, then check them against the list on the next page.

### Hepatomegaly with cardiac failure

- Congestive heart failure (due to valvular/cardiomyopathic/pericardial tamponade) with hepatic engorgement
- Amyloidosis
- Lymphoma with cardiac involvement/tamponade
- Haemochromatosis
- Alcoholic cardiomyopathy
- Sarcoidosis

Which of these is the likely cause? In this instance, the cardiac failure is due to a disease causing a restrictive cardiomyopathy or tamponade (Kussmaul's sign is positive). Which of these can cause nephrotic syndrome? You will find this list later in the book. In the meantime, your general knowledge ought to tell you.

**A34**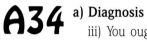

a) **Diagnosis**

iii) You ought to be left with a differential diagnosis lying between amyloidosis A, amyloidosis secondary to chronic rheumatoid arthritis, and haemochromatosis. In the absence of any features in the history pointing to haemochromatosis, amyloidosis must be the answer.

b) **Investigation**

iv) The diagnosis is made by SAP scanning or, better, organ biopsy of liver, right ventricle, or rectal tissue. A SAP scan uses a $^{123}$I-isotope-labelled amyloid precursor, which is injected and localises to areas of amyloid accumulation.

## More QT, Vicar?

A long QT interval is a marker of abnormal ventricular repolarisation and is defined as a QTc (corrected for heart rate) of >450 ms. Pathological U waves may be present. Its most significant consequence is a predisposition to torsades de pointes.

## Causes of a long QT syndrome

| | |
|---|---|
| Hereditary | Jervell and Lange–Nielsen syndrome and Romano–Ward syndrome |
| Electrolytes | Hypokalaemia, hypomagnesaemia, and hypocalcaemia |
| Endocrine disorders | Hypothyroidism, hyperparathyroidism, and phaeochromocytoma |
| Cardiac conditions | Chronic myocardial ischaemia, myocardial infarction, myocarditis, bradyarrhythmia, and atrioventricular node block |
| Intracranial disorders | Subarachnoid haemorrhage, encephalitis, and head trauma |
| Nutritional disorders | Anorexia nervosa and starvation |
| Drugs | Antiarrhythmic drugs: class IA/C, class III |
| | H1-receptor antagonists: terfenadine (no longer sold, do not combine with grapefruit juice) |
| | Cholinergic antagonists: cisapride, organophosphates |
| | Antibiotics: erythromycin, clarithromycin, trimethoprim |
| | Antifungal agents: ketoconazole, itraconazole |
| | Psychotropic agents: haloperidol, phenothiazines, thioridazine |
| | Tricyclic antidepressants (especially in overdose) |

In Jervell and Lange–Nielsen syndrome (autosomal recessive, with sensorineural deafness) and Romano–Ward syndrome (autosomal dominant), mutations are in cardiac voltage-dependent sodium/potassium channel genes: *minK*, *MiRP1*, and *KVLQT1*. Patients tend to get arrhythmias if they are startled, for example by the telephone ringing or other loud noises. They should be treated with prophylactic β-blockers. If the cause is acquired then give magnesium and avoid β-blockers, as these slow the heart and repolarisation. To speed the heart up and hence accelerate repolarisation, patients require pacing or ctecholamine treatment.

If a patient presents with anything that might suggest an overdose, remember that tricyclic antidepressants are potent anticholinergic agents. In addition to causing tachycardias and arrhythmias, they cause a dry mouth, urinary retention, dilated pupils, and a lack of perspiration. Seizures, respiratory depression, and coma can occur. Always remember that depressed patients may also be taking other medications, such as lithium. Treatment of intractable arrhythmia in this context requires phenytoin. In examinations, beware of the patient with an overdose who has, for example, urinary retention (due to anticholinergic action from tricyclic antidepressants) and diabetes insipidus (lithium: renal toxicity).

**Q35** A 61-year-old man is diagnosed with atrial fibrillation during a routine check for health insurance. His GP requests a 24-hour tape and transthoracic echocardiogram, and refers him to the cardiology clinic. While the 24-hour tape shows persistent atrial fibrillation with a heart rate of between 80 and 100 beats/minute, the echocardiogram is normal. His cardiovascular and systemic examinations are also normal.

### a) What would be your next step in terms of management?

i) commence aspirin and digitalise

ii) commence warfarin and arrange a transoesophageal echocardiogram

iii) commence warfarin and amiodarone

iv) commence warfarin and arrange elective cardioversion

v) commence warfarin and arrange follow-up

No lists needed here! Questions regarding the management of atrial fibrillation are popular in the PACES examination and are also used in interviews for cardiology registrars. No doubt this type of question is also making guest appearances in written papers, as knowledge of the latest guidelines is being tested. This needs a thorough knowledge of the NICE guideline, which you can read up on at http://guidance.nice.org.uk. While you're there, acquaint yourself with all of the NICE guidelines that you would commonly use in clinical practice as a general medical registrar.

The first assessment to make is the stroke risk. This chap, being aged <65 years and with no previous history or structural abnormalities, is at low risk for stroke. It may be OK to commence him on aspirin, but it would be worth trying to cardiovert him. So, you should commence him on warfarin and ensure that the international normalised ratio is in the therapeutic range for at least 3 weeks prior to electrical cardioversion. There is no need to start an antiarrhythmic agent as the rate is well controlled, unless you plan pharmacological cardioversion instead. If the patient was not rate controlled then you would need to commence either a β-blocker or calcium antagonist. Amiodarone is useful if you know that the onset is recent, and will help with pharmacological cardioversion.

If the poor guy was unfortunate enough to have a stroke then warfarin should not be commenced immediately as there is a risk of haemorrhage within the infarct. Ideally, it is best to delay warfarin for 2 weeks and commence aspirin in the mean time. Remember, if the stroke is very large then warfarin should be delayed even further.

If there is a structural abnormality in the heart (e.g. mitral regurgitation and a dilated left atrium) then the chances of electrical cardioversion successfully maintaining the patient in sinus rhythm will be very low. Although some might argue that it is worth trying, NICE guidelines do not recommend this. Arrange follow-up to monitor the mitral valve and the atrial fibrillation. Knowing the triggers for referral to surgery will be useful for the PACES examination and if you have unfortunately decided to pursue cardiology as a career!

**A35** **a) Next management step**
iv) Give warfarin and arrange elective cardioversion

**Q36** A 61-year-old man presents to the emergency department with an embolic stroke. Clinical examination reveals an irregularly irregular pulse, which is confirmed as atrial fibrillation on the electrocardiogram. Carotid studies and a transthoracic echocardiogram are normal. A CT scan shows a small lacunar infarct in the corona radiata.

### a) What is the best course of action?

  i)    commence aspirin and start warfarin immediately

  ii)   commence aspirin with a view to giving warfarin in 2 weeks

  iii)  commence aspirin with a view to giving warfarin in 4 weeks

  iv)   commence heparin and start warfarin immediately

  v)    commence aspirin and heparin

This should be fairly straightforward to answer. The patient is quite similar to the previous one, the main difference being the presentation.

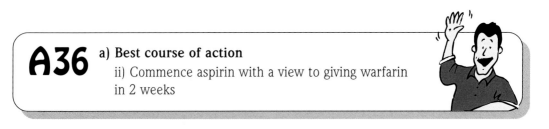

**A36** a) Best course of action
ii) Commence aspirin with a view to giving warfarin in 2 weeks

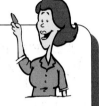

**Q37** A 72-year-old woman with non-insulin-dependent diabetes presents with gradual onset of shortness of breath over a period of a year. Over the past 2 months this has worsened dramatically, and she is unable to perform simple tasks such as going to the toilet without getting short of breath. She now presents to the emergency department. She has not seen her GP for several months and at the time of presentation she is only on metformin. She is admitted for further evaluation.

| INVESTIGATIONS | RESULTS |
|---|---|
| Haemoglobin | 12 g/dl |
| White cell count | $8 \times 10^9/l$ |
| Erythrocyte sedimentation rate | 12 mm/hr |
| Plasma sodium | 134 mmol/l |
| Plasma potassium | 3.7 mmol/l |
| Plasma urea | 4.8 mmol/l |
| Plasma creatinine | 56 μmol/l |
| Liver function tests | Normal |
| Thyroid function tests | Normal |
| HbA$_{1c}$ | 8.8% |
| Total cholesterol | 4.6 mmol/l |
| Troponin T | 0.8 μg/l |
| C-reactive protein | 5.4 mg/l |
| Electrocardiogram | Left bundle branch block |
| Chest X-ray | Mild cardiomegaly and upper lobe diversion |
| Echocardiogram | Trivial MR/trivial TR, LVEF = 25% |

HbA$_{1c}$: glycosylated haemoglobin; LVEF: left ventricular ejection fraction; MR: mitral regurgitation; TR: tricuspid regurgitation.

## a) What treatment would you give this patient in the emergency department?

    i)    aspirin, statin, angiotensin-converting enzyme (ACE) inhibitor, and β-blocker

    ii)   aspirin, statin, ACE inhibitor, and diuretic

    iii)  aspirin, statin, angiotensin-II receptor blocker, and β-blocker

    iv)   aspirin, statin, ACE inhibitor, and spironolactone

    v)    aspirin, ACE inhibitor, diuretic, and β-blocker

This type of question is appearing mainly in Part II examinations – it tests your experience, and lists aren't much help here. It is obviously also useful in the PACES examination, where it might lead to a discussion regarding subsequent management. β-Blockers are started after ACE inhibitors, and are started low and titrated upwards. Spironolactone can be added if the patient remains symptomatic despite optimal drug therapy. The discussion could go on to implantable cardioverter defibrillators (ICDs) from there, in which case it would be useful to know what NICE recommends. Anyone with an ejection fraction of $<30\%$ and a QRS duration of $>120$ ms gets an ICD; obviously, this patient needs one. There are other criteria as well, which you can look up at http://guidance.nice.org.uk.

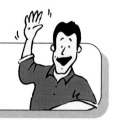

## A37   a) Treatment

    ii) Aspirin, statin, ACE inhibitor, and diuretic

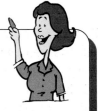

# Q38

A 63-year-old man is admitted for a coronary artery bypass graft and aortic valve replacement. The operation is uneventful, and on day 5 he is back on the ward mobilising. During the morning round, the surgical registrar advises his surgical house officer to review the patient's ECG and remove his epicardial pacing wires. The ECG obtained is shown below:

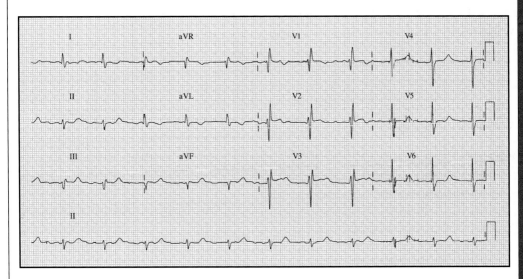

The house officer is satisfied with the ECG and is about to remove the wires when he is stopped by the astute nurse looking after the patient, who convinces him to show the ECG to his registrar. The patient is then referred to the cardiologists.

## a) What advice do you think the cardiologists give?

  i)   load up with amiodarone
  ii)  refer to the electrophysiologist
  iii) remove the epicardial wires and observe
  iv)  add onto the day list for a permanent pacemaker
  v)   administer a β-blocker

So, did you do better than the surgical house officer? Hopefully you did; if not, arrange some ECG teaching sessions with an astute cardiac nurse! ECGs appear in the MRCP examination, and you should be able to diagnose simple ECGs such as acute myocardial infarction, heart blocks, and arrhythmias (e.g. flutter, fibrillation, and junctional rhythms). The questions are never that straightforward – for example, in acute myocardial infarction, you might get asked which vessel is involved or the question might relate to a secondary complication or treatment.

This ECG shows a third-degree heart block with an accelerated escape rhythm. The arrows in the figure point to the P-waves.

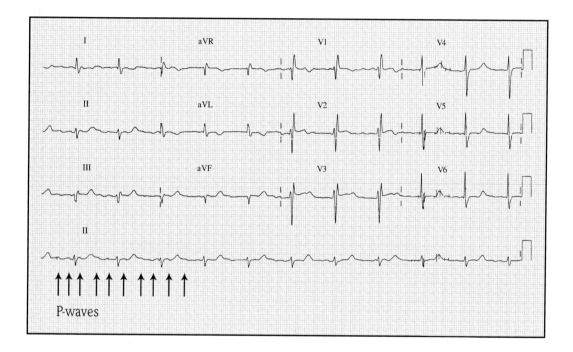

A nodal block can sometimes cause a narrow escape rhythm as the impulses for the escape beats originate within the node itself. It is likely that the conducting pathway in the heart was damaged during surgery. As a result of the heightened post-surgery adrenergic state, an accelerated rhythm superseded, maintaining the patient's blood pressure. If nothing is done, the rate may eventually slow down and the patient will subsequently become symptomatic. The safest line of action would be to insert a permanent pacemaker prior to removing the epicardial wires.

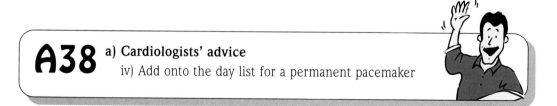

**A38** a) Cardiologists' advice
iv) Add onto the day list for a permanent pacemaker

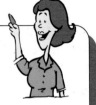

# Q39

A 35-year-old woman is referred by her GP to the cardiology clinic. She has been having palpitations for years, but they have worsened over the last 2 months. She describes an intermittent onset of rapid and regular palpitations with no precipitating factors. They are associated with presyncope and one episode of loss of consciousness. There is no other history of note. She drinks alcohol and coffee occasionally, and denies recreational drug use. All of her blood tests are normal, including thyroid function. Her ECG is shown below. An echocardiogram is performed in the clinic, which is normal.

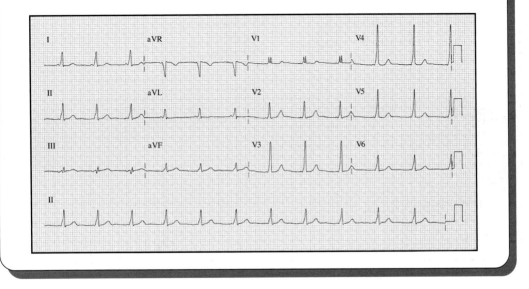

**a) What is the next step in the management of this patient?**

- i) electrophysiology studies with ablation
- ii) amiodarone
- iii) flecainide and a β-blocker
- iv) angiography
- v) exercise stress test

**b) What congenital abnormality is associated with the condition shown in her ECG?**

- i) tetralogy of Fallot
- ii) hypertrophic cardiomyopathy
- iii) atrial septal defect
- iv) Lutembacher's syndrome
- v) ventricular septal defect

In order to answer this type of question, you need to be able to unravel the abnormalities in the ECG. An obvious abnormality is the positive deflection in front of the QRS complex in V1. If you look at the other leads, you will notice a gradual upward slope immediately prior to the QRS complexes, with a shortened PR interval – the δ-wave.

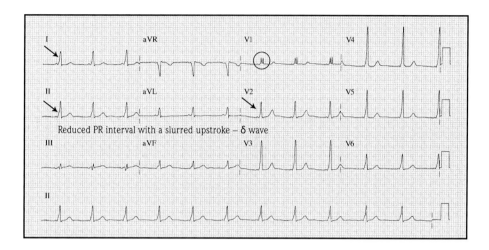

Reduced PR interval with a slurred upstroke – δ wave

The δ-wave is caused by the presence of an accessory bundle between the atria and the ventricles. The diagnosis in this case is Wolf–Parkinson–White syndrome, and the cause of the palpitations is usually a supraventricular tachycardia.

The definitive treatment for this condition is ablation, although drugs may be used in patients who refuse or are refractory to ablation. Wolf–Parkinson–White syndrome can be associated with hypertrophic cardiomyopathy or Ebstein's anomaly.

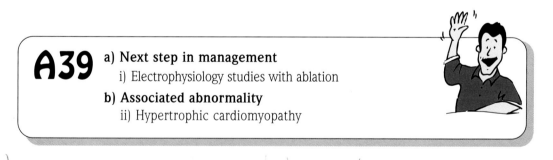

**A39**
a) **Next step in management**
 i) Electrophysiology studies with ablation
b) **Associated abnormality**
 ii) Hypertrophic cardiomyopathy

# 6

# SKINNY DIPS

DERMATOLOGICAL MRCP LISTS

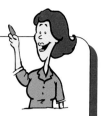

**Q40** A 27-year-old Afro-Caribbean woman presents with soreness on the anterior part of her shin. A palpable red lesion has also appeared over the area concerned. She uses a salbutamol inhaler for asthma. Three years ago she had facial palsy, which resolved spontaneously. More recently, she gave birth to her second child and has begun taking oral contraceptives. A chest X-ray is reported as normal.

| INVESTIGATIONS | RESULTS |
|---|---|
| Full blood count | Normal |
| Urinalysis and electrolytes | Normal |
| Liver function tests | Normal |
| Serum calcium | 2.75 mmol/l |
| Serum albumin | 40 g/l |
| Serum phosphate | Normal |
| Parathyroid hormone | Normal |
| Angiotensin-converting enzyme | Normal |
| Anti-streptolysin O titre | Negative |
| Mantoux test | Negative |

## a) What is the likely dermatological diagnosis?

i) erythema nodosum

ii) pretibial myxoedema

iii) varicose vein

iv) ganglion cyst

v) infected sebaceous cyst

## b) What is the most likely underlying diagnosis?

i) tuberculosis (TB)

ii) leprosy

iii) acromegaly

iv) Graves' disease

v) sarcoidosis

## c) From her history, is there another possible cause for her skin lesion?

_____

_____

The first part of this question is clearly easy, as the question gives you the clinical description of erythema nodosum. The difficult part is elucidating its cause. The patient has hypercalcaemia. Thus, the causes of erythema nodosum and hypercalcaemia need to be considered. Write down the causes of hypercalcaemia, and then compare your list with the causes of erythema nodosum given below.

### Causes of erythema nodosum

- Sarcoidosis
- TB
- Leprosy
- Inflammatory bowel disease
- Infections: streptococcal (β-haemolytic group A streptococci), histoplasmosis, coccidioidomycosis, and North American blastomycosis
- Drugs: oral contraceptive pill, sulphonamides, penicillins, bromides, and iodides

Or, put another (rather lavatorial) way, think of the stopcock: STOPCOCCiii

- sarcoidosis
- TB
- oral contraceptives
- pills
- streptococci
- inflammatory bowel disease
- infections

Or think of your own way of remembering this list, and write it in the box below.

ERYTHEMA NODOSUM

The only conditions that appear in both the hypercalcaemia and erythema nodosum lists are sarcoidosis and TB. Given that the patient's chest X-ray is normal and that her Mantoux test is negative, this makes sarcoidosis the strongest possibility. A classic feature of sarcoidosis is anergy, which explains this test result. Furthermore, she has had facial palsy in the past, again suggesting the diagnosis of sarcoidosis.

The only problem now is to find another possible cause. Again, the answer is in the question, and this would suggest that the oral contraceptive pill is responsible.

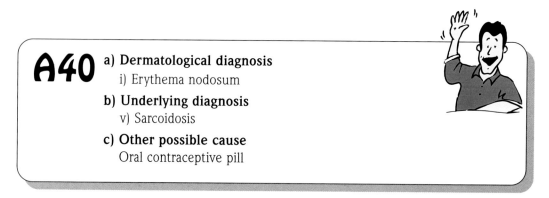

**A40**
a) **Dermatological diagnosis**
   i) Erythema nodosum
b) **Underlying diagnosis**
   v) Sarcoidosis
c) **Other possible cause**
   Oral contraceptive pill

# Quiz Spot!

**Q:** Can you complete the rhyme about cavitating lesions in the lung?

_____ cause cavities, so can _____

_____ , _____ , also PE

Think of the 'oses' of which there are three

Also of abscesses, _____

A: See page 69 for the full rhyme.

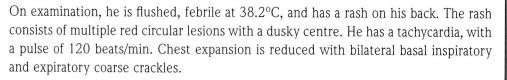

# Q41

A 23-year-old man is admitted to the emergency department with a 3-week history of shortness of breath. This has been associated with fever and a cough productive of green–yellow sputum. He has a history of asthma and hay fever. He smokes 30 cigarettes and drinks 3 pints of lager per day.

On examination, he is flushed, febrile at 38.2°C, and has a rash on his back. The rash consists of multiple red circular lesions with a dusky centre. He has a tachycardia, with a pulse of 120 beats/min. Chest expansion is reduced with bilateral basal inspiratory and expiratory coarse crackles.

| INVESTIGATIONS | RESULTS |
| --- | --- |
| Haemoglobin | $6.3 \times 10^9/l$ |
| White cell count | $6.3 \times 10^9/l$ |
| Platelets | $324 \times 10^9/l$ |
| Plasma sodium | 134 mmol/l |
| Plasma potassium | 4.2 mmol/l |
| Plasma creatinine | 89 μmol/l |
| Plasma urea | 4.3 mmol/l |
| Serum aspartate aminotransferase | 34 IU/l (normal: 5–15 IU/l) |
| Serum alanine aminotransferase | 54 IU/l (normal: 5–15 IU/l) |
| γ-glutamyl transferase | Normal |
| Serum alkaline phosphatase | Normal |
| HIV | Negative |
| Electrocardiogram | Normal |
| Chest X-ray | Bilateral basal consolidation |
| Blood cultures | Negative |
| Anti-streptolysin O titre | Normal |
| Echocardiogram | Normal |
| Autoantibodies | Negative |

## a) What is the most likely diagnosis?

i)   hepatitis B infection

ii)  *Mycoplasma pneumoniae* infection

iii) systemic lupus erythematosus

iv)  allergic bronchopulmonary aspergillosis

v)   *Legionella* pneumonia

## b) What test would you do to confirm the diagnosis?

i)  *Mycoplasma* serology

ii)  urine for *Legionella* antigen

iii)  blood cultures

iv)  hepatitis B surface antigen and hepatitis B e antigen

v)  anti-nuclear antibodies and anti-double-stranded DNA

Again, this is an easy question that we are sure you can get right by now! (Well, maybe.) This requires you to know the classic dermatological description of erythema multiforme and then correlate this with the clinical case scenario of a young man with progressive pneumonia and mild abnormalities of liver function.

## CAUSES OF ERYTHEMA MULTIFORME

- Infections: herpes simplex virus types I and II, Epstein–Barr virus, varicella zoster virus, adenovirus, hepatitis B/C viruses, *Mycoplasma*, *Streptococcus*, fungi

- Drugs: sulphonamides, sulphonylureas, nonsteroidal anti-inflammatory drugs, anticonvulsants, barbiturates

- Collagen vascular disease: systemic lupus erythematosus

- Malignancy: especially adenocarcinoma

- Sarcoidosis

**A41**

a) **Diagnosis**
   ii) *Mycoplasma pneumoniae*

b) **Investigations**
   i) *Mycoplasma* serology

Note: the white cell count is often not raised with atypical pneumonias. Cold agglutinins are a feature of *Mycoplasma* infection. Other features of *M. pneumoniae* infection include sinusitis and haemorrhagic bullous myringitis, anaemia, low platelet count, hepatitis, pancreatitis, myocarditis, encephalitis, and cranial nerve palsies/Guillain–Barré syndrome.

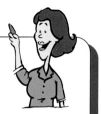

# Q42

A 42-year-old man presents to the emergency department with severe pain in the mouth and lips. He first noticed problems 2 days ago, when he developed a number of skin lesions on his body and trunk. Over the next few days these coalesced and the skin around his mouth began to peel off. He is known to suffer from HIV infection and had an episode of *Pneumocystis carinii* pneumonia 2 years ago, since when he has received chemoprophylaxis. Currently his HIV is well controlled, with a CD4 (T-helper cell) count of 390 cells/mm$^3$ and an undetectable viral load with nevirapine and a fixed-dose combination of tenofovir + emtricitabine.

On examination, he is unwell and dehydrated with a temperature of 38.5°C. The skin around his mouth is denuded, as is the skin on his tongue. Over his body there are multiple coalescing erythematous target lesions. Chest examination is unremarkable and his abdomen is soft and non-tender.

| INVESTIGATIONS | RESULTS |
| --- | --- |
| Haemoglobin | 12.6 g/dl |
| Mean corpuscular volume | 100 fl |
| White cell count | 6.9 × 10$^9$/l |
| Platelets | 360 × 10$^9$/l |
| Urinalysis and electrolytes | Normal |
| Liver function tests | Normal |
| Anti-streptolysin O titre | Negative |
| Chest X-ray | Normal |

## a) What is the most likely diagnosis?

i) herpes simplex infection

ii) pemphigus vulgaris

iii) Stevens–Johnson syndrome

iv) pityriasis rosea

v) necrotising vasculitis

**b) What two things would you do next?**

   i)   topical and oral steroids

   ii)  withdraw the offending drug, rehydrate, and give steroids

   iii) stop highly active antiretroviral therapy and give antibiotic therapy

   iv)  prescribe topical steroids and add acyclovir

   v)   prescribe steroids and empiric antibiotic therapy

The history gives a classic description of erythema multiforme, but this time it is complicated by the fact that the patient is HIV positive. This therefore requires a further list of complications of HIV therapy, and we need to cross-reference this with the list of causes of erythema multiforme. Write down the possible causes of erythema multiforme and compare it to the table of HIV-therapy-related complications below and continued on the following page:

| FUSION INHIBITORS | CCR5 INHIBITORS | INTEGRASE INHIBITORS |
|---|---|---|
| Enfuvirtide: | Maraviroc: | Raltegravir: |
| • peripheral neuropathy | • cough | • diarrhoea |
| • hypersensitivity | • dizziness | • nausea |
| • abnormal LFTs | | • headache |

| NUCLEOSIDE AND NUCLEOTIDE ANALOGUES | NON-NUCLEOSIDE ANALOGUES | PROTEASE INHIBITORS |
|---|---|---|
| Azidothymidine/ zidovudine: <br> • macrocytosis <br> • anaemia <br> • nausea <br> • mitochondrial toxicity* <br> • lipodystrophy** <br> • black nails <br> Stavudine: <br> • peripheral neuropathy <br> • mitochondrial toxicity* <br> • lipodystrophy** <br> Didanosine: <br> • pancreatitis <br> • mitochondrial toxicity* <br> • peripheral neuropathy <br> Abacavir: <br> • hypersensitivity <br> • alopecia <br> Emtricitabine: <br> • nausea <br> • fatigue <br> Tenofovir: <br> • renal dysfunction | Efavirenz: <br> • nightmares <br> • sleep disturbance <br> • rashes <br> • abnormal LFTs <br> Nevirapine: <br> • rashes including erythemamultiforme <br> • Stevens–Johnson syndrome <br> • abnormal LFTs | Lopinavir: <br> • diarrhoea <br> • hypercholesterolaemia <br> Atazanavir: <br> • raised bilirubin <br> Indinavir: <br> • renal stones <br> • nausea <br> • diarrhoea <br> Fosamprenavir: <br> • rashes |

*Mitochondrial toxicity presents with lactic acidosis and fatty liver. **Lipodystrophy presents with high cholesterol and triglycerides, diabetes, fat redistribution including a buffalo hump, abdominal distension, and facial lipodystrophy. LFT: liver function test.

## A42

a) **Likely diagnosis**

iii) Stevens–Johnson syndrome caused by either co-trimoxazole (as prophylaxis against *P. carinii* pneumonia) or nevirapine

b) **Management**

ii) Withdraw the offending drug, rehydrate, and give steroid therapy (however, none of these are thought to be helpful in nevirapine-induced Stevens–Johnson syndrome)

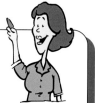

**Q43** A 21-year-old man presents to the emergency department with a large necrotic ulcer on his right shin that first appeared 3 weeks earlier. On examination, he is a thin man with digital clubbing and a colostomy. He has previously suffered from mild epilepsy and hypertension. He is not currently on any medication for these conditions. He has an elder brother who has asthma.

## a) What is the most likely cause of his skin condition?

- i) granuloma annulare
- ii) vasculitic ulcer
- iii) squamous cell carcinoma
- iv) pyoderma gangrenosum
- v) Sweet syndrome

## b) Why has he got a colostomy?

This question is easy, as long as you know the causes of pyoderma gangrenosum and clubbing. These are recorded for you below.

## CAUSES OF PYODERMA GANGRENOSUM

- Inflammatory bowel disease
- Multiple myeloma
- Acute myeloid leukaemia
- Polycythaemia rubra vera
- Immunoglobulin A paraproteinaemia
- Connective tissue diseases: systemic lupus erythematosus, rheumatoid arthritis, polyarteritis nodosa

## CAUSES OF CLUBBING

| | |
|---|---|
| Congenital | |
| Cardiac | subacute bacterial endocarditis |
| | atrial myxoma |
| | congenital cyanotic heart disease |
| Respiratory | carcinoma of bronchus |
| | bronchiectasis |
| | cystic fibrosis |
| | pulmonary fibrosis |
| | mesothelioma |
| | lung abcess |
| Gastrointestinal | inflammatory bowel disease |
| | liver cirrhosis |
| | coeliac disease |
| Endocrine | thyroid acropachy |

**A43**  **a) Likely cause of skin condition**
iv) Pyoderma gangrenosum

**b) Cause of colostomy**
Ulcerative colitis

Use the space below to come up with ways of remembering these lists. You could use mnemonics, verse, pictures, alliteration (same letters), or biological classifications.

# QUIZ SPOT!

## PRESENTATION PUZZLE

George, Michael, Sarah, Nicole, Peter, and Ruth are six members of the Job family, and all suffer from the same four presenting conditions, A–D. Some are unlucky in that they have contracted large numbers of diseases. Others are unlucky in that a single disease has led to more than one clinical presentation. Which disease states are responsible for each finding in each patient? Write one causal disease in each box. The answers are on page 349, but the following information might help:

1. Michael has one disease responsible for more than two of his clinical presentations.
2. Sarcoid causes George's bilateral hilar lymphadenopathy, and also his lung fibrosis.
3. Sarah has recent abdominal swelling and positive β-hCG.
4. Michael and Nicole share an infective cause of thenar eminence wasting.
5. Michael and Sarah share a cause of chronic sputum production.
6. Ruth does not have any infectious diseases.
7. One man has cystic fibrosis as a cause of two conditions.
8. The person with an autoimmune joint disease also has yellow nails.
9. The girl who keeps pigeons is also pregnant.
10. Sarah gave Nicole an infectious disease.
11. The girl who gave the infectious disease to Michael also has a fungal infection.
12. The man with cystic fibrosis has a GP who thinks that amiodarone is a treatment for gout.
13. The acromegalic has Kartagener's syndrome.
14. The girl with extrinsic allergic alveolitis also has rheumatoid arthritis.

| Presenting condition | A: | B: | C: | D: |
|---|---|---|---|---|
| George | | | | |
| Michael | | | | |
| Sarah | | | | |
| Nicole | | | | |
| Peter | | | | |
| Ruth | | | | |

Which two are the least infected?
In which patients may serum angiotensin-converting enzyme levels be elevated?

β-hCG: β-human chorionic gonadotrophin.

# 7

# GASTROINTESTINAL TRACTS

THE GASTROINTESTINAL MRCP LISTS

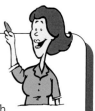

# Q44

By now, there are several list structures that you should know by heart. For instance, the causes of ascites may be divided by the nature of the ascitic tap: transudates (which are due to low plasma oncotic pressure or high capillary pressure), exudates (which can be inflammatory), and chylous (lymph fluid). Complete your own table of causes below.

| Transudates | | Exudates | Chylous |
|---|---|---|---|
| Low oncotic pressure | High capillary pressure | | |

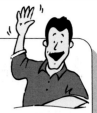

# A44

## TRANSUDATES

Transudates can be caused by a low plasma protein level due to not eating enough (such as kwashiorkor), not synthesising enough (all causes of liver failure), or losing protein. Remember that you can lose protein from the kidneys (nephrotic syndrome) and gut (protein-losing enteropathy, which may complicate any inflammation of the bowel). Or you can have high capillary pressure of cardiac origin (remember all causes of right heart failure and constrictive pericarditis) or of local origin (remember compression of the portal vein by a tumour or portal nodes, as well as destruction of the liver architecture in cirrhosis).

## EXUDATES

Meanwhile, any local infection or inflammation will produce an exudate. In particular, remember Budd–Chiari syndrome and TB as causes.

## CHYLOUS

Chylous is usually caused by lymphatic obstruction. It can result from trauma to the thoracic duct, either through surgical procedures or (rarely) from blunt force trauma and malignancies.

## JAUNDICE

Jaundice is also a common enough clinical finding, and the causes (as you also ought to know well) may be divided into prehepatic (or haemolytic), hepatic (or hepatocellular), and post-hepatic (or obstructive). You ought to be able to come up with your own list of causes for each of these. Jot them down now to remind yourself.

There are, however, one or two classic causes that might need a little neuronal refreshment. These are Gilbert's syndrome, Crigler–Najjar syndrome, Dubin–Johnson syndrome, and Rotor's syndrome. Remember that the 'i's are the 'un's: Gilbert's syndrome and Crigler–Najjar syndrome produce **un**conjugated hyperbilirubinaemia, while Rotor's syndrome and Dubin–Johnson syndrome produce conjugated hyperbilirubinaemia. As Crigler–Najjar syndrome is usually fatal in the first year of life, in adults you only need to consider the other three.

| Bilirubin | Syndrome | Inheritance | Comments |
|---|---|---|---|
| Unconjugated | Gilbert's | Autosomal dominant | UDPGT deficiency, SBR usually <35 μmol/l, fasting and intravenous nicotinic acid cause a rise in SBR, no haemolysis, normal LFTs, benign course |
| | Crigler–Najjar | Autosomal recessive | Similar to Gilbert's, but very rare and presents in neonates as kernicterus. Type I has no UDPGT, but type II has some, which can be induced with phenobarbitone |
| Conjugated | Dubin–Johnson | Autosomal recessive | Conjugated bilirubin +++, black-pigmented liver biopsy, right upper quadrant pain, malaise, fatigue, no gall bladder seen on oral cholecystogram |
| | | | Bromsulphthalein test shows early clearance at 45 min, and late rise at 90 min |
| | | Autosomal recessive | No significant clinical jaundice, normal liver biopsy |

LFT: liver function test; SBR: serum bilirubin; UDPGT: uridine diphosphate glucuronosyl transferase.

## CATCH POINT

Always remember that, whatever the case in the MRCP examination, drugs may be responsible. Don't be caught out. "It's the tablets what's doin' it, doc" is very true as far as the examiners are concerned. For example, in a case of intermittent ataxia, consider whether the child might be eating granny's phenytoin.

Jaundice may also be due to drugs, either through haemolysis (virtually anything will cause this), hepatotoxicity, or intrahepatic cholestasis. Any drug can, in theory, cause jaundice. Thus, you should think of this as a cause, and there is little point in learning an exhaustive list. But just for fun...

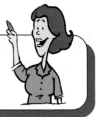

**Q45** Name four drugs that may cause intrahepatic cholestasis

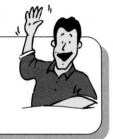

**A45** **Drugs causing intrahepatic cholestasis**
Chlorpromazine, imipramine, sulphonamides, erythromycin estolate, nitrofurantoin, chlorpropamide... and, yes, there are loads more too.

## CLASSIC CASES

### PERNICIOUS ANAEMIA

You will remember that pernicious anaemia is associated with a lack of intrinsic factor and achlorhydria. Most patients (>90%) have anti-parietal-cell antibodies. Watch out, therefore, for pernicious anaemia in any patient in which the mean corpuscular volume is high or when another autoimmune disease is present (30% of those with myxoedema have pernicious anaemia). Also watch out for the presence of other associated features:

- mild splenomegaly, mild haemolysis, a hypocellular bone marrow
- hypogammaglobulinaemia and immunoglobulin (Ig)A deficiency
- reticulocytosis with treatment
- achlorhydria
- stomach cancer (4%)
- *Salmonella* osteomyelitis (rare)

# QUIZ SPOT!

### CAUSES OF ERYTHEMA NODOSUM

Starting with the shaded square, move in any direction (single squares only, no diagonals) to find the causes of erythema nodosum. Just to muck things up, there is a sporting animal and a few beasts of burden in there too. What are they? See page 94 for the answers.

| S | T | Y | C | I | S | D | E | O | D |
|---|---|---|---|---|---|---|---|---|---|
| A | O | M | O | S | M | I | S | I | I |
| L | I | P | T | B | O | R | B | E | D |
| B | L | E | H | T | S | I | S | S | S |
| S | L | S | U | S | A | S | E | R | T |
| I | M | S | L | C | R | O | D | E | M |
| S | O | A | P | O | I | D | I | P | U |
| S | T | L | H | O | N | A | M | T | L |
| I | O | P | H | O | R | S | E | O | E |
| H | D | B | I | I | C | C | O | C | S |

### Bloody diarrhoea, again!

The presence of bloody diarrhoea can be the clue to grey cases, and is often mentioned 'in passing' if you will excuse the pun. However, all causes are associated with systemic symptoms and complications that are often laboured.

All causes may lead to renal failure due to the septic state and dehydration, and to haemolytic uraemic syndrome in the case of *Escherichia coli*.

#### Salmonella typhi

Typhoid is faeco-orally transmitted, and may be associated with pancytopenia, osteomyelitis (in pernicious anaemia and sickle cell disease), and perforation (rarely). Typhoid presents with:

- week 1: fever, malaise, constipation, headache, dry cough, confusion, abdominal pain
- week 2 (hits Peyer's patches): diarrhoea, rose spots, splenomegaly, leucopenia, and virtually any 'itis' (osteomyelitis, meningitis, myocarditis)
- week 3: gastrointestinal bleed, perforation

In week 1, 90% of patients are blood culture positive. In week 2, bone marrow/stool/urine cultures are more likely to be positive. The analytical protein index and Widal's reaction (serum agglutinins for the O and H antigens) can also be used for diagnosis.

#### Salmonella typhimurium (or S. Dublin)

*S. typhimurium* is a zoonosis. Look out for sausages, curried eggs, and frozen chicken. Watch out, as it causes a septic state and ends up anywhere; hence meningitis, pyelonephritis, splenic abscess, or skin lesions.

#### Shigella/E. coli

Note that verotoxin 0157-producing strains of *E. coli* may cause haemolytic uraemic syndrome.

#### Campylobacter

*Campylobacter* is caught from puppies and chicken. It is often associated with severe systemic symptoms, such as headache and severe myalgia.

#### Amoebiasis

Amoebiasis may 'rear' its head long (even years) after exposure, and may present with an abdominal mass, with or without obstruction, or abscess; always think of abscess in the presence of unexplained fever, malaise, and weight loss.

*Diverticulitis*

Diverticulitis may be a cause of bloody diarrhoea and, like any other sepsis, may be associated with portal pyaemia and severe illness, as well as perforation, abscess (see above), fistula, and obstruction.

*Ulcerative colitis and Crohn's disease*

Both of these conditions may be associated with malignant conversion, seronegative arthritides, mouth ulcers, iritis, autoimmune hepatitis, cholangitis, and amyloidosis. Drug treatment may be the cause of a rash or pancytopenia.

Remember that terminal ileitis may be caused by Crohn's disease and TB (the common differential) as well as *Yersinia*. It may also be mimicked by a tumour.

*Ischaemic colitis*

This should be considered in the presence of other vascular disease or mesenteric angina. Sudden onset of bloody diarrhoea should make you think of embolisation of clot (atrial fibrillation), immune complexes (subacute bacterial endocarditis), or tumour (atrial myxoma).

*Carcinoma*

This may present in a number of ways, which you should already be aware of.

## CAUSES OF CIRRHOSIS

| | |
|---|---|
| Congenital | haemochromatosis and Wilson's disease |
| | $\alpha_1$-antitrypsin (remember early emphysema) |
| | galactosaemia |
| | type IV glycogenosis |
| Infectious | chronic active hepatitis (hepatitis B and C) |
| Immunological | primary biliary cirrhosis, autoimmune hepatitis |
| Prolonged cholestasis | secondary biliary cirrhosis |
| Vascular diseases | congestive heart failure, hepatic vein thrombosis, Rendu–Osler–Weber syndrome |
| Adverse drug reactions | methotrexate, methyldopa, sulphonamides, isoniazid, carbon tetrachloride, amiodarone |
| Cryptogenic | |

## MALABSORPTION

This sneaks in under all sorts of guises, usually of the deficiency variety. This means that the presence of oedema (protein deficiency), bleeding (vitamin K deficiency), neuropathies (vitamin $B_{12}$ or folate deficiency), or anaemia (macrocytic, usually due to vitamin $B_{12}$ deficiency; iron deficiency due to malabsorption is unusual, and you should consider hookworm as a cause of a mixed deficiency picture). In addition, the case may be presented as a specific complication of one of the causes, such as one of the associated complications of Crohn's disease and ulcerative colitis (above) or of coeliac disease.

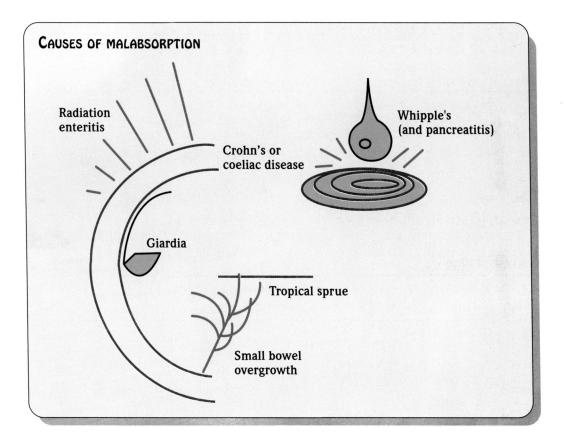

**CAUSES OF MALABSORPTION**

Radiation enteritis

Crohn's or coeliac disease

Whipple's (and pancreatitis)

Giardia

Tropical sprue

Small bowel overgrowth

## CAUSES OF MALABSORPTION

Most of these cause malabsorption through villous atrophy. Tropical sprue is a tropical form of post-enteritis villous atrophy, and is treated with tetracycline and folic acid. Coeliac disease is due to gluten insensitivity and may be associated with hyposplenism and dermatitis herpetiformis, which is characterised by symmetrical itchy urticaria on extensor aspects of the limbs, gluteal regions, and interscapular that becomes vesicular. Post-enteritis villous atrophy can occur after any infectious diarrhoea. Lymphoma of the small bowel is also a cause.

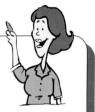

# Q46

A 35-year-old health visitor presents to the emergency department with a 6-month history of lower abdominal pain, altered bowel habit with frequent diarrhoea, and weight loss of nearly 1 stone in the same period. She came to the UK at the age of 12 years with her parents, and visited Pakistan once a year to see her grandparents until 4 years ago when they died within months of each other. She has suffered chronic constipation, strains at stool, and has recently been diagnosed as suffering from haemorrhoids. Her doctor says she 'needs vitamins'. She doesn't smoke or drink alcohol. Her husband is a regular attendee at the diabetes clinic.

## ON EXAMINATION

- Thin and pale, but not clubbed, cyanosed, or jaundiced
- Temperature = 37.5°C
- Pulse = 98 beats/min regular
- Blood pressure = 130/85 mmHg
- No lymphadenopathy
- Cardiovascular system = normal
- Respiratory system = normal
- Abdominal examination reveals a globally tender abdomen, with a mass in the right iliac fossa
- Normal rectal examination

## INVESTIGATIONS

- Haemoglobin = 9.5 g/dl
- Plasma sodium = 136 mmol/l
- Plasma potassium = 3.2 mmol/l
- White cell count = $13 \times 10^9$/l
- Platelets = $450 \times 10^9$/l
- Plasma urea = 4.5 mmol/l
- Serum albumin = 30 g/l
- Other liver function tests = normal
- ESR = 78 mm in first hour
- Stool microscopy: no ova, cysts, or parasites
- Chest X-ray: normal, clear lung fields, two calcified nodules in right hilum

ESR: erythrocyte sedimentation rate.

## a) What is the most likely diagnosis?

i) ileocaecal TB

ii) terminal ileal Crohn's disease

iii) small bowel lymphoma

iv) *Yersinia* enterocolitis

v) actinomycosis

## b) Which investigation would you perform?

    i)     colonoscopy

    ii)    biopsy and culture

    iii)   small bowel meal and follow-through

    iv)   abdominal ultrasound

    v)    all of the above

This is one of those 'you get it or you don't' questions. This scenario (or one like it) is much loved by MRCP examiners (bless their little hearts). The patient has:

- systemic features (weight loss, anaemia, fever)
- right iliac fossa mass and non-bloody diarrhoea
- hilar calcified nodules

The 'not-very-well-with-mass-in-the-right-iliac-fossa' story has three possible conclusions: cancer (especially small bowel lymphoma), ileocaecal TB, or Crohn's disease. The Indian origin and nodules are meant, in this case, to suggest TB.

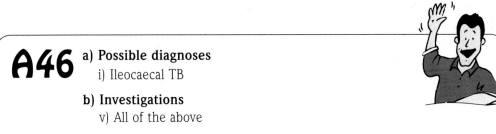

**A46**   **a) Possible diagnoses**
         i) Ileocaecal TB

         **b) Investigations**
          v) All of the above

(Stool culture for TB would be another option, but the test may be negative and takes a long time.)

### TIP

There is a rule that disease of the terminal ileum affects vitamin $B_{12}$/folate absorption more than iron absorption. The reverse is true for disease that affects the duodenum (e.g. coeliac disease) and this may be useful in helping to distinguish different disease processes.

## QUICK CHECK

Jot down the causes of:

- porphyria
- polycythaemia
- polyarthropathy
- optic atrophy

- high anion gap acidosis
- lung cavitation
- erythema nodosum

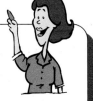

# Q47

A 55-year-old company director presents with a 4-month history of weight loss and abdominal pain. The pain is intermittent and is associated with what the patient describes as the passage of "putty coloured" stools. Despite this, he has a good appetite and is surprised that he has lost almost 8 kg in weight. On direct questioning he admits to sweating more of late, but not possessing a thermometer he is unaware of whether he has had a fever. He travels often with his work, primarily to New York, Tokyo, and Lagos, but insists that he has had all of the requisite immunisations, and denies extra-marital liaisons or the use of illicit drugs. He smokes 10 cigarettes per day and restricts his alcohol intake to 1–2 whiskeys with clients. His only other medical problem is a 10-year history of recurrent painless swelling of his wrists, knees, and ankles, which seems to settle spontaneously. He has never sought medical advice regarding this.

## ON EXAMINATION

- Very tanned but anaemic, with cervical and supraclavicular lymphadenopathy
- Temperature = 37.5°C
- Pulse and blood pressure = normal
- Early clubbing
- Joints normal
- Abdominal examination reveals diffuse tenderness, but no organomegaly or masses

## INVESTIGATIONS

- Haemoglobin = 9.5 g/dl
- Plasma sodium = 138 mmol/l
- Plasma potassium = 3.3 mmol/l
- Plasma glucose = 5.3 mmol/l
- Plasma urea = 6.5 mmol/l
- Serum albumin = 25 g/l
- Plasma creatinine = 95 μmol/l
- White cell count = 7.5 × 10⁹/l
- Platelets = 212 × 10⁹/l
- ESR = 80 mm in first hour
- Mean corpuscular volume = 105 fl
- Serum ACE = 100 U/l
- Stool microscopy negative for ova, cysts, and parasites
- Jejunal biopsy shows jejunal villous atrophy
- CT scan of the abdomen shows para-aortic lymphadenopathy

ACE: angiotensin-converting enzyme, CT: computed tomography; ESR: erythrocyte sedimentation rate.

### a) What is the diagnosis?

i)    coeliac disease

ii)   familial Mediterranean fever

iii)  Whipple's disease

iv)   inflammatory bowel disease

v)    chronic active hepatitis

### b) How would you confirm this?

i)    anti-endomysial IgA antibodies

ii)   periodic acid-Schiff (PAS) staining of jejunal biopsy

iii)  hepatitis serology

iv)   submucosal rectal biopsy

v)    colonoscopy

### c) What treatment would you give?

i)    oral and rectal steroids with anti-inflammatory agents

ii)   interferon-γ

iii)  cotrimoxazole for 6–24 months, with or without steroid therapy

iv)   radical pancreaticoduodenectomy

v)    colchicine

The patient has:

- systemic features (weight loss, fever, sweating)
- lymphadenopathy
- small bowel malabsorption secondary to jejunal villous atrophy (steatorrhoea, weight loss, macrocytic anaemia)
- large joint arthropathy (preceding the onset of gastrointestinal upset)

Remember Occam's razor and the principle of scientific parsimony and try to find *one* unifying diagnosis, rather than making additional assumptions about the relevance of clearly pathological findings.

Start with a list you have already learned: the causes of polyarthropathy.

# QUIZ SPOT!

**Q:** Can you complete the rhyme about polyarthropathy?

*Joint attacks are done by three –*

_____ , _____ , *and* _____

_____ , _____ ,

*And* _____

_____ , _____ , _____ ,

_____ , _____ , _____

*Spread by* _____ *(and not by* _____ *)*

*Is the dreaded* _____

_____ , _____ ,

_____

*Coming over* _____

*With widespread* _____

_____ *and* _____ *do*

*Chronic* _____ *, too*

_____ *and* _____ *, never fear!*

_____ *shall bring up 'the rear'!*

A: See page 5 for the full rhyme.

## WHICH OF THESE IS ASSOCIATED WITH BOWEL DISEASE?

Five patterns fit the bill:

- inflammatory bowel disease (IBD: ulcerative colitis or Crohn's disease) plus ankylosing spondylitis (not related to disease activity)
- IBD plus enteropathic synovitis (related to disease activity)
- autoimmune chronic active hepatitis (CAH) plus bilateral symmetrical small joint arthropathy
- Whipple's disease plus large joint arthropathy (often precedes gastrointestinal symptoms)
- familial Mediterranean fever (FMF) plus monoarticular arthritis

The diagnosis has been narrowed down to FMF, Whipple's disease, CAH, or IBD.

## SMALL BOWEL MALABSORPTION

Earlier it was established that there are few causes of small bowel malabsorption. Most of the causes are through villous atrophy. Tropical sprue is a tropical form of post-enteritis villous atrophy, which can occur after any infectious diarrhoea and is treated with tetracycline and folic acid. Coeliac disease is due to gluten insensitivity and may be associated with hyposplenism and dermatitis herpetiformis (symmetrical itchy urticaria on extensor aspects of the limbs, gluteal regions, and interscapular that becomes vesicular). Lymphoma of the small bowel is also a cause.

Thus, the differential diagnosis of jejunal villous atrophy is:

- coeliac disease
- infectious enteritis
- gastrointestinal lymphoma
- Whipple's disease
- tropical sprue
- HIV infection

Thus, the only overlap on the lists for polyarthropathy, bowel disease, and jejunal villous atrophy is Whipple's disease. IBD, FMF, and CAH have been excluded.

**A47**   a) **Diagnosis**
   iii) Whipple's disease

b) **Tests**
   ii) PAS staining of jejunal biopsy sample: the macrophages
   in the section stain strongly with PAS and contain the intracellular
   bacilli of *Tropheryma whippelii*. Alternatively, polymerase chain reaction
   may detect *T. whippelii* DNA on biopsy samples.

c) **Treatment**
   iii) Cotrimoxazole for 6–24 months, with or without steroids

## WHIPPLE'S DISEASE

Whipple's disease is a rare (except in the MRCP examination!) multi-system disorder that is more common in those who are HLA-B27 (human leucocyte antigen B27) positive. It most commonly affects the small bowel, but extra-intestinal features frequently precede the malabsorption. Other associated features of Whipple's disease include:

- joints: large joint arthropathy
- heart: endocardial, myocardial, pericardial involvement with heart failure
- lungs: pleural effusion, pulmonary oedema
- central nervous system: cranial nerve palsies, aseptic meningitis, ataxia, dementia
- skin: hyperpigmentation, photosensitivity
- other: splenomegaly, glossitis, lymphadenopathy

On the next page, draw yourself a cartoon of a classic patient with Whipple's disease. Learn to draw it repeatedly so that you remember the features.

Whipple's disease also shares several features with sarcoidosis, frequently leading to confusion. Such features include elevated serum angiotensin-converting enzyme levels, the appearance of epithelioid granulomas on lymph node biopsy, and an occasional improvement with steroids.

Note that all causes of small bowel malabsorption may cause hyperpigmentation. (In this question, for 'tanned' read 'hyperpigmented'.) The 'hyperpigmented' list, therefore, includes: malabsorption, haemochromatosis, copper storage diseases, amiodarone treatment, Addison's disease, and Nelson's syndrome.

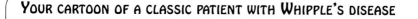

Y**OUR CARTOON OF A CLASSIC PATIENT WITH** W**HIPPLE'S DISEASE**

## E**XTRA BITS:** **AUTOIMMUNE LIVER DISEASE**

Examiners will often try to catch you out by making the presenting complaints (or dominant pathological findings) due not to the liver disease itself, but to the sequelae of chronic liver disease. These include the 'medical student' list (e.g. gynaecomastia, liver flap, Dupuytren's contracture), but also HePatic COMAX:

- hyponatraemia
- peripheral neuropathy from vitamin deficiency
- coagulopathies
- osteomalacia from malabsorption
- malabsorptive diarrhoea
- ascites
- xanthelasmata

You have to be especially alert for the association of autoimmune liver disease with other autoimmune diseases, which may have a greater focus in the question. The two most common autoimmune diseases to focus on for examinations are primary biliary cirrhosis and chronic active hepatitis.

## Primary biliary cirrhosis

- Histologically: periportal fibrosis, Mallory bodies, and liver granulomata (see 'other causes of liver granulomata', below). The mention of copper deposition is meant to fool you into diagnosing Wilson's disease (in which Mallory bodies and granulomata are not seen)
- Associated with rheumatoid arthritis, CREST (calcinosis, Raynaud's disease, oesophageal motility disorder, sclerodactyly, and telangiectasia) syndrome, systemic sclerosis, Sjögren's syndrome, Hashimoto's disease, coeliac disease, dermatomyositis, and renal tubular acidosis
- Clinically may be associated with peptic ulcer and may be triggered by the pill or pregnancy
- Also associated with very high levels of alkaline phosphatase, γ-glutamyl transferase, cholesterol, and IgM anti-mitochondrial antibodies

## Chronic active hepatitis

- Histologically: macronodular cirrhosis, periportal inflammation, piecemeal necrosis (the latter is not seen in primary biliary cirrhosis)
- Associated with viral hepatitis (hepatitis B, particularly if e antigen is positive), Wilson's disease
- Associated with drug use, such as methyldopa or isoniazid
- Associated with autoimmunity (50% of cases of ulcerative colitis)

The presence of anti-smooth-muscle, anti-nuclear, and anti-mitochondrial antibodies is common in both primary biliary cirrhosis and chronic active hepatitis. The presence of anti-centromere antibodies suggests systemic sclerosis as a cause, whereas speckled anti-nuclear antibodies suggest mixed connective tissue disease.

## Other causes of liver granulomata

- Classic granulomatous disease: sarcoidosis, TB, Wegener's granulomatosis, *Brucella*, berylliosis
- Other autoimmune disease: IBD, polyarteritis nodosa, giant cell arteritis
- Infections ($T^2AG$ along and $C^4$): tropical (leprosy, schistosomiasis), toxocariasis, ascariasis, giardiasis, and *Coxiella*, cytomegalovirus, coccidioidomycosis, clap (syphilis)
- Malignancies, drugs, and the chronic granulomatous diseases

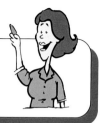

**Q48** A 15-year-old girl presents to the clinic with weight gain and nausea for the last 2 months. A number of investigations are ordered.

| INVESTIGATIONS | RESULTS |
|---|---|
| Haemoglobin | $11.1 \times 10^9/l$ |
| White cell count | $3.8 \times 10^9/l$ |
| Platelets | $234 \times 10^9/l$ |
| Plasma calcium | Normal |
| Serum bilirubin | 6 µmol/l (normal: 3–17 µmol/l) |
| Serum alanine aminotransferase | 9 IU/l (normal: 5–15 IU/l) |
| Serum alkaline phosphatase | 860 IU/l (normal: 0–95 IU/l) |

**a) What is a possible cause of the raised alkaline phosphatase level?**

    i)    pregnancy
    ii)   alcohol abuse
    iii)  vitamin D deficiency
    iv)   Paget's disease
    v)    osteosarcoma

**b) What investigation would you arrange next?**

    i)    serum γ-glutamyl transferase levels
    ii)   pregnancy test
    iii)  serum vitamin D levels
    iv)   X-ray of the skull and pelvis
    v)    abdominal ultrasound

The sources of a raised alkaline phosphatase level are either liver or bone. The uterus can also make large amounts when it is growing during pregnancy. Always remember to think of these different sources.

### CAUSES OF A RAISED ALKALINE PHOSPHATASE LEVEL

- Biliary obstruction, cholangiocarcinoma, alcoholic liver disease
- Pregnancy, growing children, Paget's disease
- Temporal arteritis
- Metastatic bone disease, vitamin D deficiency, etc.

Thus, in a young person such as this, a raised alkaline phosphatase level may be part of the normal growth spurt associated with puberty. However, in this particular case, with the history of weight gain with nausea, the possibility of uterine-derived alkaline phosphatase should be investigated.

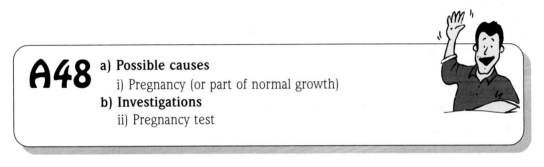

**A48**    **a) Possible causes**
         i) Pregnancy (or part of normal growth)
     **b) Investigations**
         ii) Pregnancy test

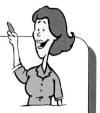

**Q49** A 50-year-old market data manager presents to the emergency department with pain in her hips and increasing difficulty standing. She says that this has been building up over the last 2 months and that apart from occasional abdominal pain she has noticed nothing else unusual. She has a history of mild hypothyroidism, for which she takes thyroxine. She has no drug allergies, although she has recently tried buying different washing powders and soaps as she seems prone to itching. She is a nonsmoker and drinks only socially.

## ON EXAMINATION

- Icteric
- Afebrile
- Several bruises over back and upper arms
- Abdominal examination reveals 3 cm hepatomegaly
- Neurological examination reveals 4/5 weakness in the quadriceps muscles

- Haemoglobin = 12.4 g/dl
- White cell count = $8.5 \times 10^9$/l
- Platelets = $165 \times 10^9$/l
- Plasma sodium = 136 mmol/l
- Plasma potassium = 4.5 mmol/l
- Plasma urea = 6.0 mmol/l
- Plasma creatinine = 89 μmol/l
- Plasma calcium = 1.9 mmol/l
- Plasma phosphate = 0.6 mmol/l
- Serum albumin = 38 g/l
- Serum bilirubin = 80 μmol/l
- Serum aspartate aminotransferase = 100 IU/l
- Serum alkaline phosphatase = 850 IU/l
- Prothrombin time = 20 s
- APTT = 34 s
- Plasma glucose = 5.2 mmol/l

APTT: activated partial thromboplastin time.

### a) What is the underlying diagnosis?

   i) undertreated hypothyroidism

   ii) primary biliary cirrhosis

   iii) systemic lupus erythematosus

   iv) coeliac disease

   v) primary sclerosing cholangitis

**b) What one investigation would you do to confirm this?**

   i)    liver biopsy

   ii)   upper gastrointestinal endoscopy with biopsy

   iii)  anti-mitochondrial antibodies

   iv)   anti-smooth-muscle antibodies

   v)    anti-nuclear antibodies

**c) What is the cause of her presenting symptoms?**

   i)    osteomalacia secondary to vitamin D deficiency

   ii)   proximal myopathy

   iii)  polyneuropathy

   iv)   all of the above

   v)    none of the above

**d) What management steps would you instigate immediately?**

   i)    calcium supplements

   ii)   vitamin D supplements

   iii)  intravenous vitamin K

   iv)   all of the above

   v)    none of the above

OK. What are the key abnormal features?

   •   Obstructive jaundice plus hepatomegaly

   •   Osteomalacia

   •   Prolonged prothrombin time

In a middle-aged woman with itching and other evidence of autoimmune disease... you've pretty much got a full house here, short of some weight loss, clubbing, and xanthelasma! If this chick hasn't got primary biliary cirrhosis, then I'm Cleopatra!

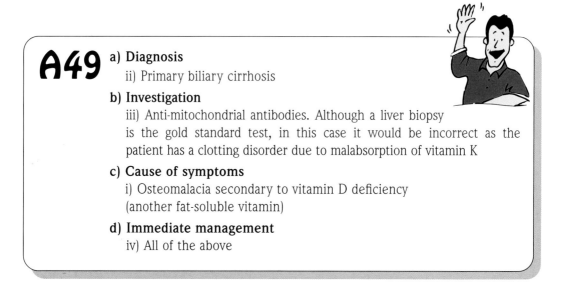

**A49**
a) **Diagnosis**
   ii) Primary biliary cirrhosis
b) **Investigation**
   iii) Anti-mitochondrial antibodies. Although a liver biopsy is the gold standard test, in this case it would be incorrect as the patient has a clotting disorder due to malabsorption of vitamin K
c) **Cause of symptoms**
   i) Osteomalacia secondary to vitamin D deficiency (another fat-soluble vitamin)
d) **Immediate management**
   iv) All of the above

## MORE ABOUT PRIMARY BILIARY CIRRHOSIS

Other extra-hepatic features of primary biliary cirrhosis are:

- arthralgia

- connective tissue diseases; 75% have Sjögren's syndrome or limited systemic sclerosis

- renal disease: membranous glomerulonephritis or renal tubular acidosis

- cholecystitis: don't forget that people with primary biliary cirrhosis are more prone to pigment gallstones

- dermatitis or neuropathy related to malabsorption of vitamin E

## EXTRA BITS: DIFFERENTIAL DIAGNOSIS OF OSTEOMALACIA

| EFFECT | EFFECT |
| --- | --- |
| Lack of vitamin D | Poor diet |
| | Low sun exposure |
| Vitamin D malabsorption | Post-gastrectomy, small bowel surgery, coeliac disease |
| | Biliary disease, such as primary biliary cirrhosis (vitamins A, D, E, and K are fat-soluble) |
| Renal disease | Chronic renal failure |
| | Vitamin D-resistant rickets (due to reduced renal tubular phosphate reabsorption) |
| | All causes of renal tubular acidosis (proximal and distal) |
| Miscellaneous | Phenytoin-induced osteomalacia |
| | Sclerosing haemangiomas |
| | Hypophosphataemic rickets |
| | End-organ resistance to 1,25-dihydroxy-vitamin D |

*Remember:*

- Type I hereditary vitamin D-dependent rickets is caused by mutations of the 1α-hydroxylase receptor in the kidneys and responds to physiological quantities of 1,25-dihydroxy-vitamin D.

- Type II hereditary vitamin D-dependent rickets is due to mutations in the 1,25-dihydroxy-vitamin D receptor. Some patients may respond to very high doses of 1,25-dihydroxy-vitamin D.

- Familial hypophosphataemic (vitamin D-resistant) rickets is an X-linked dominant disorder with low plasma phosphate level.

- Type I disease has low plasma levels of 1,25-dihydroxy-vitamin D; the other two diseases have high endogenous levels because of end-organ resistance.

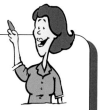

# Q50

A 30-year-old nurse presents after returning to the UK from travelling in the Far East for 8 months. Whilst in Thailand, she received a course of cotrimoxazole for *Shigella* dysentery. Two days after her return flight from Bangkok, she developed abdominal cramping pains with distension and flatulence. She also developed bloodless diarrhoea, which, although initially quite mild, became pale, foul smelling, and difficult to flush away over the course of 2–3 weeks. Her flatmates took her to the emergency department, as they were increasingly worried about her poor appetite and the fact that she had lost a considerable amount of weight since her return.

## ON EXAMINATION

- Thin, dehydrated, and with increased pigmentation on arms and feet
- Weight = 46 kg (previously 51 kg)
- Temperature = 36.6°C
- No clubbing, lymphadenopathy
- Pulse = 110 beats/min regular
- Blood pressure = 95/60 mmHg
- Cardiovascular examination = normal
- Respiratory examination = normal
- Abdominal examination: active bowel sounds, nil else

## INVESTIGATIONS

- Haemoglobin = 11.5 g/dl
- Plasma sodium = 143 mmol/l
- Plasma potassium = 4.0 mmol/l
- Serum albumin = 28 g/l
- Serum bilirubin = 8 μmol/l
- Plasma urea = 8.2 mmol/l
- White cell count = 6.5 × 10⁹/l
- Platelets = 410 × 10⁹/l
- Rigid sigmoidoscopy = normal
- Faecal fat = 120 mmol/l
- Urinalysis unremarkable

## a) What is the most likely diagnosis?

i)   tropical sprue

ii)  strongyloidiasis

iii) gastrointestinal lymphoma

iv) adult coeliac disease

v) amoebiasis

## b) What is the most appropriate investigation?

i)    barium meal and follow-through

ii)   stool for ova, cysts, and parasites

iii)  jejunal biopsy

iv)   duodenal aspirate and biopsy

v)    small bowel enema

We know that the patient has:

- systemic symptoms (weight loss, anorexia, tachycardia)
- textbook malabsorption (steatorrhoea, high faecal fat, bloodless diarrhoea)

The causes of malabsorption have been learned before. Write them down...

_____

_____

Now check them against the picture below:

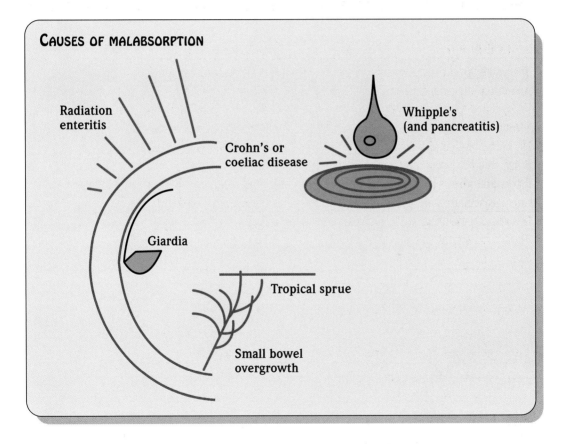

**CAUSES OF MALABSORPTION**

Radiation enteritis

Crohn's or coeliac disease

Whipple's (and pancreatitis)

Giardia

Tropical sprue

Small bowel overgrowth

Small bowel lymphoma is also a cause. The tendency is to think of exotic diseases. However, both amoebiasis and shigellosis are associated with bloody diarrhoea, and do not usually cause classic small bowel malabsorption, which is why they do not appear on the list. The same applies to strongyloidiasis, particularly as there is no preceding history of either skin or pulmonary involvement.

From the list, gastrointestinal lymphoma is unlikely without more systemic upset. The same would be true for Crohn's disease, particularly as there is an absence of other pointers from the examiners in this direction.

The two remaining diagnoses – tropical sprue and coeliac disease – have very similar initial presentations, but, given the history of recent travel, tropical sprue is the most likely. You would have to exclude this before making a diagnosis of adult coeliac disease.

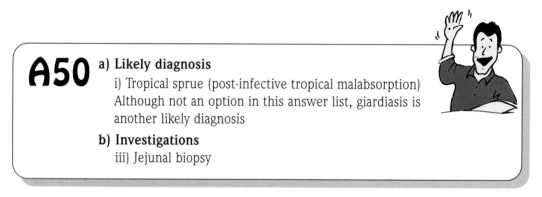

**A50**  **a) Likely diagnosis**
   i) Tropical sprue (post-infective tropical malabsorption)
   Although not an option in this answer list, giardiasis is
   another likely diagnosis

**b) Investigations**
   iii) Jejunal biopsy

## SCHILLING TEST

An alternative strategy that is increasingly being used in the assessment of tropical sprue is to perform a Schilling test, which shows a low vitamin $B_{12}$ uptake in the presence of tropical sprue, then treat with a short course of antibiotics and repeat the Schilling test. In tropical sprue, vitamin $B_{12}$ uptake should improve after antibiotic treatment.

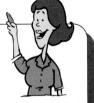

# Q51

A 30-year-old nurse presents after returning to the UK from travelling in the Far East for 8 months. Whilst in Thailand, she received a course of cotrimoxazole for *Shigella* dysentery. Two days after her return flight from Bangkok, she developed cramping abdominal pains and distension, associated with an itchy rash on her back and feet. She also developed bloodless diarrhoea, which, although initially quite mild, became pale, foul smelling, and difficult to flush away over the course of 2–3 weeks. Her flatmates took her to the emergency department, as they were increasingly worried about her poor appetite and the fact that she had lost a considerable amount of weight since her return.

## ON EXAMINATION

- Thin, dehydrated, and with increased pigmentation on arms and feet
- Vesicular rash on back and extensor surfaces
- Angular stomatitis with intraoral ulceration
- Weight = 46 kg (previously 51 kg)
- Temperature = 36.6°C
- No clubbing, lymphadenopathy
- Pulse = 110 beats/min regular
- Blood pressure = 95/60 mmHg
- Cardiovascular examination = normal
- Respiratory examination = normal
- Abdominal examination: active bowel sounds, nil else

## INVESTIGATIONS

- Haemoglobin = 9.5 g/dl
- Mean corpuscular volume = 105 fl
- Vitamin $B_{12}$ = 400 pg/ml
- Plasma sodium = 143 mmol/l
- Plasma potassium = 4.0 mmol/l
- Serum albumin = 28 g/l
- Serum bilirubin = 8 μmol/l
- Plasma urea = 8.2 mmol/l
- Plasma creatinine = 115 μmol/l
- White cell count = 6.5 × 10⁹/l
- Platelets = 210 × 10⁹/l
- Rigid sigmoidoscopy = normal
- Faecal fat = 120 mmol/l
- Urinalysis unremarkable

## a) What is the diagnosis?

   i)    cholera

   ii)   adult coeliac disease

   iii)  typhoid fever

   iv)  amoebiasis

   v)   giardiasis

## b) How would you confirm your suspicions?

i)    stool for ova, cysts, and parasites

ii)    blood cultures

iii)    jejunal biopsy and anti-endomysial antibodies

iv)    bone marrow aspirate and culture

v)    duodenal aspirate and biopsy

## c) What two therapeutic measures would you initiate?

i)    gluten-free diet and dapsone

ii)    intravenous fluids and chloramphenicol

iii)    oral rehydration therapy and tetracycline

iv)    metronidazole and diloxanide furoate

v)    intravenous fluids and metronidazole

A very similar question to the previous one! She has:

- systemic features: weight loss, anorexia, tachycardia, mouth ulcers
- malabsorption: steatorrhoea, high faecal fat, macrocytic anaemia – probably due to folate loss
- vesicular, itchy rash on extensor surfaces – dermatitis herpetiformis

In this case, the examiner has given you a strong clue. The presence of dermatitis herpetiformis makes coeliac disease the most likely diagnosis.

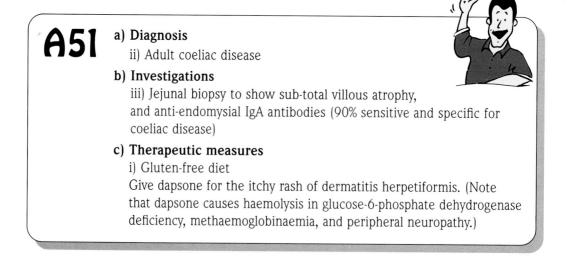

**A51**

a) **Diagnosis**
ii) Adult coeliac disease

b) **Investigations**
iii) Jejunal biopsy to show sub-total villous atrophy, and anti-endomysial IgA antibodies (90% sensitive and specific for coeliac disease)

c) **Therapeutic measures**
i) Gluten-free diet
Give dapsone for the itchy rash of dermatitis herpetiformis. (Note that dapsone causes haemolysis in glucose-6-phosphate dehydrogenase deficiency, methaemoglobinaemia, and peripheral neuropathy.)

## EXTRA BITS: COELIAC DISEASE

Coeliac disease can crop up in the MRCP examination in a number of disguises.

*Cancers*
- small/large bowel adenocarcinomas
- small bowel T-cell lymphoma

*Diarrhoea/weight loss*
- plus mixed blood film: folate and iron-deficiency anaemia
- plus hyposplenic picture: Howell–Jolly bodies, target cells – Pappenheimer bodies, acanthocytes
- plus malabsorption of fat-soluble vitamins:
  - A – visual disturbance
  - D – osteomalacia
  - E – dermatitis, neuropathy
  - K – bleeding, bruising
- plus tetany – a rare complication of coeliac disease
- plus neurological disturbance: long-tract signs and cerebellar ataxia; rare again
- plus other autoimmune diseases (beware the patient with life-long insulin-dependent diabetes mellitus!)

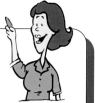

**Q52** A 60-year-old woman presents with sharp epigastric pain that is worse on lying down. This is accompanied by regurgitation of a greenish foul liquid. After 2 weeks of treatment with a histamine ($H_2$) receptor antagonist, her symptoms are unchanged. Her only other medical history is of an underactive thyroid gland for which she took thyroxine 50 μg daily.

## ON EXAMINATION

- High body mass index
- Clinical anaemia

## INVESTIGATIONS

- Haemoglobin = 9.5 g/dl
- Mean corpuscular volume = 108 fl
- White cell count = 6.5 × $10^9$/l
- Platelets = 180 × $10^9$/l
- Schilling test without intrinsic factor: urinary radioactive cobalamin excretion = 2%
- Schilling test with intrinsic factor: urinary radioactive cobalamin excretion = 13%

### a) What is the diagnosis?

- i) Barrett's oesophagus
- ii) pernicious anaemia
- iii) adult coeliac disease
- iv) myxoedema
- v) tropical sprue

### b) What is the cause of her symptoms?

- i) subacute intestinal obstruction
- ii) bile oesophagitis
- iii) reflux oesophagitis
- iv) duodenal ulcer and stricture
- v) hiatus hernia

Again, this is a 'case you should know', rather than a list question. The essence here is that she has:

- vitamin $B_{12}$ deficiency anaemia due to lack of intrinsic factor
- evidence of autoimmune disease (hypothyroidism)
- oesophagitis unresponsive to antacids

**A52** a) **Diagnosis**
  ii) Pernicious anaemia

b) **Symptom cause**
  ii) Bile oesophagitis (a feature of pernicious anaemia)

## MORE ABOUT PERNICIOUS ANAEMIA

As pernicious anaemia has such an insidious onset, this question comes in a variety of forms:

- the elderly woman with megaloblastic anaemia and peripheral sensory neuropathy
- the patient with autoimmune disease, painful glossitis, and ataxia (due to dorsal column disease)
- the patient with vitiligo, and any of the above factors

## QUICK CHECK

Write the lists of causes of:

- bloody diarrhoea
- loss of ankle jerks and upgoing plantars
- eosinophilia
- pyoderma gangrenosum
- cerebrospinal fluid lymphocytosis

And the features of:

- Gilbert's syndrome, Crigler–Najjar syndrome, Dubin–Johnson syndrome
- Friedreich's ataxia

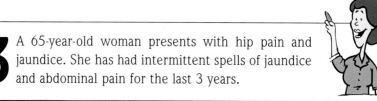

**Q53** A 65-year-old woman presents with hip pain and jaundice. She has had intermittent spells of jaundice and abdominal pain for the last 3 years.

| INVESTIGATIONS | RESULTS |
| --- | --- |
| Haemoglobin | 9.8 g/dl |
| White cell count | $3.9 \times 10^9/l$ |
| Platelets | $179 \times 10^9/l$ |
| Serum calcium | 1.9 mmol/l |
| Serum phosphate | 0.7 mmol/l |
| Serum albumin | 32 g/l |
| Serum alanine aminotransferase | 7 IU/l (normal: 5–15 IU/l) |
| Serum alkaline phosphatase | 350 IU/l (normal: 0–95 IU/l) |
| Serum bilirubin | 32 μmol/l (normal: 3–17 μmol/l) |
| Clotting INR | 1.4 |
| Thrombin time | Normal |
| Abdominal ultrasound | Normal |
| Liver biopsy | Liver granulomas with copper deposition |

INR: international normalised ratio.

### a) What is the most likely cause of her jaundice?

i) cholangiocarcinoma

ii) Wilson's disease

iii) sarcoidosis

iv) primary biliary cirrhosis

v) choledocholithiasis

### b) What test would you do to confirm this diagnosis?

i) serum caeruloplasmin levels

ii) anti-mitochondrial antibodies

iii) serum angiotensin-converting enzyme levels

iv) chest X-ray

v) CT scan of the abdomen

## c) What is the cause of her low calcium level?

i) chronic renal failure

ii) osteomalacia

iii) hypoparathyroidism

iv) calcium malabsorption

v) none of the above

The causes of liver granulomata on biopsy are:

- primary biliary cirrhosis

- classic granulomatous disease: sarcoidosis, TB, Wegener's granulomatosis, *Brucella*, berylliosis

- other autoimmune diseases: IBD, polyarteritis nodosa, giant cell arteritis

- infections? $T^2AG$ along and $C^4$: tropical (leprosy, schistosomiasis), toxocariasis, ascariasis, giardiasis, *Coxiella*, cytomegalovirus, coccidioidomycosis, clap (syphilis)

- malignancies, drugs, and the chronic granulomatous diseases

The answer ought to scream out at you from this list.

This is a classic MRCP examination question that can appear in many formats. Given that the patient has intermittent jaundice with a raised alkaline phosphatase level, you should immediately be alerted to the diagnosis. The question has been deliberately made easy by the liver biopsy result. The mention of copper deposition is meant to fool you into diagnosing Wilson's disease (in which granulomas are not seen – see question 27, page 120).

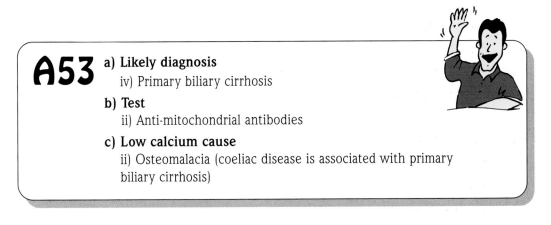

**A53**

a) **Likely diagnosis**
iv) Primary biliary cirrhosis

b) **Test**
ii) Anti-mitochondrial antibodies

c) **Low calcium cause**
ii) Osteomalacia (coeliac disease is associated with primary biliary cirrhosis)

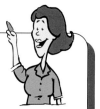

# Q54

A 60-year-old man attends your outpatient clinic with a 1-month history of indigestion. He has been seeing his GP three times a week and is frustrated to be told that he should lose weight. He smokes 50 cigarettes per day, but hardly drinks any alcohol. There are no other gastrointestinal or systemic symptoms. He has been taking nifedipine for his hypertension. His blood tests (including full blood count, renal, and liver function tests) are all normal.

## a) Which of the following would not be your initial management?

i)    refer for endoscopy

ii)   advise the patient to continue to lose weight

iii)  prescribe a proton-pump inhibitor

iv)  conduct *Helicobacter pylori* testing

v)   review his antihypertensive medication

NICE sets out the criteria for urgent specialist endoscopic investigation. Patients of any age who present with dyspepsia and alarm symptoms (gastrointestinal bleeding, weight loss, dysphagia, persistent vomiting, iron-deficiency anaemia, epigastric mass, or a suspicious barium meal) should be referred for urgent endoscopy.

In this patient, the initial management should include:

- addressing his lifestyle, including weight reduction and smoking cessation
- medication check – review nifedipine! Other culprits include steroids, nitrates, bisphosphonates, and nonsteroidal anti-inflammatory drugs
- proton-pump inhibitors or *H. pylori* testing and eradication are recommended in dyspepsia without alarm symptoms

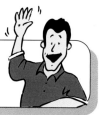

# A54
**a) Management**
i) Refer for endoscopy

# QUIZ SPOT!

## SIADH PUZZLE

Fill in the letters for four causes of SIADH, beginning each cause at the 'P'. If right, the numbered circles will complete a well-known seaside phrase. The solution is on page 335.

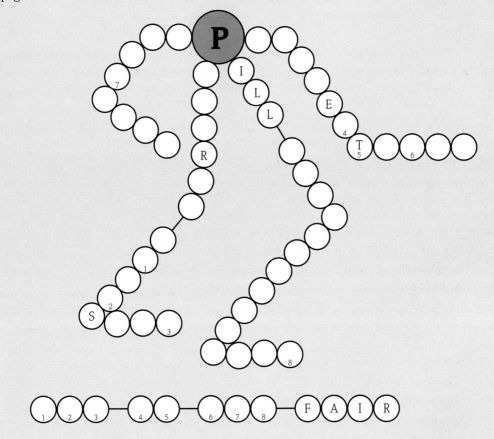

# 8

# A BLOODY HELL

Haematological MRCP lists

Abnormal haematological results or findings in the reticuloendothelial system are often the key to grey cases and data interpretation questions. If you know nothing else, you must know your haematology lists.

*Seen any good films lately?*

## TOP HAEMATOLOGY SONGS

1) You're So Vein (Carly Simon)
2) Lady in Red (Chris de Burr Cell)
3) Whiter Shade of Pale (Procul Harum)

## TOP HAEMATOLOGY FILMS

Any MRCP candidate should know these backwards

1) The Three Colours Trilogy (Red, Blue, and White)
2) Marrowed to the Mob
3) The Cell
4) Spurtigo
5) *Leucoerythroblastosis*
6) *Pancytopenia*
7) *Neutropenia*
8) *Thrombocytopenia*
9) *Polycythaemia*
10) *Eosinophilia*

Reviews of the latter six can be found in this chapter.

## Q55

You are asked to see a 6-year-old maladjusted child in a residential home. He presents with a 2-week history of decreasing visual acuity on the right side with the recent onset of blurring of the right eye. Examination reveals the presence of enlarged axillary and cervical lymph nodes. Fundoscopy shows white macular plaques with some retinal detachment.

| INVESTIGATIONS | RESULTS |
| --- | --- |
| Haemoglobin | 11.4 g/dl |
| White cell count | $6.5 \times 10^9/l$ |
| Eosinophils | 20% |
| Platelets | $156 \times 10^9/l$ |

### a) What is the most likely diagnosis?

- i) Hodgkin's lymphoma
- ii) lymphoblastic lymphoma
- iii) toxocariasis
- iv) retinoblastoma
- v) acariasis

### b) What two investigations would you do next?

- i) blood film and lymph node biopsy
- ii) bone marrow and lymph node biopsy
- iii) stool for ova, cysts, and parasites and lymph node biopsy
- iv) CT scan of the orbits and lymph node biopsy
- v) *Toxocara* serology and lymph node biopsy

This question is pretty straightforward, using the method we have described. There is only one major list to know, and that is for the causes of eosinophilia. We have done this before (see page 58): eoS$^4$I$^3$N$^3$oP$^6$hI$^5$lia. Try writing down the causes, then check against the list over the page.

## CAUSES OF EOS⁴I³N³OP⁶HI⁵LIA

Skin:          rheumatoid arthritis (RA) with cutaneous manifestations

               dermatitis herpetiformis

               scabies

               atopic eczema

Immune:        asthma

               atopy

               any drug reactions

Neoplastic:    Hodgkin's lymphomas

               acute lymphoblastic lymphoma

               all solid malignancies

Pulmonary:     increases in sputum and peripheral blood eosinophil counts are caused by:

- allergic bronchopulmonary aspergillosis (asthma, cough, sputum plugs, proximal bronchiectasis)
- Löffler's syndrome (cough, fever, yellow sputum, malaise, fluffy X-ray infiltrates)
- tropical eosinophilia (microfilaraemia, ascariasis, ankylostomiasis, toxocariasis, strongyloidiasis)
- drug reactions (cotrimoxazole, busulphan, methotrexate, nitrofurantoin, or anything at all!)
- Churg–Strauss syndrome (small/medium-vessel vasculitis, asthma, eosinophilia)
- adult asthma

Infective:     nematodes – roundworms (e.g. *Toxocara, Ascaris lumbricoides*)

               cestodes – tapeworms (e.g. *Echinococcus*)

               trematodes – flukes

               *Schistosoma* and other parasites

               Whipple's disease

You now need to sift through and see which cause fits best with the history. With the added recurrent eye problems with retinal detachment and retinal plaques then, against your better judgement, it is time to come up with a weird and wonderful diagnosis. In this case you can exclude nearly all of them, leaving one major contender – and that is *Toxocara* infection.

The additional investigations are difficult. However, in the MRCP examination, if you suggest an infectious disease as a potential cause of anything then we would recommend going for serology. Given that the patient has enlarged lymph nodes then a biopsy is always indicated (a fine needle aspiration is also acceptable).

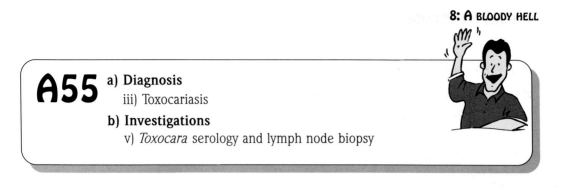

**A55** a) **Diagnosis**
iii) Toxocariasis
b) **Investigations**
v) *Toxocara* serology and lymph node biopsy

*T. canis* (puppy poo in soil) causes visceral larva migrans, spreading via haematogenous or lymphatic routes to all organs. Systemic inflammation, eosinophilia, itch, breathlessness, and an enlarged liver are all seen, as are all the usual features of end-organ inflammation of, for example, brain, lung, and heart. *T. canis* infection is treated with antiparasitic drugs such as albendazole, usually in combination with anti-inflammatory medications.

## Leucoerythroblastic film

Immature erythroid and myeloid stem cells appear in the peripheral blood film. This is most commonly due to marrow infiltration causing 'overspill', in which case a high erythrocyte sedimentation rate, normochromic, normocytic anaemia with anisopoikilocytosis, and raised white cell count shift to the left are seen. Alternatively, it may be due to a sudden 'switch on' and outpouring from a marrow 'on the roll'.

*M$^5$arrow infiltrations$^2$ (or 'M$^5$o ss grows fast on rolling bone')*

- metastases
- malignancies: multiple myeloma, myeloid leukaemias (chronic myeloid leukaemia [CML] and acute myeloid leukaemia [AML])
- myelofibrosis
- myeloproliferative (polycythaemia rarely)
- mycobacteria: tuberculosis (TB)
- osteopetrosis and Paget's disease
- sarcoidosis
- storage: Gaucher's disease – a recessive β-glucocerebrosidase deficiency causing glucocerebroside accumulation, and hence cutaneous pigmentation, hypersplenism, splenomegaly, and skeletal deformity; also Niemann–Pick disease – autosomal recessive, hepatosplenomegaly, hypersplenism

*Switch on*

Massive sepsis, massive haemolysis, or massive haemorrhage leads to pancytopenia.

## CAUSES OF PANCYTOPENIA

'VD that c$^2$lim$^4$bs$^2$ p$^2$retty f$^2$ast'

- viral infections, drug reactions*
- thymic tumours, hypersplenism**, alcohol, TB
- carcinoma/chemotherapy, lymphoproliferative disease, irradiation, myelofibrosis, multiple myeloma, megaloblastic anaemia, myelodysplasia, *Brucella*, systemic lupus erythematosus (SLE), sideroblastic anaemia
- paroxysmal nocturnal haemoglobinuria (PNH), parvovirus with sickle cell/ haemolytic disease
- Fanconi's syndrome***, Felty's syndrome****

*Drug reactions can be divided into:

| PROPORTIONAL TO DOSE | IDIOSYNCRATIC |
|---|---|
| Benzene | Sulphonamides/streptomycin |
| TNT (2,4,6-trinitrotoluene) | Gold/penicillamine/phenoxybenzamine |
| 6-Mercaptopurine | Hydralazine |
| Busulphan | Arsenic |
| | Acetazolamide |
| | DDT (dichloro-diphenyl-trichloroethane) |

**See 'Causes of hypersplenism' list, on the next page.

***Fanconi's syndrome: hyperpigmentation, mental retardation, microcephaly, short stature, small thumb/radius/carpus, microsomia, cryptorchidism, hypogonadism.

****Felty's syndrome: splenomegaly, lymphadenopathy, cutaneous pigmentation/ulcers, stomal ulcers in the presence of rheumatoid factor-positive arthritis.

Answers to Criteria Connections (see page 16):

Major criteria: Aschoff nodules, erythema marginatum, pancarditis, polyarthropathy, Sydenham's chorea.

Minor criteria: high ESR/CRP, leucocytosis, long PR interval.

You need two major criteria, or one major criterion and at least two minor criteria, to make the diagnosis. Missing are past rheumatic fever (minor) and arthralgia (minor, if polyarthropathy is absent).

## CAUSES OF HYPERSPLENISM

6 infections:

- TB
- *Brucella*
- syphilis
- malaria
- subacute bacterial endocarditis
- kala azar

5 haematological:

- lymphoma
- chronic lymphocytic leukaemia (CLL)
- CML
- myelofibrosis
- thalassaemia/haemoglobinopathies

4 connective tissue:

- RA
- Still's disease
- Felty's syndrome
- SLE

3 other:

- congestion
- sarcoidosis
- idiopathic

2 metabolic:

- Gaucher's disease
- Niemann–Pick disease

## Causes of Neutropenia

That may seem a lot to learn, but you can use this list as the basis for another list. You might have thought that PIES[2] could cause bovine spongiform encephalopathy. But who would have thought that they were the cause of *neutropenia*?

| | |
|---|---|
| Pancytopenia: | all causes in the list above |
| Infection: | typhoid, typhus, TB, any type of viral infection, *Brucella*, kala azar, malaria |
| Endocrine: | hypopituitarism, and both hypothyroidism and hyperthyroidism |
| SLE | |
| Specific drugs: | alcohol and alcoholic cirrhosis, thiouracil |

## Causes of Thrombocytopenia

The causes can be divided into decreased production, increased destruction, and toxic suppression. Hopefully these terms are not on your appraisal forms!

| | |
|---|---|
| Decreased production: | megaloblastic anaemia, liver failure, bacterial or viral infection (TB, typhoid, typhus, kala azar, malaria, *Brucella*, parvovirus with sickle cell/haemolytic disease), malignancy (lymphoproliferative disease, myelodysplasia, thymic tumours, sideroblastic anaemia, myelofibrosis, multiple myeloma) |
| Increased destruction: | hypersplenism, Felty's syndrome, Fanconi's syndrome, SLE, paroxysmal nocturnal haemoglobinuria, thrombotic thrombocytopenic purpura, haemolytic–uraemic syndrome, idiopathic thrombocytopenic purpura |
| Toxic suppression: | chemotherapy, irradiation, drugs |

Also think of hypopituitarism, hypothyroidism, and hyperthyroidism.

## Causes of Polycythaemia

We're bored now. Make up your own way of remembering the causes. Here they are:

| | |
|---|---|
| Relative: | dehydration, Gaisböck's syndrome (stress) |
| Primary: | polycythaemia rubra vera (splenomegaly, raised platelets) |
| Secondary: | hypoxia, chronic obstructive pulmonary disease, altitude, abnormal haemoglobin, sleep apnoea |
| Excess erythropoietin: | cerebellar haemangioma, hepatoma, phaeochromocytoma, hypernephroma, polycystic/transplant kidneys, uterine leiomyomata/fibromata |

**Q56** What do target cells, Howell–Jolly bodies, siderocytes, microspherocytes, and a high platelet and neutrophil count signify?

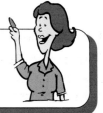

**A56** Hyposplenism. Learn these features – hyposplenism is a common finding in the MRCP examination and can crop up in a number of different guises.

## FASCINATING FACT

Auer rods are seen in acute promyelocytic leukaemia as rod-shaped inclusions in white blood cells. Not many people wanted to know that.

## SIZE AND SHAPE DO MATTER

Sorry. But they do. And nowhere more so than in the haematology question. You can get clues to the diagnosis of short and grey cases by looking for abnormal red blood cell features.

*Macrocytosis*

Macrocytosis is a common finding that usually represents the release into the circulation of immature (and therefore large) red blood cell precursors. Most candidates can think of very few causes – namely liver disease and vitamin $B_{12}$ deficiency. Pause here, and write yourself a list of 15 other causes. When you have finally had enough, learn the list below:

$L^3EG \; CR^3A^3M^4P^2S = 17$

- liver disease, leukoerythroblastosis, lead poisoning
- cytotoxic chemotherapy
- reticulocytosis, renal failure, respiratory failure
- alcohol ingestion, aplastic anaemia, azathioprine treatment
- megaloblastic anaemia (vitamin $B_{12}$/folate deficiency), myeloma, myxoedema, malaria
- pregnancy, pellagra
- sideroblastic anaemia

*Spherocytosis*

Spherocytes have a round, uniform shape, just as their name suggests. As usual, this finding can be hereditary or acquired. As a rule of thumb, structural defects are usually dominant, and metabolic defects are usually recessive. Thus, hereditary spherocytosis (a structural defect caused by defects in membrane-stabilising proteins) is transmitted as an autosomal dominant condition and is not associated with haemolysis. However, just like injured cattle, injured red blood cells are rounded up. Thus, any red blood cell injury can cause haemolysis, and all causes of haemolysis can produce spherocytes.

*Target cells*

Take the stuffing out of a cushion and sit on it and it will look like a target. Similarly, any very thin red blood cell will look like a target. How do you knock the stuffing out of a red blood cell? Quite simply, by mucking up its haemoglobin. The causes are, therefore, sickle cell disease, sickle/haemoglobin C, haemoglobin C disease, haemoglobin C/thalassaemia, thalassaemia (major and minor), and iron deficiency. Easy, isn't it? Oh, by the way, post-splenectomy patients may also have target cells.

*Howell–Jolly bodies*

These are tiny granules of damaged DNA in red blood cells. Normally, the spleen would filter out these cells. Thus, you see them when the spleen isn't there (i.e. in any cause of hyposplenism, including post-splenectomy and sickle cell disease) or when the spleen is overwhelmed with damaged cells, such as in haemolysis, toxic anaemias, and the lymphoid leukaemias.

*Siderocytes*

These contain granules of nonhaemoglobin iron (Pappenheimer bodies), which stain blue at the edge of the cell with Wright stain. Think metals (haemochromatosis, lead poisoning), prematurity, pernicious anaemia (PA), thalassaemia, myelodysplasia/proliferation, and haemolysis. It may also be caused by RA and some drugs (e.g. chloramphenicol). The most common cause, however, is alcoholism. We can't think of an easy way to remember this list. Feel free to try!

# MAHA

MAHA, or microangiopathic haemolytic anaemia to its friends, can be recognised by the presence of fragmented red blood cells and burr cells. The causes are:

- growths: cancers, foetuses (eclampsia, abruption, intrauterine death, amniotic fluid embolus)
- damage to small vessels (malignant hypertension, vasculitides, burns, sepsis, and disseminated intravascular coagulation [DIC])
- renal-failure association: thrombotic thrombocytopenic purpura, haemolytic uraemic syndrome, acute glomerulonephritis
- drugs: such as cytotoxics, cyclosporin

Note: thrombotic thrombocytopenic purpura is another name for Moschcowitz disease. This is the same as haemolytic uraemic syndrome, but with added fever, neurological impairment, and mild abnormalities of clotting, with haemolysis and renal impairment. It is associated with infection (especially verotoxin-producing *Escherichia coli*), SLE, and cancers. Remember that the causes of MAHA overlap with those of standard haemolytic anaemia (see next).

## HAEMOLYTIC ANAEMIA

We couldn't think of a funny mnemonic for these, but the causes are relatively well known so we will just list them. If you can come up with something that is amusing then we would be pleased to hear from you.

Congenital:

- membrane defects: hereditary spherocytosis/elliptocytosis
- haemoglobinopathies: sickle cell anaemia, thalassaemia
- enzyme problems: glucose-6-phosphate dehydrogenase deficiency, pyruvate kinase deficiency

Acquired

- immune: autoimmune, lymphoma, RA, drug-induced (e.g. methyldopa, penicillin), post-transfusion, PNH
- MAHA: mechanical injury, malaria, prosthetic valves, burns, clostridial sepsis (*Clostridium perfringens*), snake bites, march haemoglobinuria
- DIC
- hypersplenism

Remember that hyposplenic patients, particularly children, are susceptible to infections with *Klebsiella, E. coli, Streptococcus pneumoniae, Haemophilus influenzae* type B, and *Neisseria meningitidis*. These patients should be given prophylactic penicillin (erythromycin for allergic patients).

## Hepatomegaly

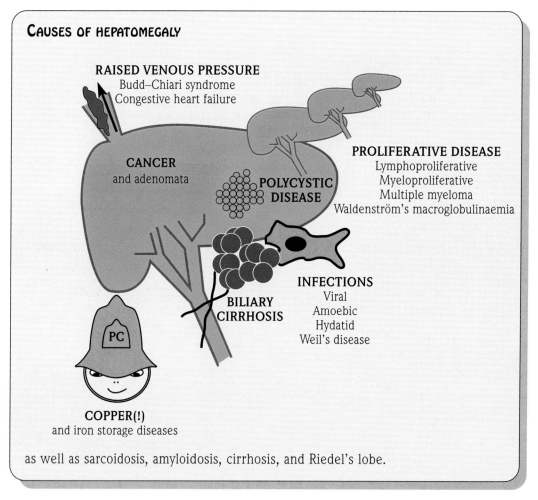

### CAUSES OF HEPATOMEGALY

**RAISED VENOUS PRESSURE**
Budd–Chiari syndrome
Congestive heart failure

**CANCER**
and adenomata

**POLYCYSTIC DISEASE**

**PROLIFERATIVE DISEASE**
Lymphoproliferative
Myeloproliferative
Multiple myeloma
Waldenström's macroglobulinaemia

**BILIARY CIRRHOSIS**

**INFECTIONS**
Viral
Amoebic
Hydatid
Weil's disease

PC

**COPPER(!)**
and iron storage diseases

as well as sarcoidosis, amyloidosis, cirrhosis, and Riedel's lobe.

Learn to draw the picture above, or invent your own.

Remember that:

- the top three common causes are cirrhosis, congestive heart failure, and malignancy
- hard and knobbly suggests malignancy, cirrhosis (particularly after hepatitis B infection), polycystic disease, hydatid cyst, or syphilis.

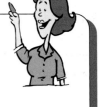

# Q57

A 23-year-old man is admitted for the investigation of anaemia. It is noted that he has a palpable spleen. There is no hepatomegaly or lymphadenopathy, and the patient is otherwise well, except that he has recently suffered a mild upper airway infection.

| Investigations | Results |
| --- | --- |
| Haemoglobin | 8.9 g/dl |
| White cell count | 6.5 × 10⁹/l |
| Platelets | 234 × 10⁹/l |
| Reticulocytes | 9% |
| Spherocytes | Present |

## a) What three steps would you take to investigate this patient further?

i) travel history, thick and thin blood smears, and liver function tests

ii) Epstein–Barr virus serology, cytomegalovirus serology, and hepatitis B serology

iii) Family history, bone marrow aspirate, and CT scan of the thorax and abdomen

iv) Coomb's test, glucose-6-phosphate dehydrogenase levels, and red blood cell pyruvate kinase level

v) Family history, sickling test, and haemoglobin electrophoresis

This sort of question is always a good one, and an example of why the MRCP examination is in love with haematology. It's just so easy to mix up a few good clinical signs with a few odd blood tests.

Here we could go for several lists, but the obvious one is for the causes of splenomegaly. Again, try to jot down as complete a list as you can before looking at the summary overleaf.

## CAUSES OF SPLENOMEGALY

| MASSIVE | MODERATE | MILD |
|---|---|---|
| • CML<br>• Myelofibrosis<br>• Malaria<br>• Kala azar<br>• Gaucher's disease | • All causes of massive splenomegaly<br>• Myeloproliferation<br>• Cirrhosis and portal hypertension<br>• Leukaemia<br>• Haemolysis | • All causes of massive/moderate splenomegaly<br>• Infection<br>• Lymphoproliferative disorders<br>• Immunoproliferative disorders |

*Other causes*

- *Brucella*, typhoid, TB, trypanosomiasis, subacute bacterial endocarditis, viral infections (infectious mononucleosis [IMN], hepatitis B)
- sarcoidosis, amyloidosis
- SLE, Felty's syndrome
- idiopathic thrombocytopenic purpura, haemolysis, iron deficiency, PA

We know that the patient is anaemic with a high reticulocyte count, and must therefore be bleeding or haemolysing. The chances of a young man bleeding *and* having a big spleen are small, unless you want to invoke DIC with a lymphoma or liver disease with an impalpable liver, no other signs, and portal hypertension. The likelihood is that he is haemolysing – a conclusion that you should have reached even without the presence of spherocytes on the film. Now combine the splenomegaly list with the haemolytic anaemia list and... hey presto!

**A57** a) Tests
iv) Coomb's test, glucose-6-phosphate dehydrogenase level, and red blood cell pyruvate kinase level

## HEPATOSPLENOMEGALY WITH LYMPHADENOPATHY

Well, at last it gets easier. The causes are simply all those of splenomegaly, plus thalassaemia and all the causes of hepatomegaly, with the exception of biliary cirrhosis and proliferative disease.

Here we hit the **WALL**:

- Waldenström's macroglobulinaemia
- acute lymphoblastic leukaemia
- lymphoma
- (and think of the other lymphoproliferative disorders)

## Common tests

### ESR IN THE BASEMENT

Think of:

- polycythaemia
- afibrinogenaemia
- hypofibrinogenaemia

### ESR THROUGH THE ROOF

Think of:

- first line – temporal arteritis, polymyalgia rheumatica, SLE, multiple myeloma
- second line – carcinoma and chronic infection

### LAP DANCING

*What the hell is LAP?* OK, so it stands for leucocyte alkaline phosphatase. But a score? I ask you! OK, if you *really* want to know… it's found in neutrophils. The earlier the neutrophil precursor or the younger the cell, the higher the LAP score. So anything that causes you to increase the production of young or immature neutrophils will cause a rise in the LAP score. Make a list of these causes below, and then check it against ours.

*Causes of high LAP scores*

- myeloproliferative disorders: polycythaemia rubra vera, myelofibrosis, Hodgkin's lymphoma

- steroids: Cushing's syndrome, treatment with steroids, the oral contraceptive pill, pregnancy

It is also:

- *up* in *Down's* syndrome

- *up* when protein levels are *down* (e.g. in kwashiorkor when serum levels are low!)

*Causes of low LAP scores*

The LAP score is low in things with letters in:

- CML

- PA

- IMN or Epstein–Barr virus (EBV)

- PNH

as well as in:

- rickets

- hypophosphataemia

## OSMOTIC FRAGILITY

In the presence of an osmotic challenge, some cells are resistant to bursting and are said to show decreased osmotic fragility. These are best remembered as being the cells with abnormal haemoglobin: haemoglobin C, sickle cells, thalassaemia, and iron and vitamin $B_{12}$ deficiencies. Increased fragility is seen in all haemolytic states: it is the classic test for spherocytosis.

# Q58

An 8-year-old girl of Nigerian origin, recently arrived in the UK, presents to her local emergency department with a 10-day history of fever and malaise. She lives with her parents and she has a 5-year-old brother who has been in complete remission from acute lymphoblastic leukaemia for 1 year. Her mother is a primary school teacher and her father is in the diplomatic service, necessitating the family to move to different countries twice a year. Ten days before the onset of her symptoms, she had a 1-week course of antibiotics from her GP for a throat infection. In addition to her fever, she complains of several days' pain and swelling in both hands. She has had no gastrointestinal disturbance or overt signs of blood loss. She has had similar attacks before.

## ON EXAMINATION

- Temperature = 37.5°C
- Pulse = 98 beats/min regular
- Blood pressure = 105/70 mmHg
- No rashes or lymphadenopathy
- Mild icterus
- Mouth clear
- Jugular venous pressure not elevated
- Heart sounds 1 + 2 + soft ejection systolic murmur at the left sternal edge
- Chest clear
- Abdomen soft, no hepatosplenomegaly
- Painful dactylitis of the right index and ring fingers, and the left middle and ring fingers

## INVESTIGATIONS

- Haemoglobin = 9.0 g/l
- Reticulocytes = 8%
- White cell count = $13 \times 10^9$/l
- Neutrophils = 85%
- Platelets = $450 \times 10^9$/l
- Urinalysis and electrolytes = normal
- Bilirubin = 40 µmol/l
- Aspartate aminotransferase = 45 IU/l
- ESR = 130 mm in the first hour
- C-reactive protein = 76 mg/l
- Urinalysis: normal dipstick, no casts/cells, negative cultures
- ECG: sinus rhythm, PR interval 0.18 s, QRS 0.12

ECG: electrocardiogram; ESR: erythrocyte sedimentation rate.

a) **The most likely diagnosis is:**

    i)     polyarticular Still's disease

    ii)    acute rheumatic fever

    iii)   sickle cell disease with hand-and-foot syndrome

    iv)   Lyme disease

    v)    juvenile rheumatoid arthritis

b) **Which one investigation will confirm your diagnosis?**

    i)     rheumatoid factor

    ii)    haemoglobin electrophoresis

    iii)   anti-*Borrelia burgdorferi* immunoglobulin M antibodies

    iv)   acute and convalescent serum anti-streptolysin O titres

    v)    X-ray of the joints

c) **What is the appropriate management?**

    i)     intravenous ceftriaxone

    ii)    penicillamine

    iii)   opiate analgesia

    iv)   acetylsalicylate

    v)    immunosuppressive agents

You have seen a similar question before (at least we hope that you can recognise it!) – in **Chapter 1** (The strategy). The history here, however, is slightly different: in this case there is a preceding infection followed by a painful dactylitis of the hands and haemolytic anaemia in a younger child of African origin. This alone must make sickle cell disease scream out to be diagnosed. But let us suppose that you are blinded by fear in the examination. The key features with a limited list of causes are:

- polyarthralgia in the hands: remind yourself of the causes (AGAIN!) on the next page
- haemolysis or blood loss: again, check that you know these by writing them down

*Causes of polyarthralgia*

---
---
---
---
---
---
---
---

*Causes of haemolysis*

---
---
---
---
---
---
---
---

The absence of abdominal or bowel symptoms excludes (for the examination) the whole of the last verse of the polyarthralgia poem. None of the first or second verses are associated with anaemia and a high reticulocyte count (suggesting haemolysis or blood loss). But remember, we had two causes at the bottom that were not part of the verse. We said, "Remember the haematological causes such as sickle cell disease, which can give rise to hand-and-foot syndrome." In addition, "Remember that septic polyarthritis can occur when joints are seeded with organisms such as *Neisseria gonorrhoeae* or *Staphylococcus*."

This leaves septic polyarthritis (excluded on the same grounds) or sickle cell disease.

**A58**

a) **Diagnosis**
iii) Sickle cell disease with hand-and-foot syndrome

b) **Investigation**
ii) Haemoglobin electrophoresis

c) **Management**
iii) Opiate analgesia

A blood transfusion and family screening and counselling would also be appropriate.

# QUIZ SPOT!

**Q:** What are the six pulmonary causes of peripheral (circulating) eosinophilia?

A: See page 58 for the list of causes.

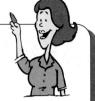

# Q59

A 30-year-old Caucasian man presents to the emergency department with a 10-day history of wrist-drop. He did some heavy lifting recently while helping a friend to move house and wonders whether this could have contributed. He suffers from asthma and chronic rhinitis, which are currently well controlled on regular inhaled steroids. On direct questioning he recalls having had foot-drop some years ago, but this was somewhat overshadowed by an acute exacerbation of asthma at the same time, for which he required hospital admission. On his discharge from hospital the foot-drop had resolved and he thought nothing more about it.

## ON EXAMINATION

- Looks well apart from obvious left radial nerve palsy and some adductor weakness of the right thumb. He cannot stand on the tips of his toes
- 3–4 tender subcutaneous nodules on dorsum of arm
- Remainder of examination, including full neurological examination = normal

## INVESTIGATIONS

- Skin nodule biopsy shows noncaseating granuloma
- Haemoglobin = 14 g/dl
- White cell count = $12 \times 10^9$/l
- Eosinophils = $2.0 \times 10^9$/l
- Platelets = $281 \times 10^9$/l
- Plasma sodium = 135 mmol/l
- Plasma potassium = 4.9 mmol/l
- Plasma urea = 8.1 mmol/l
- Plasma creatinine = 160 μmol/l

a) **What is the underlying diagnosis?**

 i)   rheumatoid arthritis

 ii)  Churg–Strauss syndrome

 iii) Guillain–Barré syndrome

 iv)  polyarteritis nodosa

 v)   sarcoidosis

b) **What is the mechanism of this patient's wrist-drop?**

 i)   trauma

 ii)  polyneuropathy

 iii) mononeuritis multiplex

 iv)  tendon rupture due to long-term steroid use

 v)   granulomas in the nerve

## c) What would you do next?

i) discontinue steroids

ii) start oral steroids

iii) refer to physiotherapy for splinting

iv) nerve biopsy

v) nerve conduction study

The key features here are:

* eosinophilia
* noncaseating granuloma
* atopic background

You already know the list of causes of eosinophilia (see Pants chapter, page 58).

## CAUSES OF POLYNEUROPATHY

You might want to add in a list of causes of acquired polyneuropathy, which you also learned earlier (see page 42).

| Born unlucky | Friedreich's ataxia, Refsum's disease, Charcot–Marie–Tooth disease |
| --- | --- |
| Three dejected | alcoholics due to the effects of alcohol; vitamin $B_1$, $B_6$, and $B_{12}$ deficiencies; isoniazid used to treat TB – which is why people receiving TB treatment must receive pyridoxine supplements |
| Two infected | leprosy, Guillain–Barré syndrome |
| Two injected | paraneoplasia in cancer patients, or the effects of its treatments, such as vincristine and isoniazid; diabetes mellitus |
| One connected | connective tissue disease, such as RA/SLE/polyarteritis nodosa |
| Granuloma suspected | sarcoidosis, Churg–Strauss syndrome |
| Hypothyroid | which just refuses to rhyme |

This should leave you with two likely answers; lymphoma or Churg–Strauss syndrome. Only one gives rise to granulomata...

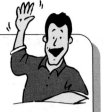

**A59** a) **Diagnosis**
ii) Churg–Strauss syndrome

b) **Cause of wrist-drop**
iii) Mononeuritis multiplex

c) **Treatment**
ii) Start oral steroids, reducing the dose over the course of 2 weeks
according to symptoms

## CHURG–STRAUSS SYNDROME

This is characterised by:

- asthma (typically males in their thirties)
- *medium* vessel vasculitis
- extravascular granulomas
- history of atopy/asthma/rhinitis that usually preceded granuloma
- peripheral blood eosinophilia
- mild renal impairment
- mononeuritis multiplex
- perinuclear anti-neutrophilic cytoplasmic antibody positivity in 50%
  (as opposed to Wegener's granulomatosis, see below).

## WEGENER'S GRANULOMATOSIS

This is characterised by:

- *small* vessel vasculitis
- extravascular granulomas
- any two of upper respiratory, lower respiratory, or renal involvement
- upper respiratory tract: stuffiness, sinusitis, nasal bridge collapse, nasal mucosa
  granulomas, conductive deafness
- lower respiratory tract: haemoptysis, pulmonary cavitating lesions, pleuritic pain
- renal: acute renal failure, rapidly progressive glomerulonephritis
- occasional but rare involvement of skin and nervous system
- anti-neutrophilic cytoplasmic antibody positivity

### EXTRA BITS: VARIATIONS TO QUESTION

This question may appear in a similar format, but with a few changes:

- young man + wheeze/asthma + eosinophilia + history of ulcerative colitis = eosinophilic alveolitis secondary to sulphasalazine
- young woman + wheeze + eosinophilia + recurrent urinary tract infections = eosinophilic alveolitis secondary to nitrofurantoin

### CAUSES OF GRANULOMATA

- Sarcoidosis
- TB (caseating)
- Langerhans cell histiocytosis
- Wegener's granulomatosis
- Churg–Strauss syndrome
- Fungal and helminthic infections
- Hypersensitivity reactions (e.g. dust)
- Malignancy (primary or secondary to colon, kidney, germ-cell, bone, prostate, melanoma)

# Q60

A 35-year-old woman is referred to her local gastroenterologist for investigation of recurrent abdominal pain. She denies any diarrhoea or mucus or slime in the stool. (By the way, who would want to be a gastroenterologist?) She is otherwise fit and well, apart from having had a left tibial vein thrombosis 3 years ago and a right deep vein thrombosis 8 months ago. On direct questioning she complains of intermittent pain and swelling of her fingers, but this has not been severe enough for her to be worried. On examination she is clinically anaemic, but findings are otherwise unremarkable.

| INVESTIGATIONS | RESULTS |
| --- | --- |
| Haemoglobin | 8.5 g/dl |
| White cell count | $2.1 \times 10^9/l$ |
| Platelets | $85 \times 10^9/l$ |
| Reticulocytes | 10% |
| Serum bilirubin | 21 μmol/l |
| Serum aspartate aminotransferase | 16 IU/l |
| Serum alkaline phosphatase | 75 IU/l |
| Prothrombin time | 14 s |
| Activated partial thromboplastin time | 38 s |

## a) What is the diagnosis?

i)   Crohn's disease

ii)   ulcerative colitis

iii)   rheumatoid arthritis

iv)   sarcoidosis

v)   SLE

## b) How would you confirm this with only two tests?

i)   sigmoidoscopy and small bowel biopsy

ii)   small bowel follow-through with colonoscopy

iii)   rheumatoid factor and X-ray of the joints

iv)   anti-nuclear antibodies and anti-double-stranded DNA antibodies

v)   serum angiotensin-converting enzyme levels and chest X-ray

This is a 'just know it' question. The key features are:

- recurrent venous thromboses
- pancytopenia (with haemolytic anaemia)
- small joint arthropathy

You might consult your list of causes of polyarthropathy – it must be on there. Run through the poem and add-ons (see page 5) and the causes are:

- RA, Still's disease, osteoarthritis, seronegative arthritides, pyrophosphate arthropathy, and SLE (Henoch–Schönlein purpura, sarcoidosis, and serum sickness are also included in the poem)
- infections: parvovirus, *Neisseria gonorrhoeae*, *Streptococcus*, TB, German measles, hepatitis, Lyme disease, chickenpox, HIV, and subacute bacterial endocarditis are also included in the poem
- bowel-associated: familial Mediterranean fever, inflammatory bowel disease, and Whipple's disease
- sickle cell anaemia
- Behçet's syndrome

Which of these can cause thrombotic tendency? Well, Crohn's disease and ulcerative colitis can. So, too, can SLE (lupus anticoagulant). The absence of altered bowel habit is meant to point you towards SLE.

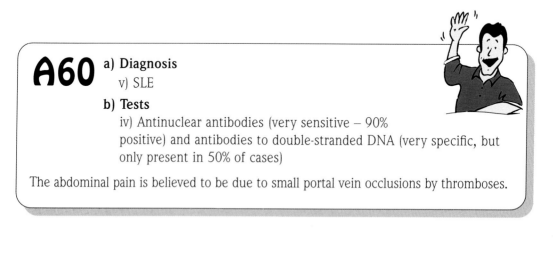

**A60**
a) **Diagnosis**
  v) SLE
b) **Tests**
  iv) Antinuclear antibodies (very sensitive – 90% positive) and antibodies to double-stranded DNA (very specific, but only present in 50% of cases)

The abdominal pain is believed to be due to small portal vein occlusions by thromboses.

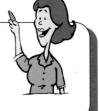

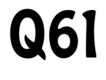 **Q61** A 30-year-old man is investigated for recurrent venous thrombosis. Apart from the intermittent passage of dark urine, he is a fit person and regularly plays five-a-side football on Saturday mornings.

| INVESTIGATIONS | RESULTS |
| --- | --- |
| Haemoglobin | 9.5 g/dl |
| White cell count | $2.5 \times 10^9/l$ (normal differential) |
| Reticulocytes | 12% |
| Platelets | $90 \times 10^9/l$ |

**a) What is the diagnosis, and what tests would you perform?**

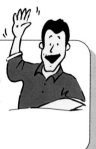

**A61** a) **Diagnosis and test**
This is a classic case. No lists here, then! You just have to know that this is PNH. Diagnosis is with Ham's acid lysis/acidified serum test; cells from patients with PNH readily lyse in acidified serum.

Red cells are especially sensitive to complement lysis as pH lowers. Thus, anything that makes the blood more acid (including intense exercise, operative stress, and hypoventilation during sleep) can cause continued intravascular haemolysis. It may be associated with abdominal pain, pancytopenia, all of the features of haemolysis (including reticulocytosis and slight jaundice), dark urine (from haemoglobin, often in the morning), and a tendency to thrombosis (arterial or venous); Hence, the sudden accumulation of ascites and severe abdominal pain in a patient with PNH should alert you to the complication of portal vein thrombosis.

## Quick refresher

List the causes of:

- cerebellar syndromes
- splenomegaly
- pulmonary eosinophilia

And the causes of:

- spherocytosis
- erythema multiforme
- pancytopenia
- hepatomegaly

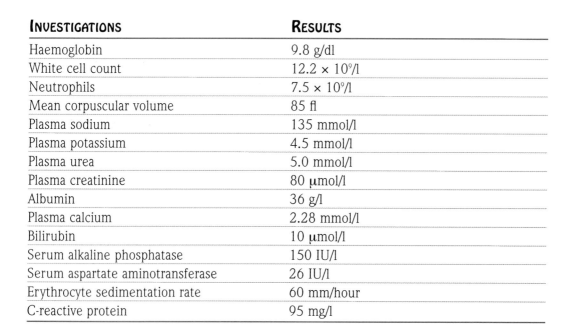

**Q62** A 67-year-old man presents with a 2-month history of easy bruising, bleeding, weight loss, and fatigue. His younger sister (59 years old) has recently been diagnosed with leukaemia. His blood film shows immature lymphocytes, and cytogenetic studies identify internal tandem duplications of Flt3.

| INVESTIGATIONS | RESULTS |
|---|---|
| Haemoglobin | 9.8 g/dl |
| White cell count | 12.2 × 10⁹/l |
| Neutrophils | 7.5 × 10⁹/l |
| Mean corpuscular volume | 85 fl |
| Plasma sodium | 135 mmol/l |
| Plasma potassium | 4.5 mmol/l |
| Plasma urea | 5.0 mmol/l |
| Plasma creatinine | 80 µmol/l |
| Albumin | 36 g/l |
| Plasma calcium | 2.28 mmol/l |
| Bilirubin | 10 µmol/l |
| Serum alkaline phosphatase | 150 IU/l |
| Serum aspartate aminotransferase | 26 IU/l |
| Erythrocyte sedimentation rate | 60 mm/hour |
| C-reactive protein | 95 mg/l |

## a) What is the diagnosis?

   i)    AML

   ii)   acute promyelocytic leukaemia

   iii)  acute lymphoblastic leukaemia

   iv)  myelodysplastic syndrome

   v)   myeloproliferative disease

Information can sometimes throw you. It doesn't matter if you don't know the implication of internal tandem duplications of Flt3 – you can still work out the answer from the remaining information. You've been told that the patient has anaemia, thrombocytopenia, leucocytosis consisting of immature cells, and an affected relative. So the answer is...

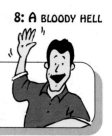

## A62  a) Diagnosis
i) AML

### SOME FACTS ABOUT MYELOID LEUKAEMIA

- AML represents 80% of all acute adult leukaemias.
- It is classically characterised by the presence of Auer rods.
- There is an increased risk in first-degree relatives of sufferers.
- The cause is unknown, but several risk factors have been identified. These include radiation exposure, chemotherapy (alkylating agents), and several congenital conditions, in particular Down's syndrome.
- CML, the myelodysplastic syndromes, and the myeloproliferative syndromes can all progress to AML.
- The peripheral blast count is directly related to prognosis.
- Distinct morphologic subtypes exist with overlapping clinical presentations. There are, however, important differences:
  - Acute promyelocytic leukaemia (FAB3) has a tendency for DIC (due to the release of procoagulants), particularly on commencing chemotherapy, and is sensitive to all-*trans* retinoic acid (a vitamin A analogue). It is associated with t(15;17).
  - FAB M6 stains positive for periodic acid-Schiff.
- Patients with a very high white cell count ($>100 \times 10^9$/l) may present with complications secondary to leucostasis syndrome (e.g. cerebrovascular accident, pulmonary embolism).

Just so you know, internal tandem duplications of Flt3 are associated with a poorer prognosis in AML. Flt3 binds to CD135, a proto-oncogene important in lymphocyte development.

A little mnemonic to help... **AM³L**

- **A**uer rods
- CML, **m**yelodysplastic syndromes, and **m**yeloproliferative syndromes can all progress to AML
- **l**eucostasis

As for the others, remember they have malignant potential. The myeloproliferative diseases cause 'too much of a good thing': polycythaemia vera, essential thrombocytosis, and myelofibrosis. On the other hand, the myelodysplastic syndromes result in 'too little of everything': pancytopenia. If they transform they have a very poor prognosis.

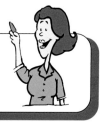

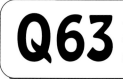 **Q63** A 60-year-old man presents with fatigue, malaise, and increasing abdominal girth. His blood film shows an abundance of all granulocytes.

| INVESTIGATIONS | RESULTS |
| --- | --- |
| Haemoglobin | 9.8 g/dl |
| Mean corpuscular volume | 76 fl |
| White cell count | $240 \times 10^9$/l |
| Platelets | $872 \times 10^9$/l |
| Plasma sodium | 140 mmol/l |
| Plasma potassium | 5.7 mmol/l |
| Plasma urea | 8.0 mmol/l |
| Plasma creatinine | 74 µmol/l |
| Urate | 4 mg/dl |
| Bilirubin | 11 µmol/l |
| Serum alkaline phosphatase | 60 IU/l |
| Serum alanine aminotransferase | 24 IU/l |
| Plasma glucose | 3.0 mmol/l |
| Total protein | 70 g/l |
| Serum albumin | 32 g/l |
| Leucocyte alkaline phosphatase score | Low |
| Lactate dehydrogenase | 1240 IU/l |
| Vitamin $B_{12}$ | Normal |

## a) What is the diagnosis?

- i) leucoerythroblastic reaction
- ii) CML
- iii) lymphoma
- iv) PA
- v) acute promyelocytic leukaemia (M3)

**A63** a) Diagnosis
ii) CML

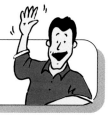

**ALL YOU NEED TO KNOW ABOUT CHRONIC MYELOID LEUKAEMIA FOR THE MRCP**

- CML has an insidious onset in patients aged >60 years old.

- It causes unregulated proliferation of myeloid cells; hence there is abundance of all granulocytes.

- Clinical signs include anaemia and splenomegaly.

- >90% of cases are associated with the Philadelphia chromosome, resulting from a reciprocal translocation between chromosome 9 and 22 and producing the fusion gene product BCR–ABL. Its action as a tyrosine kinase has become a therapeutic target (see the next point).

- Imatinib targets the tyrosine kinase domain of BCR–ABL and has become the mainstay of treatment.

Take time to see if you can remember the causes of a leucoerythroblastic blood film. Jot them down here.

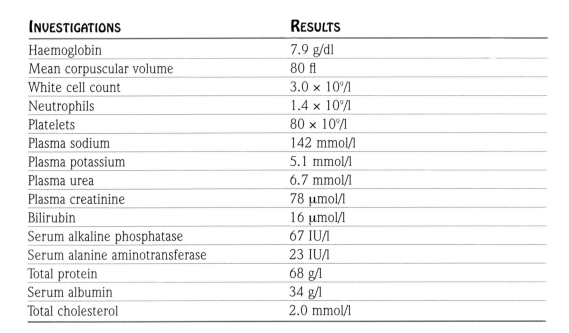

**Q64** A 50-year-old hairdresser presents with fatigue. Over the preceding 9 months he has suffered from recurrent bacterial and viral infections and epistaxis. On examination he is pale, with massive splenomegaly. His blood film stains positive with tartrate-resistant acid phosphatase.

| INVESTIGATIONS | RESULTS |
| --- | --- |
| Haemoglobin | 7.9 g/dl |
| Mean corpuscular volume | 80 fl |
| White cell count | $3.0 \times 10^9/l$ |
| Neutrophils | $1.4 \times 10^9/l$ |
| Platelets | $80 \times 10^9/l$ |
| Plasma sodium | 142 mmol/l |
| Plasma potassium | 5.1 mmol/l |
| Plasma urea | 6.7 mmol/l |
| Plasma creatinine | 78 µmol/l |
| Bilirubin | 16 µmol/l |
| Serum alkaline phosphatase | 67 IU/l |
| Serum alanine aminotransferase | 23 IU/l |
| Total protein | 68 g/l |
| Serum albumin | 34 g/l |
| Total cholesterol | 2.0 mmol/l |

## a) What is the diagnosis?

    i)    chronic lymphocytic leukaemia

    ii)    AML

    iii)    acute promyelocytic leukaemia

    iv)    hairy-cell leukaemia

    v)    CML

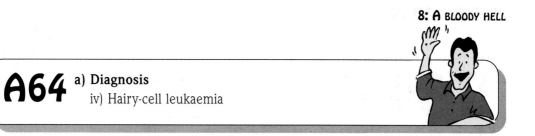

# A64 a) Diagnosis
## iv) Hairy-cell leukaemia

You may not know anything about hairy-cell leukaemia, but you should know the characteristics of the others and it then becomes a process of elimination. As for the 'spot the right answer' facts: hairy-cell leukaemia stains positive with tartrate-resistant acid phosphatase and is associated with low cholesterol.

See if you can come up with your own list for the others in the space below.

___

## DID YOU KNOW...

...Patients with hairy-cell leukaemia have an increased risk of developing other unrelated malignancies.

**Q65** A 65-year-old man working in a plastics factory presents with increasing tiredness and recurrent infections – pneumonia and skin abscesses. He's sure it's not his age. Bloods show haemoglobin 8.8, MCV 106. A blood film shows scanty ringed sideroblasts. His bone marrow shows 15% blasts.

## a) What is the diagnosis?

    i)      vitamin B$_{12}$ deficiency

    ii)     aplastic anaemia

    iii)    AML

    iv)    myelodysplastic syndrome

    v)     a myeloproliferative disorder

You may have known this answer straight away. If not, think laterally – what information have you been given? A 65-year-old man, recurrent BACTERIAL infections (hope you spotted that clue – pneumonia and skin abscesses)... he must be immunosuppressed! Macrocytic anaemia; can you remember the causes of macrocytosis? Jot them down now....

...and finally, his bone marrow shows 15% blasts. Now look at the options. In a nutshell:

Vitamin B$_{12}$ deficiency:

- Yes it causes macrocytic anaemia and fatigue, but what about all those other problems he's got. It's clearly not the answer. So exclude it! But just a reminder:
  - Causes: PA, poor diet, small bowel disease (bacterial overgrowth, terminal ileal resection)
  - Symptoms: fatigue, shortness of breath, neurological symptoms, psychiatric disturbances

Aplastic anaemia:

- Everything's low (anaemia, thrombocytopenia, leucopenia), so exclude it! But just so you know:
  - Marrow is replaced by fat: hypoplastic
  - Can be inherited or acquired
  - Equal sex distribution
  - Bimodal age distribution; patients are typically in their twenties or sixties
  - Symptoms as you'd guess: infections, bruising, bleeding, fatigue, and shortness of breath

AML: Remember those facts, list them here...

_____

_____

_____

_____

_____

_____

_____

_____

_____

_____

As far as differentiating acute leukaemia from the myelodysplastic syndromes, remember: those myelodysplastic syndromes are preleukemic – they have fewer blasts. It depends on which classification you use as to how the myelodysplastic syndromes are defined. According to the WHO classification >20% BM blasts is classified as transformation to acute leukaemia. The FAB system classes >30% BM blasts as transformation to acute leukaemia. This man has 15% blasts in his bone marrow, so you've excluded AML.

Myeloproliferative disorders

- Remember 'too much!' This man has anaemia, so this option can be excluded.

So that leaves myelodysplastic syndrome. Oh, those myelodysplastic syndromes, we're all confused. Remember:

- Patients have hyperactive bone marrow, but low peripheral counts.
- 25% of cases transform to AML.
- Treatment is mainly with blood product support and granulocyte colony-stimulating factor.
- Patients may suffer complications from long-term treatment, such as iron overload from repeated transfusions.
- Patients are typically in their sixties.
- The myelodysplastic syndromes are more common in men.
- The cause is unknown, although risk factors include chemotherapy and radiation: beware the patient who was previously treated for cancer..

So the answer is:

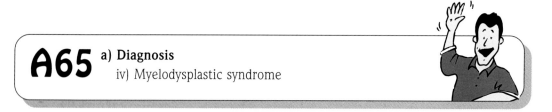

**A65** **a) Diagnosis**
iv) Myelodysplastic syndrome

**Q66** A 64-year-old woman presents with a 2-week history of fatigue, drenching night sweats, and weight loss. Two months previously she had returned from a tour of central Africa with her husband. On examination, you find an enlarged lymph node in her left axilla.

**a) Which of the following tests would be the least useful in making a diagnosis?**

   i)     lymph node biopsy

   ii)    fine-needle aspiration

   iii)   CT scan of the chest, abdomen, and pelvis

   iv)   PET scan

   v)    bone marrow aspiration and trephine

**b) The pathologist rings you with the histology results: "classical Reed–Sternberg cells are not seen." What is the diagnosis?**

   i)     Hodgkin's lymphoma

   ii)    non-Hodgkin's lymphoma

   iii)   Burkitt's lymphoma

   iv)   follicular lymphoma

   v)    Waldenström's macroglobulinaemia

A lymph node biopsy is the key investigation for diagnosis. A CT scan, PET scan, and bone marrow aspiration and trephine are required to determine the disease stage. Fine-needle aspiration is not adequate! If there is bone marrow involvement then the patient will also require a lumbar puncture to exclude meningeal disease.

This is one of those answers that you just need to know. One way of remembering is: no Reed–Sternberg cells = non-Hodgkin's. Simple, but effective!

**A66**  a) **Least useful test**
  ii) Fine-needle aspirate

b) **Diagnosis**
  ii) Non-Hodgkin's lymphoma

## More non-Hodgkin's lymphoma facts

- Non-Hodgkin's lymphoma represents approximately 80% of all lymphomas.
- It is increasing in incidence.
- There are >20 different types.
- Although the cause is unknown, it is associated with increased age, reduced immunity (e.g. HIV infection, inherited immunodeficiencies), viruses (e.g. Epstein–Barr virus, human T-cell lymphoma virus-1), previous chemotherapy and radiotherapy, and certain diseases (e.g. coeliac disease).
- Patients may be asymptomatic, have lymphadenopathy or extranodal disease, or present with complications.

Below is a table of possible clinical presentations, depending on the site of disease:

| MEDIASTINAL DISEASE | RETROPERITONEAL DISEASE | ABDOMINAL DISEASE | BONE INVOLVEMENT | CNS INVOLVEMENT |
|---|---|---|---|---|
| Pericardial tamponade | Hydronephrosis | Ascites | Fracture | Confusion |
| | | Obstruction | Pain | Cranial nerve defects |
| SVCO | | Pain | | Headache |
| | | Perforation | | Seizure |

CNS: central nervous system; SVCO: superior vena cava syndrome.

# Q67

A 23-year-old woman presents with acute right ear pain and paralysis of the right side of her face. On examination, you find a right lower VIIth motor neuron palsy and vesicles in her ear. You tell her she has Ramsay Hunt syndrome caused by herpes infection, and recommend treatment with steroids and aciclovir. She asks what other diseases are associated with herpes infection.

## a) Which of the following is not associated with a herpes virus?

i)   primary effusion lymphoma

ii)  Castleman's disease

iii) hairy leucoplakia

iv)  nasopharyngeal carcinoma

v)   Sutton's disease

Sutton's disease is a rare disease characterised by recurrent aphthous ulcers. Its aetiology is unknown. The rest are associated with positive herpetic serology. The rare ones first...

- Primary effusion lymphoma is an aggressive B-cell lymphoma. It is associated with human herpesvirus (HHV)-8 and HHV-4. It does, as it sounds, accumulate in body cavities.

- Castleman's disease, an atypical lymphoproliferative disorder, is as rare as hens' teeth. It is sometimes classed as a benign disorder, but this is not always so. It may be complicated by infections, haemophagocytic syndrome, or POEMS (polyneuropathy, organomegaly, endocrinopathy, M protein, skin changes), or progress to lymphoma. It is associated with HHV-8.

- Hairy leucoplakia presents with white plaques on the lateral aspect of the tongue, which usually resolve spontaneously. Treatment depends on the symptoms, although most patients are asymptomatic. It is associated with HIV infection, irrespective of the patient's CD4 count, and HHV-4.

- Nasopharyngeal carcinoma, as it sounds, is a malignancy of the nasopharynx. It can present with cranial nerve palsies, hearing problems, or symptoms of nasal obstruction. It is associated with HHV-4 and Asian ancestry.

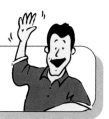

**A67** a) Not associated with a herpes virus
v) Sutton's disease

### HERPES VIRUS ASSOCIATIONS

That 'kissing disease' virus has much to answer for. Here are a few other diseases that it's involved in:

- Alice in Wonderland syndrome – distorted visual perception
- certain non-Hodgkin's lymphomas, such as primary cerebral lymphoma and Burkitt's lymphoma
- common variable immunodeficiency – a group of primary immunodeficiencies resulting from various gene defects causing impaired cellular and humoral defence systems
- IMN... we've all had it!
- Kikuchi's disease – a rare, benign, self-limiting, necrotising lymphadenitis that is predominantly found in young women
- post-transplant lymphoproliferative disorder – a B-cell lymphoma that can occur, as it's name suggests, post-transplant
- Stevens–Johnson syndrome

Remember, to 'spot' Epstein–Barr virus you need to do the 'monospot' test, or find >10% atypical cells. The presence of Paul–Bunnell heterophile antibodies is diagnostic.

Other well known associations are human T-cell lymphotrophic virus-1 with adult T-cell leukaemia, and *Helicobacter pylori* with gastric mucosa-associated lymphoid tissue lymphoma, a form of non-Hodgkin's lymphoma.

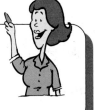

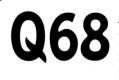 A 70-year-old man presents with fatigue. He has a positive Coomb's test, and clonal lymphocytes and many 'broken' or 'smudge' cells are found on his blood film.

| Investigations | Results |
| --- | --- |
| Haemoglobin | 11.0 g/dl |
| White cell count | $45.5 \times 10^9$/l |
| Platelets | $236 \times 10^9$/l |
| Plasma sodium | 145 mmol/l |
| Plasma potassium | 5.0 mmol/l |
| Plasma urea | 4.3 mmol/l |
| Plasma creatinine | 51 μmol/l |
| Bilirubin | 14 μmol/l |
| Serum alkaline phosphatase | 56 IU/l |
| Serum alanine aminotransferase | 21 IU/l |
| Total protein | 53 g/l |
| Serum albumin | 37 g/l |

Differential: neutrophils $7.6 \times 10^9$/l, lymphocytes $37 \times 10^9$/l, monocytes $0.6 \times 10^9$/l, basophils $0.2 \times 10^9$/l, eosinophils $0.1 \times 10^9$/l

### a) What is the diagnosis?

- i) CLL
- ii) B-cell prolymphocytic leukaemia
- iii) hairy-cell leukaemia
- iv) Richter's syndrome
- v) mantle-cell lymphoma

### b) How should the patient be treated?

- i) systemic chemotherapy
- ii) watch and wait
- iii) intravenous immunoglobulin
- iv) leucophoresis
- v) radiotherapy

You may never have heard of some of these options, but work out what you know from the question: elderly man, positive Coomb's test, blood film shows clonal lymphocytes and smudge cells. This means that there are many abnormal lymphocytes, which are more fragile than normal cells, and hence they 'smudge' when they are spread on a glass slide. All of this points to CLL. Remember, **CLL**:

- Coomb's positive
- lymphocytosis
- lots of infection

Like all of the leukaemias, however, it's more complicated than that. CLL is officially staged according to two systems, Binet and Rai. A simplified approach would be: CLL is lymphocytosis; the associated features of lymphadenopathy, hepatomegaly and/or splenomegaly, anaemia, and thrombocytopenia each contribute to a more aggressive form of disease.

Treatment options for CLL depend on the patient's haematological count and symptoms. Based on our simplified approach, this man has low-grade disease and mild symptoms. He does not require treatment at present, but should be monitored.

- As in this case, chemotherapy is often not needed initially.
- Those who are symptomatic, with a high white cell count may require immediate chemotherapy.
- Despite very high counts (well in excess of $100 \times 10^9/l$), they rarely suffer symptoms of hyperviscosity.
- Radiotherapy may be used for symptomatic lymphadenopathy or splenomegaly.
- Hypogammaglobulinaemia resulting in frequent infections may respond to intravenous immunoglobulin.

There are a many great mimics of CLL, some more obscure than others – ever heard of mantle cell lymphoma? Make sure you know how to differentiate the more common ones! Make a list now...

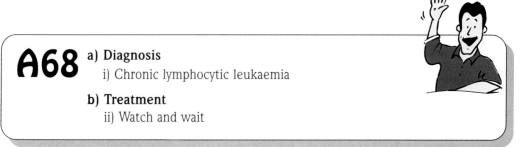

**A68** a) **Diagnosis**
    i) Chronic lymphocytic leukaemia

    b) **Treatment**
      ii) Watch and wait

# Q69

A 47-year-old sun worshipper is admitted from the emergency department following a seizure. He has a past history of melanoma, which was excised with lymph node dissection 13 years previously. He has not attended follow-up for some years. A chest X-ray demonstrates multiple opacities. CT brain shows multiple lesions that enhanced post-contrast.

| INVESTIGATIONS | RESULTS |
|---|---|
| Haemoglobin | 14.3 g/dl |
| White cell count | $9.6 \times 10^9/l$ |
| Platelets | $350 \times 10^9/l$ |
| Plasma sodium | 141 mmol/l |
| Plasma potassium | 3.7 mmol/l |
| Plasma urea | 5.6 mmol/l |
| Plasma creatinine | 73 μmol/l |
| Bilirubin | 7 μmol/l |
| Serum alkaline phosphatase | 56 IU/l |
| Serum alanine aminotransferase | 31 IU/l |
| Plasma calcium | 2.2 mmol/l |
| C-reactive protein | 51 mg/l |

## a) Which tumour marker may be elevated in this patient?

i) none

ii) chromogranin A

iii) human chorionic gonadotrophin

iv) α-fetoprotein

v) cancer antigen 19-9

## b) Which of the following would indicate a better prognosis?

i) Breslow's depth >4 mm

ii) ulceration

iii) tumour-infiltrating lymphocytes

iv) macrometastases

v) nodular melanoma

### TUMOUR MARKERS

Tumour markers are used to stage, indicate prognosis, and monitor treatment and recurrence. They are not specific enough to diagnose cancer, as most are associated with benign diseases as well as cancer. No tumour marker test is 100% sensitive and specific.

| MARKER | COMMENT |
|---|---|
| α-Fetoprotein | Elevated in hepatocellular carcinomas, germ-cell tumours, and pregnancy |
| Human chorionic gonadotrophin | Elevated in germ-cell tumours, gestational trophoblastic disease, pregnancy, and marijuana users |
| Carcinoembryonic antigen | Elevated in colorectal, gastrointestinal-tract, breast, lung, and ovarian cancers |
| CA 15-3 | Elevated in breast cancer, benign breast disease, cirrhosis, pregnancy, advanced ovarian, cervical, and endometrial cancers |
| CA 125 | Elevated in ovarian cancer. Also breast, bronchus, and gastrointestinal-tract cancers |
| CA 19-9 | Elevated in pancreatic and colorectal cancers |
| Lactate dehydrogenase | Elevated in germ-cell tumours, Ewing's sarcoma, non-Hodgkin's lymphoma, and some types of leukaemia |
| Chromogranin A | Elevated in neuroendocrine tumours |

CA: cancer antigen.

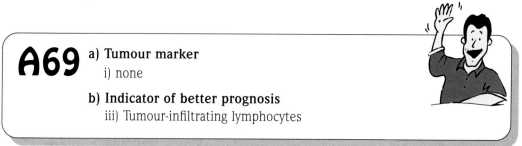

**A69**  **a) Tumour marker**
  i) none

**b) Indicator of better prognosis**
  iii) Tumour-infiltrating lymphocytes

We're sure that you guessed that this patient has melanoma. Melanoma cells can masquerade as any poorly differentiated tumour. Thankfully, the histopathologists are always close to hand. A simple test is the identification of melanin on the hematoxylin and eosin stain but this is often not enough. Immunocytochemistry is often used, with antibodies against HMB-45 and S-100 being the most frequently used markers for melanoma. In practice, remember to always examine the testicles of young men with evidence of metastases – germ-cell tumours are curable!

Just to remind you:

- Breslow's depth – tumour thickness in millimetres: <1 mm = good prognosis, >4 mm = bad
- Clark's level – depth related to skin structures: II–III = good prognosis, V–VI = bad
- nodular melanoma is the most aggressive form of melanoma

Features that are associated with a poor prognosis include:

- ulceration
- satellite lesions
- a large number of lymph nodes involved and greater degree of disease involvement within the node
- metastases

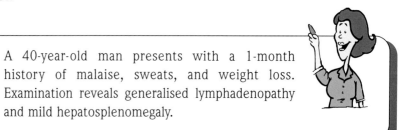

**Q70** A 40-year-old man presents with a 1-month history of malaise, sweats, and weight loss. Examination reveals generalised lymphadenopathy and mild hepatosplenomegaly.

| INVESTIGATIONS | RESULTS |
| --- | --- |
| Haemoglobin | 10.8 g/dl |
| White cell count | $205.2 \times 10^9/l$ |
| Peripheral blast count | $201 \times 10^9/l$ |

### a) He is diagnosed with acute lymphoblastic leukaemia. Which of the following is not standard chemoprophylaxis?

   i)   allopurinol

   ii)  cotrimoxazole

   iii) aciclovir

   iv)  penicillin V

   v)   fluconazole

Allopurinol is used for prophylaxis of hyperuricaemia associated with chemotherapy. It is a xanthine oxidase inhibitor. Remember that allopurinol and azathioprine should not be co-prescribed! Allopurinol interferes with the metabolism of azathioprine, increasing plasma levels of 6-mercaptopurine (its active metabolite), which may result in potentially fatal blood dyscrasias. In those at high risk of tumour lysis syndrome (e.g. those with a high disease burden, as in this case, or with renal impairment), rasburicase may be used. It is a biosynthetic urate oxidase enzyme. It works by catalysing the conversion of uric acid to allantoin, a more soluble, inactive metabolite.

Aciclovir, fluconazole, and cotrimoxazole are all standard chemoprophylaxis. Penicillin V is routinely prescribed for those who have undergone a splenectomy or are functionally hyposplenic, such as those with sickle cell anaemia.

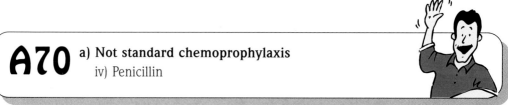

**A70** a) Not standard chemoprophylaxis
iv) Penicillin

# ALL IN ONE: EVERYTHING YOU WANTED TO KNOW ABOUT HAEMATOLOGY...

You may want to cut this out and put it on your wall, or carry it around with you.

| Group | Diagnosis | Liver | Spleen | Nodes | Haematological comments | Other comments |
|---|---|---|---|---|---|---|
| Chronic myelo-proliferative disorders | Essential thrombocythaemia | + | + (leading to atrophy) | | | LAP high; Philadelphia chromosome negative; may have high vitamin $B_{12}$ and urate |
| | PVR | + | + | | NN anaemia if phlebotomy is prescribed; WCC high in 60%; platelet count high in 50% | LAP high; low iron; high total iron-binding capacity; may have high vitamin $B_{12}$ and urate |
| | Myelofibrosis | + | ++ | | May have features of hypersplenism or pancytopenia; WCC high or low; platelet count high or low | LAP high; high SBR concentration and LDH; low folate; may have high vitamin $B_{12}$ and urate |
| | CML | + | ++ | | +/- NN anaemia; WCC +++; platelet count high or low; neutrophils ++, myelocytes ++, blasts ++ | LAP low; may have high vitamin $B_{12}$ and urate |
| Lympho-proliferative disorders | Prolymphocytic leukaemia | | + | +/- | Prolymphocytes >100 × $10^3$ cells/mm³; variant of CLL, but no nodes and a big early spleen | Systemic symptoms +++ |
| | CLL | + | +/- | + | Lymphocytosis 100–500 × $10^3$ cells/mm³; NN anaemia; platelet count low; smear cells with or without haemolysis | Reduced Igs +/- IgM or light chain band |
| | Hairy-cell leukaemia | + | + | +/- | BM involvement or hypersplenism lead to pancytopenia | |
| | HMR | + | + | | Pancytopenia | |
| | Infectious mononucleosis | + (20%) | + (50%) | + | Lymphocytes <30 × $10^3$ cells/mm³; platelet count may be low; haemolysis possible | IgM high; cold agglutinin; heterophil antibodies react with beef but not guinea pig; LFTs abnormal |
| | Non-Hodgkin's lymphoma | + | + | + | NN anaemia in 15%–30%, BM involvement; ESR very high; leucoerythroblastic film; lymphocytes +++ (unlike Hodgkin's) | $CaPO_4$ high; urate high; LFTs abnormal; acute-phase reactants (including caeruloplasmin) raised |
| | Hodgkin's lymphoma | + | + | ++ | Often normal or NN anaemia; lymphopenia: high platelets, ESR, eosinophils, and neutrophils; leucoerythroblastic; less BM involved | $CaPO_4$ high; urate high; LFTs abnormal; acute-phase reactants (including caeruloplasmin) raised |
| Acute leukaemias | Myelodysplastic syndromes | | +/- | +/- | Pancytopenia with NN anaemia or high MCV; hypergranular cells | |
| | AML | +/- | + | +/- | WCC <4 × $10^3$ cells/mm³ in 50%, normal in 20%, high in 30%, NN anaemia; platelets low; Sudan Black positive; neutrophil Auer rod positive | Urate high; myelocyte lysozyme raised |
| | ALL | + | + | ++ | WCC high (often <10 × $10^3$ cells/mm³ in children); blasts ++; NN anaemia; platelets low | Urate high; sodium may be low; potassium may be low |
| And not forgetting… | PNH | +/- | + | | Pancytopenia with reticulocytosis | Occasional jaundice with haemosiderinuria |
| | Multiple myeloma | + (40%) | + (10%) | | NN anaemia leading to pancytopenia; high ESR; rouleaux (except pure light chain); leucoerythroblastic | |
| | Waldenström's | + | + | + | | |

ALL: acute lymphoblastic leukaemia; AML: acute myeloid leukaemia; BM: bone marrow; CLL: chronic lymphocytic leukaemia; CML: chronic myeloid leukaemia; ESR: erythrocyte sedimentation rate; HMR: histiocytic medullary reticulosis; Ig: immunoglobulin; LAP: leucocyte alkaline phosphatase; LDH: lactate dehydrogenase; LFT: liver function test; MCV: mean corpuscular volume; NN: normocytic normochromic; PNH: paroxysmal nocturnal haemoglobinuria; PVR: polycythaemia rubra vera; SBR: serum bilirubin; WCC: white cell count.

University Hospitals of Derby & Burton
NHS Foundation Trust
01332 788146

Mail: uhdb.library@nhs.net

Self Service Receipt for Borrowing

Patron: Christian Okonkwor

Title: My first MRCP book
Item: B16949
Due Back: 24/06/2024

Total Borrowing: 1
29/04/2024 15:54:41

.Thank you and see you soon

# 9

# TAKING THE P\*\*S

RENAL MRCP LISTS

Renal questions are interesting. They usually refer to oliguria or anuria, yet engender almost exactly the opposite sign (immediate loss of sphincter control with subsequent flooding) in most candidates. Renal medicine is actually, however, quite fun in the MRCP examination, even if not in real life.

Actually, scratch all of the above – it isn't fun. It's a pain. Clinical renal medicine involves obtaining urea and creatinine measurements every 2 hours, and nodding in a sage and mature fashion, as if you are really interested in active sediment. The MRCP examination medicine is just as smart-arsed.

However, there are one or two recurrent themes, which tend to revolve around the presence of nephrotic syndrome or glomerulonephritis. Occasional 'casts' are thrown in, but these are usually to confuse.

## NEPHROTIC SYNDROME

Nephrotic syndrome appears in a number of guises. The questions will involve:

- making the diagnosis of nephrotic syndrome
- identifying the likely cause
- recognising that the findings in grey cases are complications of nephrotic syndrome

In terms of making the diagnosis, provided you are alert to the classical triad of oedema, hypoalbuminaemia, and proteinuria (defined by a urinary protein level of $>3.5$ g/1.73 m$^2$ of body surface area per day) then you shouldn't get caught out. Causes are best remembered by the following verse.

### NEPHROTIC SYNDROME

*SBE and SLE*
*RA treatment\* – cloudy pee*
*Murky water in the area?*
*Think, as ever, of malaria*

*Amyloid and sickle too*
*Piss neat protein down the loo*
*Remember, too, that cancer\*\* can*
*Give frothy urine in the PAN*

*Nephrotic diabetic piss*
*Isn't something one should miss*
*With water, sugar, protein – think*
*It makes a fortifying drink!*

\*Gold, penicillamine, nonsteroidal anti-inflammatory drugs, captopril, interferon-α, and heroin.
\*\*Especially lymphoma.
Amyloid: amyloidosis; PAN: polyarteritis nodosa; RA: rheumatoid arthritis; SBE: subacute bacterial endocarditis; sickle: sickle cell disease; SLE: systemic lupus erythematosus.

Other rare causes include bee stings. Renal vein thrombosis is also a cause, as is pre-eclampsia. Infectious causes include HIV, hepatitis B/C, syphilis, and parasites such as schistosomiasis. Despite the verse above, glomerulonephritis is the underlying cause of nephrotic syndrome in 80% of cases.

Finally, cases are sometimes dressed up by presentation with one of the complications of nephrotic syndrome, which are $TH^2ROMB^2otI^3c$:

- thrombosis
- hyperlipidaemia, hyponatraemia
- renal vein thrombosis
- osteomalacia
- malnutrition
- vitamin $B_{12}$ deficiency, Budd–Chiari syndrome
- iron deficiency, infection, immunodeficiency

As we have said, the most common cause of nephrotic syndrome is actually glomerulonephritis, and this diagnosis itself has many potential causes; glomerulonephritis is always a tricky issue. Here, therefore, is a quick summary.

### IMMUNOGLOBULIN A GLOMERULONEPHRITIS/BERGER'S DISEASE

- Histology: mesangial expansion/hypercellularity (hyperplasia)
- Aetiology: unknown – possible immunoglobulin (Ig)A dysregulation and abnormal sialidation (glycosylation)
- Associations: cirrhosis, dermatitis herpetiformis, gluten-enteropathy, mycosis fungoides (T-cell lymphoma), other malignancies, ankylosing spondylitis, Wiskott–Aldrich syndrome, chronic liver/lung disease, human leucocyte antigen DQw7/B35
- Epidemiology: the most common primary glomerulonephritis. Increased incidence in the Far East and in men
- Presentation: varied: microscopic or macroscopic haematuria triggered by prodromal infection (upper respiratory tract infection [URTI]), proteinuria or overt nephrotic syndrome, rapidly progressive glomerulonephritis with crescents, hypertension, chronic renal failure
- Prognosis: 20% develop end-stage renal failure after 20 years. Prognosis is better in those who initially present with episodic macroscopic haematuria, well-controlled blood pressure and little proteinuria

- Treatment:
  - asymptomatic – leave alone
  - mild disease – fish oils
  - acute nephritis (rapidly progressing glomerulonephritis) – possibly immunosuppression with cyclophosphamide, corticosteroids, and plasma exchange

## MINIMAL CHANGE GLOMERULONEPHRITIS

- Histology: normal under light microscopy ('minimal change!'), but epithelial foot process effacement under electron microscopy; selective proteinuria
- Aetiology: unknown, possibly immune
- Associations: human leucocyte antigen B12, URTIs, vaccinations, Hodgkin's lymphoma, rifampicin, nonsteroidal anti-inflammatory drugs, gold, Epstein–Barr virus/HIV infection, atopy, obesity, heroin use, Fabry's disease, sialidosis
- Epidemiology: the most common primary cause of nephrotic syndrome in children (90%) and causes 20%–30% of nephrotic syndrome cases in adults
- Presentation: nephrotic syndrome, hyperlipidaemia, acute renal failure (especially if volume-depleted)
- Prognosis: very good in children, most are steroid-responsive; thus, biopsy is only indicated when disease is unresponsive to steroids, when cyclosporin can be used. In adults, about 40% of cases are steroid-responsive and, as there is a spectrum of other diseases causing nephrotic syndrome, they should all be biopsied

## FOCAL SEGMENTAL GLOMERULOSCLEROSIS

This is characterised by an accumulation of hyaline/proteinaceous material in parts (segments) of glomeruli, affecting <50% of glomeruli in any given biopsy. Many nephrologists feel that this is an advanced form of minimal change disease that has progressed to protein deposition and glomerular distortion. Aetiologically, it arises from a similar range of factors as minimal change disease and other sustained protein deposition in the kidneys. It is as if the kidneys have been chronically exposed to a clogging influence and the filter is dirty. Again, associations include sickle cell disease, HIV infection, diabetes, heroin use, sialidosis, and Fabry's disease, and also excess filtering through a limited number of glomeruli due to congenital reductions in glomeruli number (oligonephropathies, renal agenesis, and surgical resection). Unlike minimal change disease, up to 60% of these patients develop end-stage renal disease and are generally steroid unresponsive. Even if a patient receives a kidney transplant, the new kidney also eventually becomes clogged in about 50% of cases.

## Membranous glomerulonephritis

- Histology: thickened glomerular basement membrane with subepithelial deposits, but no proliferative changes
- Aetiology: primary idiopathic and secondary (see associations)
- Pathogenesis: immune-complex deposition
- Associations:
  - cancer of the bowel and bronchus
  - penicillamine, captopril, gold, heavy metals (mercury and cadmium)
  - infections such as hepatitis B virus, *Schistosoma mansoni*, malaria
  - autoimmune disease such as systemic lupus erythematosus, rheumatoid arthritis; sickle cell anaemia
  - epidemiology: more common in adults, with a slight male preponderance
- Presentation:
  - spectrum from asymptomatic proteinuria to nephrotic syndrome
  - chronic renal failure
  - hypertension
  - hyperlipidaemia
- Prognosis:
  - one-third of patients have spontaneous remission
  - one-third remain nephrotic
  - one-third progress to chronic renal failure

## MESANGIOCAPILLARY GLOMERULONEPHRITIS/MEMBRANOPROLIFERATIVE GLOMERULONEPHRITIS (RARE IN CHILDREN AGED <5 YEARS)

|  | TYPE I | TYPE II |
|---|---|---|
| Histology | Subendothelial immune deposits of IgG, IgM, IgA, C3, and C4 | Dense immune deposit disease with C3 along capillary loops, but no Ig |
| Aetiology | Primary idiopathic | Primary idiopathic |
|  | Secondary to endocarditis, SLE, hepatitis C virus, shunt nephritis | |
| Associations | C3 nephritic factor (20%–30%) | C3 nephritic factor (70%) |
|  | Hypocomplementaemia with low C3 and C4 | Partial lipodystrophy Normal C4, but low C3 |
| Presentation | Mixed nephritic and nephrotic picture in either type | |
| Prognosis | Gradual deterioration to end-stage renal failure over 10 years Type II prognosis worse than type I | |
|  | Prognosis worse if crescents found on biopsy or initial presentation with nephrotic syndrome | |

Note: Type III is also recognized; this has features of membranoproliferative glomerulonephritis Type I and membranous nephropathy.
C: complement; Ig: immunoglobulin; SLE: systemic lupus erythematosus.

## (ACUTE) POST-STREPTOCOCCAL GLOMERULONEPHRITIS

- Part of the spectrum of mesangiocapillary glomerulonephritis
- Histology: subepithelial 'humps' on electron microscopy and discontinuous granular deposition of complement (C)3, IgM, and IgG on immunofluorescence
- Aetiology: follows a nephritogenic streptococcal infection of the throat or skin with a latent period of 7–40 days. This helps to distinguish it from IgA disease, which causes renal disease to develop at the same time as an URTI
- Epidemiology: mainly affects children, primarily in developing countries
- Presentation: 90% of cases are subclinical. The remaining 10% of patients develop an acute nephritic syndrome with haematuria, hypertension, oliguria, and oedema. Rarely (<0.5% of cases), patients develop hypertensive encephalopathy with consequent coma and convulsions. Moderate proteinuria may occur, but overt nephrotic syndrome is rare
- Investigations: elevated anti-streptolysin O titres, IgM, IgG, cryoglobulinaemia, low C3 (90%), low C4 and C2 (more rarely)
- Prognosis: 90% have a full recovery from their acute nephritic illness, but the remainder progress to chronic renal failure

**OTHER INFECTIONS THAT MAY GIVE RISE TO GLOMERULONEPHRITIS**

These include:

- *Plasmodium malariae*
- HIV (usually focal segmental glomerulosclerosis)
- hantavirus
- *Schistosoma mansoni* (not *S. japonicum*)
- *Mycobacterium leprae*

Note that diagnosis of rapidly progressive glomerulonephritis is by presentation rather than histology; it requires an active sediment in the urine (i.e. red cell casts) and systemic features such as oliguria (i.e. a fall in glomerular filtration rate) and hypertension. The histological correlate is often the presence of crescents – a feature of heavy inflammation. It can occur with any glomerulonephritis. It is associated with vasculitides, particularly Wegener's granulomatosis, microscopic polyarteritis, systemic lupus erythematosus and Henoch–Schönlein purpura, and anti-glomerular basement membrane (anti-GBM) disease, which is isolated to the kidneys, especially in nonsmokers. The prognosis varies depending on the initial severity and crescent formation, but in general all patients progress to end-stage renal failure. A renal biopsy is imperative unless contraindicated, such as in cases of a single functioning kidney, bleeding diathesis, and uncontrolled hypertension.

## OK, if you encyst!

Remember that there are two types of polycystic kidney disease:

1) the childhood type, which is usually acquired as an autosomal recessive form and is associated with cysts in the liver
2) the adult type, which is acquired as an autosomal dominant condition and is associated with cysts in organs other than the kidneys, including the pancreas. It has a 10%–15% association with intracranial berry aneurysms and hence a marked increased risk of subarachnoid haemorrhage

*OK. Now let's look at some cases.*

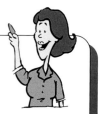

# Q71

A 41-year-old man presents to the emergency department with progressive haematuria. He and his partner have just returned from a 2-week trekking holiday in Thailand, where they both had a bout of transient gastroenteritis. Just over 1 year ago he had a renal transplant, but he is unclear as to "what had gone wrong" with his kidneys. He is aware, however, that at a recent follow-up appointment he had no sign of infection, and a letter states that his tacrolimus levels were adequate. He has needed a hearing aid since his early twenties and is currently on the waiting list to have a cataract operation. His mother and grandfather were also deaf. He never knew his grandfather as he died before he was born. He works in the Department of Social Services and champions several charities for people with both physical and mental disabilities.

## ON EXAMINATION

- Bilateral hearing aids
- Bilateral cataracts and corpuscular pigmentation of right retina
- CVS normal, except blood pressure = 175/100 mmHg
- Urine dipstick: blood +++, protein +, no leucocytes/glucose

## INVESTIGATIONS

- Haemoglobin = 10.8 g/dl
- White cell count = $7.8 \times 10^9$/l
- Platelets = $145 \times 10^9$/l
- Plasma urea = 31 mmol/l
- Plasma creatinine = 560 μmol/l
- Urine microscopy: red cell casts
- Anti-GBM antibody positive

CVS: cardiovascular system; GBM: glomerular basement membrane.

## a) What renal disease has this man developed in his transplanted kidney?

i) acute tubular necrosis

ii) anti-GBM disease

iii) rapidly progressive glomerulonephritis

iv) tacrolimus toxicity

v) malignancy

## b) How do you explain his retinal findings?

i) central retinal vein occlusion

ii) hypertensive retinopathy

iii) retinitis pigmentosa

iv) side effect of tacrolimus

v) cancer-associated retinopathy

## c) What is the underlying condition?

i) Goodpasture's syndrome

ii) Kearns–Sayre syndrome

iii) Alport's syndrome

iv) Haemolytic uraemic syndrome

v) Refsum's syndrome

Renal physicians are a funny lot. Quite why one should develop a fascination with urine (or lack of it) mystifies us. The big problem for renal physicians – and hence for you – is that there is often little to find to aid a diagnosis. Only rarely can you feel a massive kidney, and the diagnosis of polycystic kidney disease is usually obvious by then.

No; to make the right diagnosis, you generally have to depend on the history, particularly family history and drug/toxin exposure, and a few tests, particularly urine microscopy and the presence of autoantibodies.

As always, seek out the abnormalities for which there are limited lists of causes. In this case, the obvious abnormal findings are of corpuscular pigmentation of the right retina, acute renal failure, haematuria, red cell casts, and a positive anti-GBM antibody test.

'Corpuscular pigmentation' is the examiners' way of saying 'retinitis pigmentosa', for which you have already learned a list of causes. As usual, write this down now on scrap paper, then check it against the reminder below:

## RETINITIS PIGMENTOSA

- Friedreich's ataxia: spinal cord atrophy with degeneration of the spinocerebellar tracts, corticospinal tracts, and dorsal columns; peripheral neuropathies; cardiomyopathy; scoliosis and pes cavus

- Refsum's disease: polyneuritis, nerve deafness, cerebellar ataxia, and high cerebrospinal fluid protein concentration

- Laurence–Moon–Biedl syndrome

- Alport's syndrome: hereditary nephritis

- Kearns–Sayre syndrome

- Usher's syndrome

- abetalipoproteinaemia and vitamin E deficiency

Which of these is the cause? Well, it ought to be pretty obvious. Nonetheless, if you really want confirmation, you might think of the causes of red cell casts. The answer ought to appear on the list below.

## CAST AWAYS!

There are three sorts of casts that offer some help: red cell, white cell, and fatty.

- Red cell casts mean the kidneys are ravaged – in other words, they have had a major insult that is damaging them, causing both protein and red cell leak. The causes are, therefore, 'generally inflammatory and harmful':

  | generally | glomerulonephritis* |
  | inflammatory | interstitial nephritis* |
  | and | accelerated hypertension |
  | harmful | haemolytic uraemic syndrome |

- Fatty casts are due to nefrotic syndrome, for which there is a limited list of causes (see below).

- Neutrophil (white cell) casts go with nephritis. The causes are those starred* above, and pyelonephritis.

The other sorts of casts are pretty useless in making a diagnosis. Hyaline casts are very nonspecific, and broad waxy casts are the hyaline casts of chronic renal failure, which are easily fragmented. Granular casts are similarly nonspecific, and are found in all renal diseases regardless of severity or chronicity.

In this case, the lists of causes of red cell casts do not help much. They narrow it down to an interstitial nephritis or glomerulonephritis. At least this helps to confirm Alport's syndrome as the likely cause, with further support from the fact that this seems to be a hereditary problem. Both the patient's mother and grandfather were deaf, and his grandfather died at a young age.

Alport's syndrome is a hereditary nephritis characterised by haematuria, progressive renal failure, high-tone sensorineural deafness, and a variety of ocular problems – myopia, early cataracts, and retinitis pigmentosa. Its inheritance is X-linked dominant, so there is no male-to-male transmission. Affected males pass the disease on to all female offspring, and females generally manifest a less severe form of the disease. Only males develop progressive renal failure, while females have asymptomatic haematuria with no progression to renal failure. Similarly, the ocular and auditory abnormalities are more prevalent in males. The development of renal failure in males has a bimodal age distribution of 15–35 years and 45–60 years. Some 5% of patients who are transplanted for Alport's syndrome develop anti-GBM antibodies after transplantation. AC Alport (1880–1959) was a South African renal physician who practised at St Mary's Hospital in London.

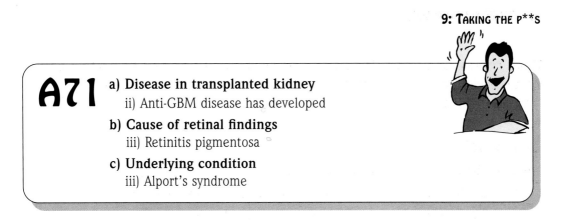

**A71**

a) **Disease in transplanted kidney**
   ii) Anti-GBM disease has developed

b) **Cause of retinal findings**
   iii) Retinitis pigmentosa

c) **Underlying condition**
   iii) Alport's syndrome

This question may appear in several forms: the examiner may show an audiogram, a retinal photograph showing retinitis pigmentosa, or a histology slide, or it may even be presented as a 'family tree' with a similar history to the above.

# QUIZ SPOT!

**UNLUCKY FOR SOME: 13 CAUSES OF PANCYTOPENIA**

Can you find the 13 causes of pancytopenia hiding in this wordsearch?

| | | | | | | | | | | | | | | | | |
|---|---|---|---|---|---|---|---|---|---|---|---|---|---|---|---|---|
| J | Q | B | W | C | E | G | L | E | V | N | B | J | U | T | Z | G | A |
| S | I | B | Z | H | J | E | Y | Z | R | T | A | S | A | S | D | U | L |
| J | R | V | U | E | R | J | V | M | L | K | L | F | R | E | P | A | R |
| P | R | I | Q | M | X | T | U | B | E | R | C | U | L | O | S | I | S |
| F | A | N | C | O | N | I | S | O | Q | Z | O | P | D | K | C | N | B |
| G | D | A | F | T | L | T | O | F | V | M | H | L | E | F | R | G | D |
| K | I | S | K | H | Z | L | S | R | U | J | O | H | K | A | A | E | L |
| A | A | G | W | E | O | D | H | T | S | E | L | S | A | K | R | T | U |
| E | T | U | H | R | T | Z | C | E | L | D | Y | U | V | E | W | D | R |
| N | I | R | A | A | V | I | R | A | L | A | J | S | R | U | W | F | O |
| C | O | D | V | P | M | D | I | S | R | F | L | N | H | T | C | I | U |
| M | N | W | T | Y | L | A | L | L | E | C | U | R | B | R | O | Y | H |
| G | T | I | H | L | W | Y | S | S | Y | Y | I | W | O | K | J | T | S |
| L | A | T | P | G | V | H | K | S | D | F | H | N | P | G | S | D | Q |
| D | M | V | K | S | U | Y | P | L | Y | M | P | H | O | M | A | J | D |
| C | F | G | T | Y | I | U | K | J | N | H | S | D | G | M | X | L | R |
| W | V | O | E | R | T | D | H | G | A | B | D | Y | I | O | A | D | T |

A: alcohol, *Brucella*, carcinoma, chemotherapy, drugs, Fanconi's, irradiation, lymphoma, PNH (paroxysmal nocturnal haemoglobinuria), SLE (systemic lupus erythematosus), thymic tumours, tuberculosis, viral

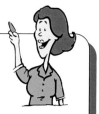

# Q72

A 35-year-old man is admitted for investigation of leg swelling and abdominal distension, which has developed over the last 6 weeks. He has also felt a little more breathless, but has not noticed any palpitations or experienced any chest pain. About 2 months ago he developed an intensely itchy rash with 'little blisters' on his knees and elbows. He was referred to a dermatologist who gave him a course of medication, which cleared the rash completely. He has had a similar rash in the past though to a lesser degree, which has usually resolved with a slight alteration of his diet. Currently, he feels somewhat tired and run-down. He works as a futures trader and has had a stressful few weeks at work. He is good friends with an advertising executive, who has recently been admitted to hospital. Together, they help fund the economies of several small South American countries, *and he can floss his nasal septum*. He denies drinking more than 10 units per week, however, and is a nonsmoker. He lives with his partner of 5 years, who also works in the City.

## ON EXAMINATION

- Facial, truncal, and limb oedema
- Leuconychia
- No anaemia, cyanosis, clubbing, jaundice, or lymphadenopathy
- Pulse = 96 beats/min
- Blood pressure = 100/55 mmHg
- Jugular venous pressure not elevated
- Heart sounds I + II + S3
- Pitting oedema of lower limbs to trunk
- Respiratory: bibasal dullness to percussion, with reduced air entry and reduced breath sounds on auscultation
- Abdomen: distended but nontender; no palpable organomegaly; shifting dullness, with a fluid thrill

## INVESTIGATIONS

- Haemoglobin = 11.8 g/dl
- White cell count = 6.2 × 10⁹/l
- Platelets = 180 × 10⁹/l
- Plasma sodium = 133 mmol/l
- Plasma potassium = 4.0 mmol/l
- Plasma urea = 1.8 mmol/l
- Plasma creatinine = 55 μmol/l
- Serum albumin = 21 g/l
- Serum bilirubin = 15 μmol/l
- Serum alanine aminotransferase = 20 IU/l
- Serum alkaline phosphatase = 105 IU/l
- Plasma glucose = 5.1 mmol/l
- Urinalysis: protein + + +; negative for blood and glucose
- 24-hour urine protein = 4.8 g
- Complement levels (C3 and C4) = normal

a) **What is the cause of this man's presenting complaint?**
   i)    nephritic syndrome
   ii)   malabsorption syndrome
   iii)  nephrotic syndrome
   iv)   acute coronary syndrome
   v)    none of the above

b) **What was the cause of his rash and what treatment did he receive?**
   i)    eczema and 2% hydrocortisone
   ii)   dermatitis herpetiformis and dapsone
   iii)  vasculitis and oral prednisolone
   iv)   seborrhoeic dermatitis and clobetasone
   v)    Kaposi's sarcoma and HAART

c) **What is his underlying diagnosis?**
   i)    AIDS and HIV-associated nephropathy
   ii)   IgA nephropathy or Berger's disease
   iii)  systemic lupus erythematosus and lupus nephritis
   iv)   coeliac disease and lymphoma
   v)    none of the above

d) **What is his likely prognosis?**

At first glance, there seems little to hang your hat on. However, the patient has ascites and widespread 'oedema', and a low albumin level. He has heavy proteinuria. Yes! He must have nephrotic syndrome!

Think of your list of causes and jot them down here:

The rash should be identified from the description as being dermatitis herpetiformis. You should remember (from the summary on page 267) that this is associated with Berger's disease. This is also associated with normal complement levels.

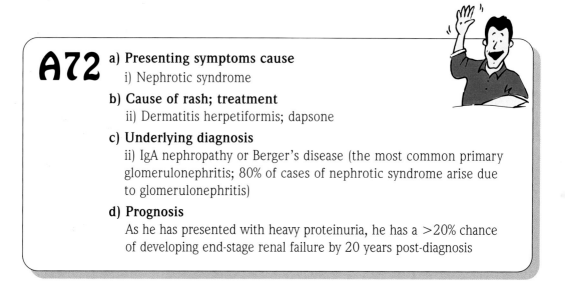

**A72**
a) **Presenting symptoms cause**
   i) Nephrotic syndrome
b) **Cause of rash; treatment**
   ii) Dermatitis herpetiformis; dapsone
c) **Underlying diagnosis**
   ii) IgA nephropathy or Berger's disease (the most common primary glomerulonephritis; 80% of cases of nephrotic syndrome arise due to glomerulonephritis)
d) **Prognosis**
   As he has presented with heavy proteinuria, he has a >20% chance of developing end-stage renal failure by 20 years post-diagnosis

And to finish this renal section...

## ANOTHER ODD RENAL LIST: RETROPERITONEAL FIBROSIS

In recent years, this has appeared as a grey case with a characteristic history of dull aching in the abdomen associated with eating and drinking, followed by progressive renal failure, with a diagnostic intravenous pyelogram showing medial deviation of the ureters and bilateral hydronephrosis. It can also cause entrapment of the aorta or inferior vena cava, causing arterial insufficiency or venous oedema in the legs.

The causes of this condition include:

- drugs such as practolol, methysergide
- aortic aneurysm
- lymphoma, radiation
- idiopathic

Treatment is surgical with either stenting of the ureters or ureterolysis, which involves dissecting out the ureters carefully from the inflammatory mass and interpositioning them with a surrounding layer of muscle or peritoneum!

# 10

# SEX!

THE MRCP LISTS OF SEXUAL MEDICINE

Sadly, given the pressures of a job and revision, this is probably as close as you're likely to get to the subject. Never mind, it'll be over pretty quickly.

There are few lists to learn and a useful one is for galactorrhoea.

## GALACTORRHOEA

Remember that dopamine is prolactin-release inhibitory factor, which is active in the hypothalamic–pituitary axis. Thus, abnormalities in this region can cause galactorrhoea, as can all dopamine-receptor antagonists. The easy ones to remember are:

- pregnancy
- excess oestrogen
- hypothalamic/pituitary lesions
- prolactinoma and ectopic prolactin secretion: bronchogenic carcinoma, hypernephroma

Antidopaminergic drugs resulting in elevated prolactin (by virtue of lack of prolactin inhibition):

- phenothiazines
- butyrophenones
- metoclopramide
- methyldopa

The three that are less easy to remember are:

- hypothyroidism
- chronic renal failure
- polycystic ovaries

Other sexy questions usually centre on weird sex-hormone levels. Such cases do not respond well to the list approach, but just have to be recognised. We shall therefore run through all of the main cases in turn. Just learn to recognise them!

## ANDROGEN INSENSITIVITY SYNDROME/TESTICULAR FEMINISATION

A defective androgen receptor means that genotypically male children (46XY) have end-organ resistance to testosterone. Some of this excess testosterone is isomerised to oestrogen, so they become phenotypically female. The groin swellings are the undescended testes, the latter being the main risk factor for the development of germ cell tumours of the testes. Therefore, patients are usually advised to have bilateral orchidectomy after 21 years of age, but not before this time as the testes are a better source of oestrogens than the oral contraceptive pill.

## Congenital adrenal hyperplasia

There are a variety of abnormalities of steroid hormone synthesis that the examiners love to throw in as a quick question. The term 'congenital adrenal hyperplasia' will make many of you groan, but never fear! Below is a simplified scheme of steroid hormone synthesis that is relatively easy to learn and from which you can work out the phenotypic appearance and relevant biochemistry!

## Steroid hormone synthesis pathways

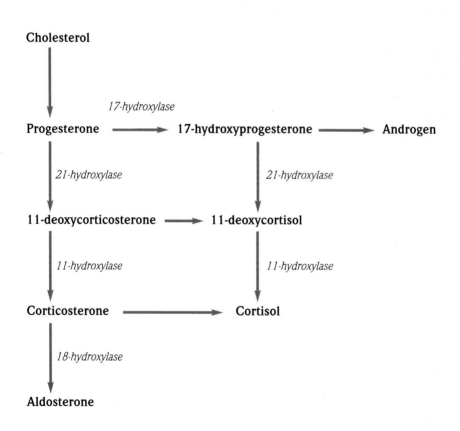

Remember this? It keeps cropping up, a bit like the coagulation casacade! It needs to be swotted up for the examination we're afraid.

## Key facts

- For the purpose of understanding the pathways, 11-deoxycorticosterone and 11-deoxycortisol behave like aldosterone and cortisol, respectively.
- All of the congenital adrenal hyperplasias are autosomal recessive, with the genes on chromosome 6, so the question may incorporate other siblings!

In terms of sexual precocity, remember the following rules:

- Breast development is very sensitive to *oestrogens*, so precocity is usually pituitary.
- Sexual hair is usually secondary to ambient *testosterone*, so precocity is usually adrenal or occasionally ovarian in origin.

Right. That is all you need to know to be able to work out the phenotypes. Practice by filling in the following table:

| Enzyme defect | Ambiguous genitalia | | Salt loss | High BP | Puberty | ACTH | Renin |
|---|---|---|---|---|---|---|---|
| | Males | Females | | | | | |
| 21-hydroxylase | No | Yes | Yes | No | Precocious | High | High |
| 17-hydroxylase | | | | | | | |
| 11-hydroxylase | | | | | | | |

ACTH: adrenocorticotrophic hormone; BP: blood pressure.

## Diagnostic investigations

The diagnostic investigations are as follows:

- 21-hydroxylase deficiency: measurement of 17-hydroxyprogesterone and cortisol after tetracosactrin
- 17-hydroxylase deficiency: measurement of 11-deoxycorticosterone:cortisol ratio
- 11-hydroxylase deficiency: as for 21-hydroxylase deficiency

The most common congenital adrenal hyperplasia is 21-hydroxylase deficiency (about 95% of cases). However, it is almost invariably a partial deficiency, as complete deficiency presents in the first day of life with a salt-losing crisis.

## Q73

A 16-year-old girl is investigated for primary amenorrhoea. At the age of 10 years she began to develop secondary sexual characteristics, but has still not started to menstruate. Both of her parents are alive and well. She is an only child. Apart from this she has never needed to see her GP, as she has always been well.

**ON EXAMINATION**

- Looks well, with well-developed breasts, scanty pubic hair and small bilateral groin swellings
- Pulse = 80 beats/min
- Blood pressure = 110/70 mmHg
- 21-Hydroxylase = normal

**INVESTIGATIONS**

- Aldosterone = normal
- Cortisol = normal
- Testosterone = elevated
- Oestradiol = low
- 17-Hydroxylase = normal

### a) What is the diagnosis?

  i)     pregnancy
  ii)    testicular feminisation syndrome
  iii)   congenital adrenal hyperplasia
  iv)    hypogonadotrophic hypogonadism
  v)     Turner's syndrome

### b) How would you confirm this?

  i)     serum β-human chorionic gonadotrophin
  ii)    buccal smear or sex chromosome analysis
  iii)   ultrasound scan of the abdomen and pelvis
  iv)    MRI scan of the pituitary
  v)     serum DHEA sulphate

### c) What management steps would you take now and in the future?

The essence of this case is that we have an apparent female with groin swelling and an elevated testosterone level.

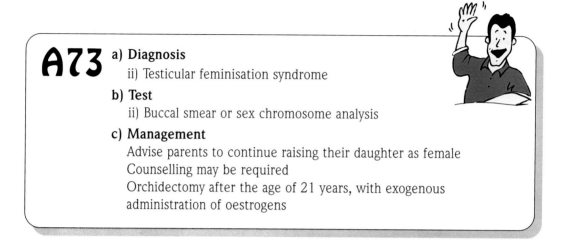

**A73**

a) **Diagnosis**
   ii) Testicular feminisation syndrome

b) **Test**
   ii) Buccal smear or sex chromosome analysis

c) **Management**
   Advise parents to continue raising their daughter as female
   Counselling may be required
   Orchidectomy after the age of 21 years, with exogenous administration of oestrogens

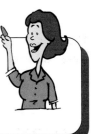

# Q74

A 16-year-old girl is being investigated for primary amenorrhoea. She has not started menstruating, and also has somewhat under-developed secondary sexual characteristics. Both of her parents are alive and well, and she is an only child.

## ON EXAMINATION

- Fundoscopy reveals scattered flame haemorrhages and exudates
- Pulse = 85 beats/min
- Blood pressure = 170/100 mmHg

## INVESTIGATIONS

- ACTH = elevated
- Renin = undetectable

ACTH: adrenocorticotrophic hormone.

## a) What is the diagnosis?

i) adrenogenital syndrome

ii) testicular feminisation syndrome

iii) congenital adrenal hyperplasia

iv) hypogonadotrophic hypogonadism

v) Turner's syndrome

## b) How would you confirm this?

i) serum 11-deoxycorticosterone levels

ii) buccal smear or sex chromosome analysis

iii) ultrasound scan of the abdomen and pelvis

iv) MRI scan of the pituitary

v) serum DHEA sulphate

This is a case of absent puberty, with low renin levels and hypertension as a result of high ACTH levels.

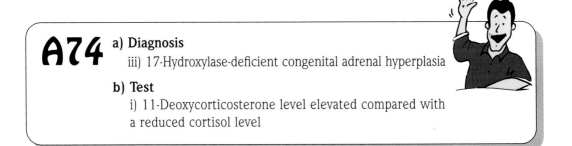

# A74

a) Diagnosis
   iii) 17-Hydroxylase-deficient congenital adrenal hyperplasia

b) Test
   i) 11-Deoxycorticosterone level elevated compared with a reduced cortisol level

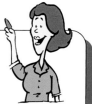

**Q75** A dermatologist sees a 19-year-old girl for treatment of her acne. She has always had slightly oily skin, but her spots have become much worse in the last year. Further questioning reveals that her menstrual periods have also become more irregular, with her cycle varying between 21 and 40 days. She has also noticed an occasional discharge from her breasts. Her 16-year-old sister has normal periods and her mother's cycle has always been regular. Both of her parents are well, although her father has taken antiepileptic drugs since he suffered a road traffic accident. The patient has never been in hospital before.

## ON EXAMINATION

- Hirsute
- Height = 1.5 m
- Weight = 67 kg
- Marked acne on face and torso
- Galactorrhoea

## INVESTIGATIONS

- Oestradiol = 500 pmol/l (normal 220–1480 pmol/l)
- Testosterone = 45 nmol/l (normal 9–35 nmol/l)
- LH = 18 IU/l (normal 1–10 IU/l)
- FSH = 0.5 IU/l (normal 1–7 IU/l)
- Prolactin = 800 mIU/l (normal 70–460 mIU/l)
- SHBG = low

FSH: follicle-stimulating hormone; LH: luteinising hormone; SHBG: sex hormone binding globulin.

## a) What is the most likely diagnosis?

i) Cushing's disease

ii) cancer of the ovaries

iii) congenital adrenal hyperplasia

iv) idiopathic hirsutism

v) polycystic ovary syndrome

## b) What other differential diagnosis would you consider?

## c) How would you best investigate this girl?

i) serum oestrogen levels

ii) serum testosterone levels

iii) ultrasound of the ovaries

iv) serum luteinising hormone (LH) and follicule-stimulating hormone (FSH) levels

v) serum prolactin levels

This woman has the following clinical features:

- hirsutism
- acne
- obesity
- galactorrhoea
- irregular menstruation
- elevated LH:FSH ratio
- elevated testosterone

There is only one answer – polycystic ovary syndrome. You just have to recognise this, we're afraid. The father's anticonvulsants, which cause hirsutism (phenytoin), have been thrown in as a red herring, but the biochemical abnormalities would not be found in such a case.

The diagnosis of polycystic ovary syndrome is primarily clinical, with the biochemistry confirming what one already suspects. In addition to a high testosterone level and LH:FSH ratio (>3), prolactin may also be elevated. This gives rise to the occasional finding of galactorrhoea in polycystic ovary syndrome. Remember that it is only the oestrogen-primed breast that can lactate, which is why men with bronchogenic carcinoma who are ectopically secreting prolactin do not experience galactorrhoea.

The only possible differential diagnosis would be mild, late-onset 21-hydroxylase-deficiency congenital adrenal hyperplasia. However, these patients would not experience galactorrhoea for the reasons outlined above.

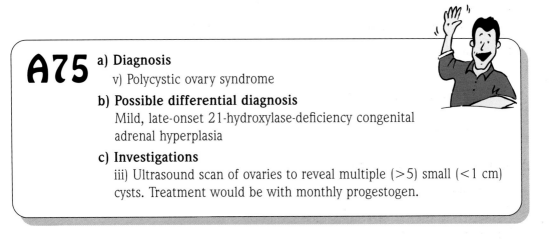

**A75** a) **Diagnosis**
v) Polycystic ovary syndrome

b) **Possible differential diagnosis**
Mild, late-onset 21-hydroxylase-deficiency congenital adrenal hyperplasia

c) **Investigations**
iii) Ultrasound scan of ovaries to reveal multiple (>5) small (<1 cm) cysts. Treatment would be with monthly progestogen.

**Q76** A 23-year-old, HIV-positive man presents with a 2-week history of a dry cough, breathlessness, headache, fever, and malaise. On examination, he has remarkably few chest signs and his saturation on air is 91%. His chest X-ray shows bilateral interstitial shadowing.

**a) Which of the following is the least likely diagnosis?**

i) *Pneumocystis jiroveci* infection

ii) cytomegalovirus pneumonitis

iii) *Toxoplasma* infection

iv) *Candida* infection

v) lymphoid interstitial pneumonitis

**b) The patient becomes pancytopenic. Which treatment has he started?**

i) pentamidine

ii) dapsone

iii) atovaquone

iv) acyclovir

v) cotrimoxazole

All of these differentials may cause bilateral interstitial infiltrates. As may:

- *Cryptococcus*
- histoplasmosis
- herpes simplex virus
- mycobacteria

Lymphoid interstitial pneumonitis is an AIDS-defining illness in children. It is rarely found in HIV-positive adults, although it can also be found in HIV-negative adults (associated with autoimmune diseases such as rheumatoid arthritis). It is a progressive disorder that is often associated with generalised lymphadenopathy and hepatosplenomegaly. It is diagnosed by finding lymphocytic and plasma cell infiltration of alveolar tissue on biopsy.

## PNEUMOCYSTIS JIROVECI PNEUMONIA

Ready for it? Take a deep breath... Here's all you need to know about *P. jiroveci* pneumonia:

- Typical history: dry cough, breathlessness (particularly on exertion), fever, malaise. Always think about *P. jiroveci* pneumonia in the immunocompromised patient who complains of headache and shortness of breath (this isn't evidence based, but clinical experience shows a strong correlation).

- There are often few clinical signs.

- Exercise-induced desaturation is very suggestive of the diagnosis.

- The characteristic chest X-ray appearance is of widespread infiltrates.

- Treatment may exacerbate symptoms; steroids are often prescribed to prevent this.

- A definitive diagnosis is made by induced sputum or bronchoalveolar lavage.

- The characteristic cysts of *Pneumocystis jirovecii* can be identified by immunofluorescence, and by various histological staining techniques including cresyl violet, Diff-Quik, and toluidine blue (to name but a few!). The fungus CANNOT be cultured in the lab!

- Never forget *P. jiroveci* pneumonia in the immunocompromised patient – it kills!

Cotrimoxazole is the standard treatment for *P. jiroveci* pneumonia, but intolerance is frequent. Alternatives include atovaquone, clindamycin, dapsone, pentamidine, primaquine, and trimetrexate. Pentamidine has many side effects, including pancreatitis, renal failure, hepatotoxicity, leucopenia, rash, fever, and hypoglycaemia.

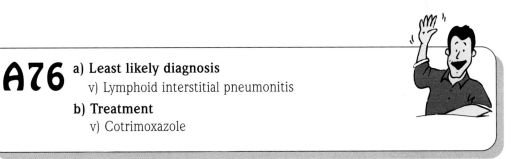

**A76**
  **a) Least likely diagnosis**
    v) Lymphoid interstitial pneumonitis
  **b) Treatment**
    v) Cotrimoxazole

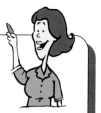

**Q77** A 46-year-old, HIV-positive man presents with double vision. He is a kennel owner, and has recently been seeing two dogs where there should only be one. Examination reveals a right sixth nerve palsy. A CT scan of the head demonstrates a single ring-enhancing lesion. An MRI scan of the brain demonstrates multiple enhancing lesions. Epstein–Barr virus serology is positive, and a PET scan shows moderate uptake (i.e. the lesion shows moderate FDG avidity on PET). He is commenced on treatment and shows radiological and clinical improvement over the next 3 weeks.

### a) What treatment has he been commenced on?

i) pyrimethamine, sulphadiazine, and folinic acid

ii) R-CHOP (rituximab, cyclophosphamide, doxorubicin, vincristine, and prednisolone) and intrathecal methotrexate

iii) spiramycin

iv) cotrimoxazole

v) amphotericin, flucytosine, and fluconazole

This question requires you to know the causes of ring-enhancing lesions. Repeat after me: metastases, demyelinating disease, and infection. In the immunocompromised, this list needs expanding and reordering:

- infection: toxoplasmosis… and all the rest (tuberculosis [TB], aspergillosis, amoebic abscesses, candidiasis, coccidioidomycosis, *Cryptococcus*, histoplasmosis, neurocysticercosis, *Staphylococcus*, and *Streptococcus*)
- cancer: primary central nervous system lymphoma
- progressive multifocal leucoencephalopathy, HIV encephalopathy, and cytomegalovirus encephalitis may all be seen as ring-enhancing lesions but do not cause mass effect

This man is immunocompromised and has responded to treatment. He has toxoplasmosis.

**A77** a) **Treatment**
   i) Pyrimethamine, sulphadiazine, and folinic acid

What do the other drug combinations treat?

- R-CHOP and intrathecal methotrexate: lymphoma

- spiramycin: toxoplasmosis therapy during pregnancy to prevent infection of the foetus – on a named patient basis only

- cotrimoxazole: *P. carinii* pneumonia

- amphotericin, flucytosine, and fluconazole: cryptosporidiosis

# Q78

A 76-year-old, HIV-positive man presents with chronic, profuse, watery diarrhoea associated with abdominal pain and significant weight loss. He has been poorly compliant with his antiretroviral therapy. His CD4+ cell count is $112 \times 10^9/l$ and his viral load is 82,000/ml.

## a) Which of the following pathogens would not cause these symptoms?

i) cryptosporidia

ii) microsporidia

iii) *Isospora belli*

iv) cytomegalovirus colitis

v) John Cunningham (JC) virus

With this CD4+ cell count, diarrhoea, abdominal pain, and wasting, the most likely causes would be:

- helminthes: *Strongyloides*
- protozoa: *Cryptosporidium*, *Entamoeba*, *Isospora*, *Microsporidia*
- bacteria: *Mycobacterium avium* complex
- viruses: cytomegalovirus

JC virus is associated with acute haemorrhagic cystitis and progressive multifocal leucoencephalopathy in immunocompromised individuals.

# A78

a) Not a diagnosis
v) JC virus

## Diarrhoea in the immunocompromised

Remember, HIV infection itself can cause chronic, watery diarrhoea. A few more facts regarding diarrhoea in the immunocompromised...

- Cryptosporidiosis causes severe, non-resolving, watery diarrhoea associated with abdominal pain, nausea, weight loss, and low-grade fever. There is no specific treatment.

- Strongyloides may present with dermatological, gastrointestinal, or pulmonary involvement. Treatment is with ivermectin.

- Microsporidia causes a chronic debilitating illness, weight loss, fatigue, and reduced fertility. There may be central nervous system, dermatological, ocular, or musculoskeletal involvement. Albendazole is the treatment of choice.

- *Mycobacterium avium* complex typically presents with disseminated disease in individuals with a CD4$^+$ count of $<50 \times 10^6$/l. Patients may present with fever of unknown origin, weight loss, diarrhoea, shortness of breath, and right upper quadrant pain. It is treated with two or three antimicrobials (macrolides, rifamycins, and ethambutol) for 12 months; it is intrinsically resistant to typical anti-TB medication. Macrolides are used as chemoprophylaxis in those with a CD4$^+$ cell count of $<50 \times 10^6$/l.

- Isosporiasis results in chronic, nonbloody diarrhoea. It is treated with cotrimoxazole.

- Cytomegalovirus colitis causes bloody diarrhoea with associated fever and abdominal pain, typically in the severely immunocompromised (a CD4$^+$ cell count of $<50 \times 10^6$/l). It is treated with ganciclovir and foscarnet.

In addition to these are the causes that are also seen in immunocompetent individuals. See if you can list them!

**Q79** A 24-year-old woman presents to your clinic having returned from a 3-month tour of Asia 2 weeks previously. She complains of fever, sweats, headache, and malaise. Examination reveals cervical and inguinal lymphadenopathy.

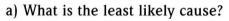

### a) What is the least likely cause?

i)     malaria

ii)    lymphoma

iii)   TB

iv)    lymphogranuloma venereum

v)     HIV seroconversion illness

Lymphogranuloma venereum it is a sexually transmitted disease. It is the only disease listed with which these symptoms don't fit. Instead, it typically presents as a painless herpetiform ulcer, progressing to tender inguinal lymphadenitis that may coalesce to form abscesses. Treatment is with doxycycline or erythromycin.

And as for TB and lymphoma, we're sure you've read enough already! Can you remember it all? Here's a bit on the others…

### MALARIA

- Prevalent in tropical and subtropical regions.
- Sickle cell disease, thalassaemia, and glucose-6-phosphate dehydrogenase deficiency all protect against malaria.
- Symptoms include fever, arthralgia, diarrhoea, vomiting, and headache.
- Serious complications include haemorrhage, pulmonary oedema, renal failure, seizures, coma, lactic acidosis, or death.
- Symptoms usually start 10–15 days following infection.
- Beware! Both the disease itself and treatment with quinine may cause hypoglycaemia.
- Examination may find lymphadenopathy and hepatosplenomegaly.
- Bloods may show anaemia due to haemolysis.
- Diagnosis depends on serial blood films. Don't always believe a negative result, especially on thin film examination.

- Side effects of antimalarial therapies:
  - chloroquine – psychosis, retinopathy
  - mefloquine – psychiatric disturbances
  - doxycycline – photosensitivity
  - primaquine – methaemoglobinaemia
- Remember to advise travellers to begin taking prophylaxis 1 week before their trip and for 4 weeks on their return.

## HIV SEROCONVERSION ILLNESS

- Usually occurs 2–4 weeks after infection.
- Symptoms include fever, rash, arthralgia, diarrhoea, headache, and lymphadenopathy.

*BHIVA guidelines*

The latest British HIV Association guidelines (2008) recommend starting antiretroviral therapy during seroconversion only within a clinical trial or if the patient has severe illness.

In those with established infection the goal posts have moved:

- If the CD4$^+$ count is <200 × 10$^6$/l, treat.
- If the CD4$^+$ count is 201–350 × 10$^6$/l, treat as soon as possible. Remember, patient acceptance is a big issue.
- Treat those with an AIDS-defining illness, regardless of the CD4$^+$ count or viral load.
- If the CD4$^+$ count is 350–500 × 10$^6$/l, the decision of whether to start treatment should take into account the patient's viral load, CD4$^+$ percentage, co-infection with hepatitis B or C, and the patient's wishes.

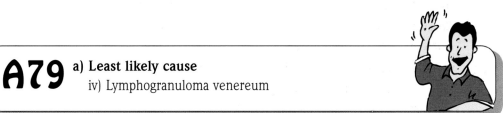

**A79** a) **Least likely cause**
iv) Lymphogranuloma venereum

# QUIZ SPOT!

## SIDE EFFECTS OF ANTIRETROVIRAL TREATMENT

There are so many side effects associated with antiretroviral treatment.
How many can you find in the wordsearch?

| W | R | R | F | L | A | T | U | L | E | N | C | E | S |
|---|---|---|---|---|---|---|---|---|---|---|---|---|---|
| D | G | J | A | N | A | L | Q | D | X | F | A | C | T |
| Y | A | K | N | S | D | H | Y | Y | S | C | S | G | E |
| S | T | L | C | W | H | L | P | A | N | U | T | A | V |
| L | I | P | O | D | Y | S | T | R | O | P | H | Y | E |
| I | T | A | N | P | I | W | P | P | V | I | E | H | N |
| P | N | N | I | E | E | O | O | H | Q | F | N | T | S |
| I | O | C | S | A | U | C | E | V | Y | P | I | A | J |
| D | I | R | S | E | E | T | I | A | H | C | A | P | O |
| A | S | E | Y | O | R | B | R | A | T | R | I | O | H |
| E | U | A | N | H | A | O | U | O | A | M | N | Y | N |
| M | F | T | D | R | M | O | L | F | P | K | H | M | S |
| I | N | I | R | R | T | B | C | L | O | E | S | K | O |
| A | O | T | O | A | H | S | E | G | R | P | N | V | N |
| Y | C | I | M | I | G | J | R | S | U | N | A | I | S |
| E | R | S | E | D | I | K | S | Y | E | O | I | D | A |
| S | O | S | O | M | N | O | L | E | N | C | E | A | W |

A: alopecia, asthenia, confusion, diarrhoea, dyslipidaemia, Fanconi's syndrome, flatulence, lipodystrophy, myopathy, neuropathy, neutropenia, nightmare, pancreatitis, rash, somnolence, Stevens–Johnson, ulcers

Now see if you can remember the table on page 170... Which side effect belongs to which drug?

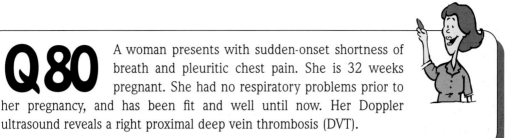

**Q80** A woman presents with sudden-onset shortness of breath and pleuritic chest pain. She is 32 weeks pregnant. She had no respiratory problems prior to her pregnancy, and has been fit and well until now. Her Doppler ultrasound reveals a right proximal deep vein thrombosis (DVT).

### a) How will you manage her pulmonary embolus (PE)?

i) admit, start on unfractionated heparin, and liaise with the obstetricians for an emergency Caesarean section

ii) proceed to ventilation/perfusion (V/Q) scan

iii) start on warfarin and continue for 2 months post-partum

iv) start on subcutaneous low molecular weight heparin (LMWH) and discuss with the patient regarding warfarin or LMWH post-partum

v) proceed to CT pulmonary angiography (CTPA) scan

### INVESTIGATION OF PULMONARY EMBOLISM DURING PREGNANCY

- A chest X-ray should be performed to assess the radiological changes of acute PE and exclude other acute respiratory problems.

- Patients with a high clinical suspicion of PE but a normal chest X-ray should undergo Doppler ultrasound scanning to look for a DVT. A diagnosis of DVT indirectly confirms a diagnosis of PE.

- Since anticoagulation treatment is the same for both conditions, Doppler ultrasound scanning has the additional advantage of reducing radiation exposure for both the mother and foetus.

- If the Doppler scan is negative and clinical suspicion remains high for PE, choosing further investigation with a V/Q or CTPA scan depends on availability, the appearance of the chest X-ray, and the radiation risk of the imaging modality. These options, with their benefits and risks, should be discussed with the patient.

- V/Q
  - advantage: high negative predictive value. In many radiology departments, the ventilation component can be omitted, which further reduces the radiation exposure.
  - disadvantage: higher risk of fatal cancer up to the age of 15 years from *in utero* exposure to V/Q (1/280,000) compared with CTPA (1/1,000,000)

- CTPA
  - advantage: more sensitive and specific than V/Q, and can identify other pathologies such as aortic dissection
  - disadvantage: increases the lifetime risk of breast cancer in mothers (13.5% following CTPA vs 0.005% background risk)

## TREATMENT OF VENOUS THROMBOEMBOLISM DURING PREGNANCY

Heparin is the treatment of choice in pregnancy because it does not cross the placenta. A weight-adjusted dose of subcutaneous LMWH is preferable to unfractionated heparin as the latter requires frequent activated partial thrombin time monitoring for maintenance treatment of venous thromboembolism, and increases the risk of haemorrhagic complications.

Warfarin crosses the placenta. It is teratogenic and can cause bleeding in the foetus, especially in the first and third trimesters. It should be avoided antenatally, but difficult situations may arise in patients who have prosthetic heart valves, atrial fibrillation, or recurrent thromboembolism. In these cases, the risks and benefits of warfarin need to be carefully considered and explained to the patient.

## TREATMENT OF VENOUS THROMBOEMBOLISM POST-PARTUM

In the post-partum period, warfarin and heparin are both safe as they are not secreted into breast milk. Warfarin is usually started 2–3 days post-partum.

 **a) Management**
iv) Start on subcutaneous LMWH and discuss with the patient regarding warfarin or LMWH post-partum

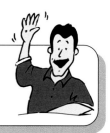

**Q81** The senior house officer in the emergency department wants your advice on a 24-year-old patient who has an unplanned pregnancy. She attended the emergency department as her GP told her that she should have her antiepileptic drug (AED) reviewed. She is currently 8 weeks pregnant and has been taking carbamazepine to control her epilepsy for the past 10 years. Her last seizure was 3 years ago. Her GP has already started her on folic acid.

## a) How would you manage this patient?

    i)    stop her carbamazepine, check her drug level, and arrange for specialist input

    ii)   continue her on carbamazepine and arrange for specialist input

    iii)  stop her carbamazepine, arrange an ultrasound scan now, and advise her to have counselling prior to her next pregnancy

    iv)  stop her carbamazepine, change to lamotrigine, and arrange for specialist input

    v)   increase her dose of carbamazepine and arrange for specialist input

## b) Which of the following AEDs has the highest rate of major congenital malformation?

    i)    carbamazepine

    ii)   lamotrigine

    iii)  sodium valproate

    iv)  phenytoin

    v)   levetiracetam

## EPILEPSY AND PREGNANCY

It can be difficult to make treatment decisions regarding AEDs during pregnancy as you need to balance the harmful effects of inadequate seizure control, especially tonic–clonic seizures, on both the mother and foetus with the adverse effects of AEDs on the foetus. It is important that the patient makes an informed decision about their epileptic treatment prior to conception. These pointers should help you:

- All AEDs increase the risk of congenital malformation. Major congenital malformations include orofacial clefts, cardiac abnormalities, and neural tube defects. Sodium valproate has the highest risk, followed by phenytoin, lamotrigine, and carbamazepine. Currently, there are limited data on levetiracetam and the newer AEDs.

- Monotherapy reduces the risk of congenital abnormalities when compared with multiple AEDs.

- Pregnant women who are taking AEDs should have an ultrasound scan at 18–20 weeks' gestation to screen for structural abnormalities.

- Withdrawal of AEDs prior to conception might be considered if the epilepsy is in remission, but should be done under specialist supervision.

## A81

a) **Management**

ii) Continue her on carbamazepine and arrange for specialist input.

In the case of this unplanned pregnancy, the patient's epilepsy is well controlled on carbamazepine and she is on the treatment of choice. She should be referred for specialist input if she wishes to adjust her medication.

b) **Highest rate of major congenital malformation**

iii) Sodium valproate

**Q82** You have been asked to see a 35-year-old woman who is 33 weeks into her first pregnancy. She was diagnosed with essential hypertension 5 years ago. Her blood pressure has been well controlled until recently. Over the last 24 hours she has vomited twice and had abdominal pain, which she attributes to a "dodgy takeaway". She has had a thumping headache since this morning and her husband is increasingly concerned. On examination, she is alert with no focal neurology. Her right upper quadrant is tender, but there are no signs of peritonism. There is minimal peripheral oedema. She is not sure if the baby has been moving as much as usual.

|  | AT BOOKING | 2 WEEKS AGO | CURRENTLY |
|---|---|---|---|
| Blood pressure (mmHg) | 130/85 | 145/95 | 170/100 |
| Urine dipstick | No protein | 1+ | 2+ |

| INVESTIGATIONS | RESULTS |
|---|---|
| Haemoglobin | 7.8 g/dl |
| White cell count | $13 \times 10^9/l$ |
| Platelets | $90 \times 10^9/l$ |
| Neutrophils | $9 \times 10^9/l$ |
| Plasma sodium | 132 mmol/l |
| Plasma potassium | 4.8 mmol/l |
| Plasma urea | 4.0 mmol/l |
| Plasma creatinine | 90 μmol/l |
| Bilirubin | 30 μmol/l |
| Serum alkaline phosphatase | 230 IU/l |
| Serum aspartate transaminase | 120 IU/l |
| Serum alanine aminotransaminase | 105 IU/l |
| Total protein | 80 g/l |
| Serum albumin | 30 g/l |
| International normalised ratio | 1.5 |
| Activated partial thrombin time ratio | 1.9 |
| D-dimer | 1.3 μg/ml |
| Fibrinogen | 0.8 g/l |
| Lactate dehydrogenase | 790 U/l |

## a) What is the likely diagnosis?

i) pre-eclampsia

ii) intrahepatic cholestasis of pregnancy

iii) eclampsia

iv) acute fatty liver of pregnancy

v) HELLP (haemolytic anaemia, elevated liver enzymes, and low platelet count) syndrome

Let's pick out the abnormal findings in this patient and consider each option:

• vomiting, abdominal pain, and headache

• possible reduced foetal movement

• hypertension

• proteinuria

• anaemia

• low platelet count

• abnormal liver function tests

• deranged clotting

• raised lactate dehydrogenase levels

i) Pre-eclampsia          **Yes   No   Maybe**

The pre-eclampsia patient may present with headache, abdominal pain, vomiting, and reduced foetal movement. A significant rise in blood pressure compared to booking blood pressure, new-onset proteinuria, and oedema are indicators of pre-eclampsia.

ii) Intrahepatic cholestasis of pregnancy      **Yes   No   Maybe**

This is characterised by pruritus in the third trimester, with a cholestatic liver function test. Symptomatic patients are treated with cholestyramine, but it usually subsides after delivery.

iii) Eclampsia           **Yes   No   Maybe**

Patients with the symptoms and signs of pre-eclampsia are closely monitored as they are at risk for developing eclampsia. Our patient has not displayed seizures or entered a coma, so the diagnosis here is not eclampsia.

iv) Acute fatty liver of pregnancy **Yes  No  Maybe**

Acute fatty liver of pregnancy is rare. Patients present with fulminant liver failure. The condition can lead to acute renal failure, hypoglycaemia, hepatic encephalopathy, disseminated intravascular coagulation, and pancreatitis. Bilirubin is markedly raised, with increases in aspartate transaminase and alanine transaminase levels.

v) HELLP syndrome **Yes  No  Maybe**

In this patient, her pre-eclampsia is complicated by HELLP syndrome: haemolytic anaemia (the elevated lactate dehydrogenase level points towards haemolysis), elevated liver enzymes, and low platelet count, as well as evidence of disseminated intravascular coagulation. The only effective treatment for HELLP syndrome is delivery of the baby. Supportive management for disseminated intravascular coagulation is required.

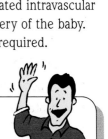

**A82** a) Diagnosis
v) HELLP syndrome

# 11

# MOPPING UP

MOPPING UP **MRCP** LISTS

This section is designed to provide you with 'cannon fodder' for practice. It should allow you to practice using your lists. We will also try to cover a few more of the 'just recognise it' classic cases, and any of the other general bits and bobs that we have so far missed out. Once you have done all of these, we suggest that you quickly run through all of the lists once more to make sure that you know them all. We have printed them all at the back of the book for you to remove so that you can carry them with you as an *aide-mémoire*. We strongly recommend that you now get hold of a selection of the other 'MRCP books' on the shelves, and use their questions for practice.

The MRCP examination is not easy, and can be a bit demoralising. However, the strategies you learn *will* be useful to you in the future: there really is no better doctor than the general medical registrar who has just passed the MRCP examination. Such a being is certainly our choice of doctor when we get poorly.

Good luck!

# Q83

A 35-year-old man returning from the tropics presents with breathlessness. Examination demonstrates dullness to percussion at the right lower zone, decreased breath sounds, and sparse crackles. His chest X-ray shows an elevated right hemidiaphragm and atelectasis. An ultrasound scan shows a large hypoechogenic mass in the liver.

## a) Which treatment should be commenced?

i) intravenous metronidazole

ii) oral metronidazole

iii) tetracycline

iv) paromomycin

v) albendazole

The clinical findings are all too common. The key fact is he has returned from the tropics so your differential diagnosis changes. The investigations then give you the answer; they're classic.

- *E. histolytica* is an anaerobic protozoa.
- Symptoms can include abdominal pain or fullness, diarrhoea, dysentery, fatigue, malaise, and weight loss.
- Bloods may show leucocytosis, normochromic, normocytic anaemia, and a raised erythrocyte sedimentation rate (typically >100 mm/hr).
- Chest X-ray may show a raised diaphragm, right basal effusion, or consolidation.
- Trophozoites may be identified in fresh faeces, while cysts can be found in a normal stool sample.

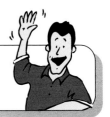

# A83

**a) Treatment**
ii) Oral metronidazole

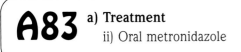

Revision munchies – how does a little anchovy sauce sound? Here are a few accompaniments...

- Sago spleen – splenic amyloidosis
- pepperpot skull – hyperparathyroidism
- nutmeg liver – chronic hepatic venous congestion
- pizza pie retina – cytomegalovirus retinitis
- beefy tongue – vitamin $B_{12}$ deficiency
- peaches and cream complexion – hypothyroidism
- ox heart – aortic valve disease, chronic hypertension
- eggshell calcification – silicosis, coal worker's pneumoconiosis

A few others...

- slapped cheek – parvovirus B19
- owl's eye cells – cytomegalovirus inclusion bodies
- Howell–Jolly bodies – hyposplenism, sickle cell anaemia, myelodysplastic syndromes, hereditary spherocytosis
- geographical tongue (appearance of the tongue's surface) – vitamin $B_2$ deficiency
- bamboo spine – ankylosing spondylitis
- lead-pipe colon – chronic ulcerative colitis
- pulmonary snowstorm – pulmonary alveolar microlithiasis
- tramline calcification – von Hippel–Lindau disease

Can you think of any more?

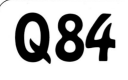

# Q84

A 45-year-old woman presents with breathlessness and lethargy. She has a history of treated hypertension. On examination, she appears anaemic and her chest is clear.

| INVESTIGATIONS | RESULTS |
| --- | --- |
| Haemoglobin | 7.6 g/dl |
| White cell count | $3.6 \times 10^9/l$ |
| Platelets | $235 \times 10^9/l$ |
| Plasma sodium | 134 mmol/l |
| Plasma potassium | 4.6 mmol/l |
| Plasma urea | 6.7 mmol/l |
| Plasma creatinine | 65 µmol/l |
| Serum bilirubin | 28 µmol/l |
| Serum aspartate aminotransferase | 12 IU/l |
| Serum alanine aminotransferase | 9 IU/l |
| Serum alkaline phosphatase | 121 IU/l |
| Reticulocyte count | 11% |
| Chest X-ray | Slight cardiomegaly |
| Electrocardiogram | Voltage criteria for LVH |

LVH: left ventricular hypertrophy.

## a) What is the diagnosis of her recent problem?

i) coeliac disease

ii) haemolytic anaemia (secondary to methyldopa used to treat her hypertension)

iii) hemolytic uraemic syndrome

iv) systemic lupus erythematosus (SLE)

v) glucose-6-phosphate dehydrogenase deficiency

## b) What would you expect to find in the urine?

i) red cell casts

ii) haemosiderin

iii) raised urobilinogen

iv) all of the above

v) none of the above

**A84**   a) **Diagnosis**
         ii) Methyldopa-induced haemolytic anaemia
       b) **Urine test**
         iv) All of the above

This question should have been easy for you by now. The only problem is to discover the cause of her haemolysis. As we have previously stated in this book, think of the drugs. In this case, the patient has been treated long term with methyldopa. It sounds as though it is time for a change. Bring her hypertension treatment up to date.

Remember the classic laboratory features associated with haemolytic anaemia:

- raised serum unconjugated bilirubin
- methaemoglobinaemia
- raised urinary urobilinogen
- raised faecal stercobilinogen
- haemosiderinuria
- absent serum haptoglobins

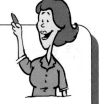

# Q85

An 82-year-old man presents with general lethargy and weakness. He was reasonably well until 3 months ago, although he has suffered with nose bleeds for the last 4 years. His brother, who lives with him, has been treated for hypertension with nifedipine for many years. Two months ago the patient had an episode of coughing up clotted blood and has felt short of breath since then, although he has a good exercise tolerance. There is no significant medical history except for an episode of typhoid fever whilst in the army in North Africa in 1942. He smokes five cigarettes per day. On examination, he is pale and appears short of breath, with dry skin and mucous membranes.

| INVESTIGATIONS | RESULTS |
| --- | --- |
| Haemoglobin | 9.9 g/dl |
| White cell count | $12.6 \times 10^9/l$ |
| Platelets | $123 \times 10^9/l$ |
| Plasma sodium | 131 mmol/l |
| Plasma potassium | 6.7 mmol/l |
| Plasma urea | 32 mmol/l |
| Plasma creatinine | 290 μmol/l |
| Serum bilirubin | 9 μmol/l |
| Serum aspartate aminotransferase | 9 IU/l |
| Serum alanine aminotransferase | 18 IU/l |
| Serum alkaline phosphatase | 65 IU/l |
| Hepatitis B serum antigen | Negative |
| Serum creatinine kinase | 120 IU/l |
| Urinalysis | Red cell casts |
| Chest X-ray | Cavitating lesions in left upper zone and right lower zone |
| Anti-glomerular basement membrane | Negative |
| Anti-nuclear antibodies | Negative |
| Anti-double-stranded DNA | Negative |
| Rhesus factor | Negative |

### a) What is the most likely diagnosis?

    i)     tuberculosis

    ii)    Wegener's granulomatosis

    iii)   Goodpasture's syndrome

    iv)   staphylococcal infection

    v)    adenocarcinoma of the lung

### b) What test would you do to confirm the diagnosis

    i)     anti-neutrophilic cytoplasmic antibodies (ANCA)

    ii)    renal biopsy

    iii)   transbronchial biopsy

    iv)   nasal biopsy

    v)    all of the above

This question requires you to put together a number of your well-known lists; in particular, the causes of lung cavitation and the causes of renal failure with red cell casts in the urine. Cover the page and write these down now.

## CAUSES OF CAVITATION ON A CHEST X-RAY

*Cancers\* cause cavities, so can TB*
*Wegener's, rheumatoid\*\*, also PE*
*Think of the 'oses' of which there are three*
*Also of abscesses\*\*\*, klebsielli*

\*Small-cell lung cancer; \*\*progressive massive fibrosis/rheumatoid nodules associated with rheumatoid arthritis; \*\*\*think staphylococcal, *Klebsiella*, amoebic, aspiration. 'oses': histoplasmosis, coccidioidomycosis, and aspergillosis; PE: pulmonary embolism; TB: tuberculosis; Wegener's: Wegener's granulomatosis.

## CAUSES OF RENAL FAILURE

- **G**enerally      **G**lomerulonephritis
- **I**nflammatory      **I**nterstitial nephritis
- **A**nd      **A**ccelerated hypertension
- **H**armful      **H**aemolytic uraemic syndrome

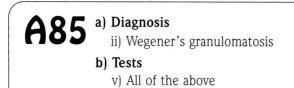

## A85   a) Diagnosis
       ii) Wegener's granulomatosis
     b) Tests
       v) All of the above

Cavitation plus casts really only leaves Wegener's granulomatosis. The presence of nasal symptoms (caused by nasal granuloma) clinches it. Always go for the least invasive site for biopsy.

At this point we will briefly discuss the various merits of the ANCA tests.

## ANCA

There are two main types of ANCA test: cytoplasmic (C)-ANCA and perinuclear (P)-ANCA.

- C-ANCA stain the cytoplasm diffusely; these antibodies are usually directed against a serine protease called proteinase 3.
- P-ANCA are usually directed against myeloperoxidase.

For C-ANCA-positive vasculitis, the level of C-ANCA, C-reactive protein, and renal function can be used to assess disease activity. As in anti-glomerular basement membrane disease, if there is pulmonary involvement, transfer coefficients can be used as a marker of the degree of pulmonary vasculitis.

Most importantly, for P-ANCA vasculitis you *cannot* use titre to monitor disease activity.

A small number of patients may be both C-ANCA and anti-glomerular basement membrane antibody positive, and these patients have a particularly poor prognosis.

### ASSOCIATIONS

C-ANCA: Wegener's granulomatosis (positive in 95% of patients).
(C-ANCA = W-ANCA; i.e. C-ANCA is positive in Wegener's granulomatosis.)

P-ANCA: unlike C-ANCA, this is a bit promiscuous and is found in many diseases, including:

- microscopic polyarteritis
- polyarteritis nodosa
- and a variety of rheumatic autoimmune diseases, including:
  - rheumatoid arthritis
  - SLE
  - Sjögren's syndrome
  - polymyositis
  - dermatomyositis

If P-ANCA is directed against myeloperoxidase then it is relatively specific to (although not sensitive for) microscopic polyarteritis and polyarteritis nodosa.

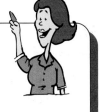

# Q86

A 43-year-old woman who was originally resident in Hong Kong presents with progressive lethargy for the last year. In addition, she has lost 2 stone in weight, felt nauseous, and been anorexic. Her husband has also noted that her eyes have appeared yellow on a number of occasions.

| INVESTIGATIONS | RESULTS |
| --- | --- |
| Haemoglobin | 11.8 g/dl |
| White cell count | 6.3 × 10⁹/l |
| Platelets | 190 × 10⁹/l |
| Erythrocyte sedimentation rate | 42 mm in first hour |
| Plasma sodium | 130 mmol/l |
| Plasma potassium | 3.9 mmol/l |
| Plasma urea | 6.9 mmol/l |
| Serum bilirubin | 37 μmol/l (normal: 3–17 μmol/l) |
| Serum alanine aminotransferase | 63 IU/l (normal: 5–15 IU/l) |
| Serum alkaline phosphatase | 83 IU/l (normal: 0–95 IU/l) |
| Clotting international normalised ratio | 1.1 |
| Thrombin time | Normal |
| Serum immunoglobulin G | 24 g/l |
| Serum immunoglobulin M | 5.3 g/l |
| Serum immunoglobulin A | 2.5 g/l |

### a) What is the most likely diagnosis?

i) primary biliary cirrhosis

ii) adenocarcinoma of the liver

iii) chronic active hepatitis

iv) autoimmune haemolytic anaemia

v) Hodgkin's lymphoma

### b) What two tests would you do to confirm your diagnosis?

i) anti-mitochondrial antibodies and ERCP (endoscopic retrograde cholangio-pancreatography)

ii) CT scan of the abdomen and liver biopsy

iii) liver biopsy and hepatitis serology

iv) Coomb's test and serum lactate dehydrogenase levels

v) CT scan of the abdomen and thorax and bone marrow aspirate

**A86**   a) **Diagnosis**
　　　　iii) Chronic active hepatitis
　　　b) **Investigations**
　　　　iii) Liver biopsy and hepatitis serology (hepatitis B, C, D)

We don't think that this question needs any explanation. We are sure that by now you will be getting these right!

# QUIZ SPOT!

### JIGSAW PUZZLE: RETINITIS PIGMENTOSA AND ANGIOID RETINAL STREAKS

Fit the following jigsaw pieces into the grid to reveal causes of retinitis pigmentosa and angioid retinal streaks. Just to make life tricky, there is one box missing. What are the diseases, and which causes which eye sign? The answers are on page 352.

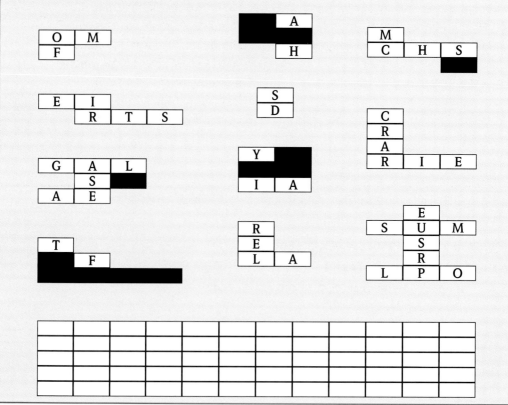

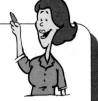

# Q87

A 58-year-old man presents to the emergency department with right-sided visual loss. He is a nonsmoker, with no previous history of ischaemic heart disease or hypercholesterolaemia. He drinks about 27 units of alcohol per week, although this may be more during weeks when he is entertaining clients. He has occasionally taken cocaine. He works in the advertising industry and has recently been headhunted to be an executive for a large, London-based firm. At that time, a medical examination found a 'muscular heart' on the electrocardiogram. On systems review, he admits to having an approximately 2-month history of intermittent left-sided loin pain and fevers, and he thinks that he has lost some weight. His GP recently started him on atenolol treatment in a well-man clinic.

## ON EXAMINATION

- He appears flushed, but has no lymphadenopathy, jaundice, cyanosis, clubbing, or oedema
- Blood pressure = 178/100 mmHg
- Pulse = 88 beats/min
- Temperature = 38.2°C
- Cardiovascular examination otherwise normal
- Respiratory examination otherwise normal
- Abdominal examination unremarkable, except for a left varicocoele
- Right homonymous hemianopia, with no other neurological deficit

## INVESTIGATIONS

- Haemoglobin = 19.2 g/dl
- White cell count = $8.2 \times 10^9$/l
- Platelets = $420 \times 10^9$/l
- ESR = 58 mm in first hour
- Plasma sodium = 138 mmol/l
- Plasma potassium = 4.5 mmol/l
- Plasma creatinine = 159 μmol/l
- Plasma urea = 7.8 mmol/l
- Urinalysis: protein ++, blood +++
- Urine 24-hour VMA elevated

ESR: erythrocyte sedimentation rate; VMA: vanillylmandelic acid.

## a) What is the haematological diagnosis?

i)   primary polycythaemia

ii)  secondary polycythaemia

iii) relative polycythaemia

iv)  thrombophilia

v)   haemolytic anaemia

### b) What is the most likely cause of this patient's presenting complaint?

i)      central retinal vein occlusion

ii)     central retinal artery occlusion

iii)    right occipital thromboembolic infarct

iv)     right temporal thromboembolic infarct

v)      left temporal thromboembolic infarct

### c) What is the underlying diagnosis?

i)      polycythaemia rubra vera

ii)     Gaisböck's syndrome

iii)    hypernephroma

iv)     phaeochromocytoma

v)      cerebellar haemangioma

### d) How do you explain the left varicocele?

Well. What do we know? This patient has some systemic illness (weight loss, fever, elevated erythrocyte sedimentation rate), neurological signs (right homonymous hemianopia), polycythaemia (haemoglobin 19.2 g/dl), and renal pathology (haematuria, proteinuria, left varicocele). He also has an elevated urinary vanillylmandelic acid (VMA) level.

Let's start with what you know already. Revise the causes of polycythaemia.

#### CAUSES OF POLYCYTHAEMIA

- Relative: dehydration, Gaisböck's syndrome (stress)
- Primary: polycythaemia rubra vera (splenomegaly, raised platelets)
- Secondary: hypoxia, chronic obstructive pulmonary disease, altitude-abnormal haemoglobin, sleep apnoea
- Excess erythropoietin: cerebellar haemangioma, hepatoma, phaechromocytoma, hypernephroma, polycystic/transplant kidneys, uterine leiomyomata/fibromata

Now exclude the unlikely ones by scoring through them with a pen. Hopefully, the list will be a lot smaller (and won't contain uterine fibromata!):

- Primary: polycythaemia rubra vera
- Secondary: hypoxia
- Excess erythropoietin: cerebellar haemangioma, hepatoma, hypernephroma

This patient has several systemic features suggestive of an underlying malignancy. The reported neurology does not fit with a cerebellar haemangioma. Hepatoma or hypernephroma seem the best choices. Which is the best fit? The varicocele is explicable on the basis that tumour invasion of the left renal vein is interfering with the drainage of the left testicular vein (the right testicular vein drains directly into the inferior vena cava).

Therefore, go with the diagnosis of hypernephroma... and you'd be right!

The elevated VMA level is thrown in as a red herring; false-positive VMA results can be seen in hypernephromas.

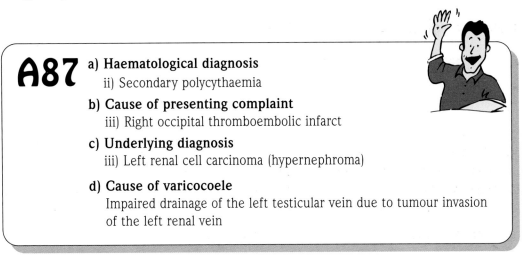

**A87**
a) **Haematological diagnosis**
   ii) Secondary polycythaemia
b) **Cause of presenting complaint**
   iii) Right occipital thromboembolic infarct
c) **Underlying diagnosis**
   iii) Left renal cell carcinoma (hypernephroma)
d) **Cause of varicocoele**
   Impaired drainage of the left testicular vein due to tumour invasion of the left renal vein

## HYPERNEPHROMA

Hypernephroma may be presented as a question in different ways.

- Pyrexia of unknown origin: renal cell carcinoma is the classic oncological cause.
- Hypercalcaemia: in addition to secreting erythropoietin, renal cell carcinoma may secrete parathyroid hormone-related peptide (PTHrP). As a result of hypercalcaemia, the patient in the case history may present with polydipsia and polyuria.
- Musculoskeletal: paraneoplastic syndromes of renal cell carcinoma are classically musculoskeletal, and patients may present with vasculitis, giant cell arteritis, myositis, or polymyalgia.

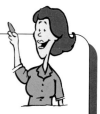

# Q88

A 75-year-old man who is under treatment for prostatic carcinoma presents with lethargy and weakness. He has been taking cyproterone acetate for the last 4 years, and his prostate-specific antigen level was <10 ng/ml when checked 6 months ago. Over the last 3 weeks he has been breathless, with reduced exercise tolerance. He used to be able to walk his dog for 3 miles, but can now only walk about half a mile. He has been a smoker for the last 60 years having started at school, but only smokes 3 cigarettes per day. He drinks 2 pints of beer per day. He does not have a cough and has not had any haemoptysis. On examination, he is pale, his chest is clinically clear, and his cardiovascular examination is unremarkable.

| INVESTIGATIONS | RESULTS |
| --- | --- |
| Haemoglobin | $7.3 \times 10^9/l$ |
| Mean corpuscular volume | 83 fl |
| Platelets | $203 \times 10^9/l$ |
| Plasma sodium | 135 mmol/l |
| Plasma potassium | 4.5 mmol/l |
| Plasma urea | 4.3 mmol/l |
| Plasma creatinine | 76 μmol/l |
| Serum bilirubin | 8 μmol/l |
| Serum aspartate aminotransferase | 12 IU/l |
| Serum alanine aminotransferase | 9 IU/l |
| Serum alkaline phosphatase | 98 IU/l |
| Chest X-ray | Normal |
| $FEV_1$ | 3.2 l |
| FVC | 3.8 l |
| Blood film | Multiple fragmented red cells and burr cells |

$FEV_1$: forced expiratory volume in 1 second; FVC: forced vital capacity.

## a) What is the diagnosis?

i)   anaemia of chronic disease

ii)  autoimmune haemolytic anaemia

iii) iron-deficiency anaemia

iv)  microangiopathic haemolytic anaemia

v)   side effect of cyproterone acetate

Again, this question may appear difficult on the surface, with multiple possible causes for the patient's shortness of breath. The anaemia is clearly pathological and could be caused by a number of factors, including bone marrow carcinomatous infiltration, drug-induced direct suppression, and intestinal bleeding. However, the blood film gives the answer away. As discussed previously, in the MRCP examination there are classic questions and classic associations. In this case, the fragmented red cells and burr cells should immediately alert you to the problem of microangiopathic haemolytic anaemia. All it then requires is for you to identify the cause from all the rubbishy information that you have been given. Of importance is the fact that he is being treated for prostatic cancer – although this has been well controlled, it must be the cause of his problem.

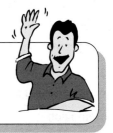

**A88**  a) Diagnosis

iv) Microangiopathic haemolytic anaemia secondary to prostatic cancer

Remind yourselves of the causes of this condition. Write them in the space below, then look at the list that follows.

_____

_____

_____

_____

_____

_____

## Causes of microangiopathic haemolytic anaemia

- Growths: cancers, foetuses (eclampsia, abruption, intrauterine death, amniotic fluid embolus)
- Damage to small vessels: malignant hypertension, vasculitides, burns, sepsis, disseminated intravascular coagulation
- Renal failure-associated: thrombotic thrombocytopenic purpura, haemolytic uraemic syndrome, acute glomerulonephritis
- Drugs: cytotoxic agents, cyclosporin

**Q89** A 26-year-old man is seen in the fertility clinic with his wife. He complains of low libido and is concerned at his lack of sexual development. He claims to shave only once every 1–2 weeks. Otherwise, he has no significant medical history and has only occasionally used arnica for chilblains.

## ON EXAMINATION

- Height = 1.96 m
- Weight = 75 kg
- Bilateral gynaecomastia
- Scanty pubic hair
- Small testes

## INVESTIGATIONS

- Serum testosterone = 7 nmol/l (normal: 9–35 nmol/l)
- Serum LH = 16 IU/l (normal: 1–10 IU/l)
- Serum FSH = 28 IU/l (normal: 1–7 IU/l)
- Serum HCG = <5 IU/l

FSH: follicle-stimulating hormone; HCG: human chorionic gonadotrophin; LH: luteinising hormone.

### a) What is the underlying diagnosis?

- i)   congenital adrenal hyperplasia
- ii)  Klinefelter's syndrome
- iii) prolactinoma
- iv)  Kallmann's syndrome
- v)   Marfan's syndrome

### b) How would you confirm this?

- i)   MRI scan of the pituitary
- ii)  serum 17-hydroxylase levels
- iii) serum 21-hydroxylase levels
- iv)  chromosomal analysis
- v)   ultrasound of the testis

Hypogonadism plus gynaecomastia plus tall and slim!

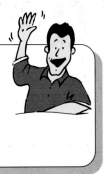

**A89** a) **Diagnosis**
  ii) Primary hypogonadism secondary to
  Klinefelter's syndrome
 b) **Test**
  iv) Chromosomal analysis (47XXY)

## FEATURES OF KLINEFELTER'S SYNDROME

- Tall
- Gynaecomastia
- Usually of normal intelligence
- Azoospermia, with small testes
- Diabetes mellitus
- Autoimmune disorders are more common
- Increased risk of breast cancer and leukaemia

# Q90

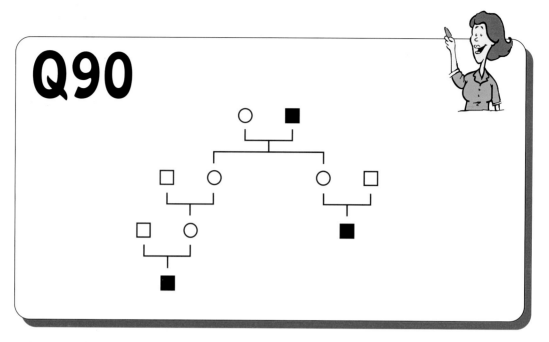

## a) What type of inheritance is shown?

i)     autosomal dominant

ii)    autosomal recessive

iii)   sex-linked recessive

iv)    Y-linked

v)     X-linked dominant

## b) Which of the following is inherited in this manner?

i)     Huntington's disease

ii)    haemophilia A

iii)   cystic fibrosis

iv)    Aicardi syndrome

v)     Marfan's syndrome

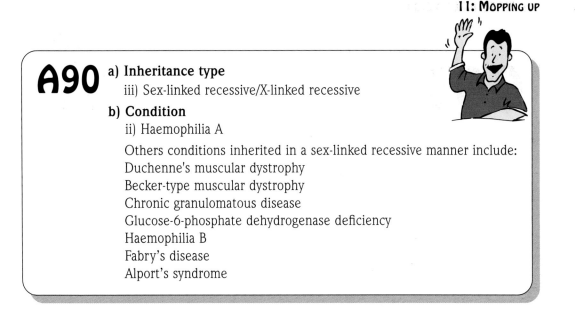

**A90**   **a) Inheritance type**
   iii) Sex-linked recessive/X-linked recessive

**b) Condition**
   ii) Haemophilia A

   Others conditions inherited in a sex-linked recessive manner include:
   Duchenne's muscular dystrophy
   Becker-type muscular dystrophy
   Chronic granulomatous disease
   Glucose-6-phosphate dehydrogenase deficiency
   Haemophilia B
   Fabry's disease
   Alport's syndrome

That came a bit out of the blue didn't it? We apologise wholeheartedly for including a genetic diagram such as this. The only problem is that this type of question has come up in the past. Just remember the patterns. We hope that this type of question will be eliminated in the future. (If you are a keen geneticist then we wish you all the best for an exciting career. No, honestly!)

# QUIZ SPOT!

**Q:** Who were the three 'born unlucky' as causes of peripheral neuropathy?
And who were the three dejected, two infected, two injected, one connected, and the granulomata suspected as causes?

A: See page 42.

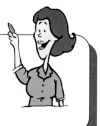

# Q91

A 13-year-old girl is seen in the emergency department with sudden onset of shortness of breath that occurred during a lesson at school. On arrival in the emergency department, an arterial blood gas is taken on air.

| INVESTIGATIONS | RESULTS |
| --- | --- |
| pH | 7.63 |
| $pCO_2$ | 2.6 kPa |
| $pO_2$ | 17.8 kPa |
| Bicarbonate | 22 mmol/l |
| Chest X-ray | Normal |
| Electrocardiogram | Normal |

## a) What is the most likely diagnosis?

- i) pneumothorax
- ii) pulmonary embolism
- iii) hyperventilation
- iv) acute/brittle asthma
- v) early stages of salicylate overdose

## b) How would you manage this girl?

- i) reassurance
- ii) nebulised and intravenous salbutamol
- iii) urgent CT scan of the chest
- iv) needle thoracocentesis
- v) transfer to the intensive care unit

This patient has respiratory alkalosis.

## CAUSES OF RESPIRATORY ALKALOSIS

- Pulmonary embolism
- Early stages of salicylate overdose
- Hysterical hyperventilation
- Any cause of a metabolic acidosis

Most are unlikely on the basis of the other investigations. This makes hysterical hyperventilation the most likely. As a point of examination technique, the examiners do not like you putting paper bags over patients' faces, so reassurance is therefore the correct answer to part b.

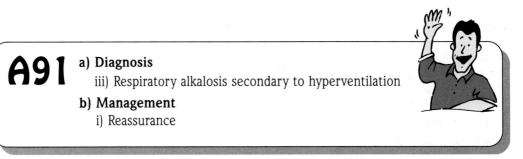

**A91** a) **Diagnosis**
   iii) Respiratory alkalosis secondary to hyperventilation
b) **Management**
   i) Reassurance

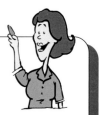

# Q92

A 27-year-old homosexual man returns from a visit to India. Prior to his visit he had been well, except for one episode of nonspecific urethritis that was treated at a sexually transmitted disease (STD) clinic 3 years ago. This settled the symptoms and he has had no further STDs. Before travelling to India, he contacted his local travel clinic and was vaccinated for hepatitis A, hepatitis B, typhoid, and cholera. Furthermore, he took antimalarial drugs as prescribed. During the visit, he was careful about hygiene and only ate in hotels, drank bottled water, and swam in the hotel pool. Two days after his return, he developed a febrile illness, associated with a diffuse rash and sore throat. He went to see his GP, who noticed that in addition to the maculo-papular rash he had diffuse lymphadenopathy and a smooth, 1 cm enlargement of the liver. His throat was reddened, with a white exudate. In addition, he was febrile with a temperature of 37.4°C.

| INVESTIGATIONS | RESULTS |
|---|---|
| 3 × malarial screens | Negative |
| Haemoglobin | 12.3 g/dl |
| White cell count | $12.5 \times 10^9/l$ |
| Lymphocytes | 90% |
| Platelets | $140 \times 10^9/l$ |
| Urinalysis and electrolytes | Normal |
| Monospot | Negative |
| Cytomegalovirus | Negative |
| TPHA | Negative |
| FTA-ABS | Negative |
| HIV I/II | Negative |
| Anti-streptolysin O titre | Negative |
| Chest X-ray | NAD |
| Blood culture | Negative |
| Urine culture | Negative |
| Throat culture | Negative |

FTA-ABS: fluorescent treponemal antibody absorbed test; NAD: no abnormality detected; TPHA: *Treponema pallidum* haemagglutination.

a) **What is the most likely diagnosis?**

    i)     typhoid

    ii)    syphilis

    iii)   HIV seroconversion illness

    iv)   hepatitis E

    v)    infectious mononucleosis

b) **What test would you perform to confirm your diagnosis?**

    i)     P24 antigen test

    ii)    blood cultures

    iii)   bone marrow aspirate

    iv)   lymph node biopsy

    v)    liver biopsy

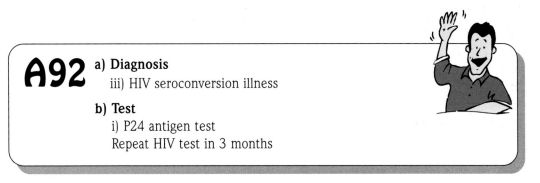

**A92**  a) **Diagnosis**
          iii) HIV seroconversion illness

        b) **Test**
          i) P24 antigen test
          Repeat HIV test in 3 months

This is one of the classic MRCP examination questions and this type of question is difficult to cover easily in a text of this size. You are faced with a patient who has been abroad and who, to all intents and purposes, has glandular fever, and yet every test that you are given is negative. This should therefore alert you to the fact that this is a 'catch-question'. If you work through the possible causes of a glandular-fever-like illness – cytomegalovirus, Epstein–Barr virus, or HIV – then there really isn't any problem. You are left with only one possible diagnosis, so treat yourself and write it down!

We are sorry that we couldn't cover how to answer this question within the book before now. But now you have seen it!

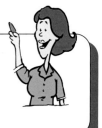

# Q93

A 53-year-old man presents to the respiratory outpatient clinic with increasing shortness of breath. He has never smoked. His lung function tests are recorded below.

| TEST | PATIENT | PREDICTED |
| --- | --- | --- |
| $FEV_1$ | 2.2 l | 4.5 l |
| FVC | 2.8 l | 5.2 l |
| TLC | 4.5 l | 6.0 l |
| DLCO | 14 ml/min/mmHg | 24 ml/min/mmHg |

DLCO: diffusing capacity for carbon monoxide; $FEV_1$: forced expiratory volume in 1 second; FVC: forced vital capacity; TLC: total lung capacity.

### a) What does this test reveal?

### b) What is the most likely diagnosis?
    i)   cryptogenic fibrosing alveolitis (usual interstitial pneumonia – UIP)
    ii)  pulmonary emboli
    iii) asthma
    iv)  myasthenia gravis
    v)   bronchiectasis

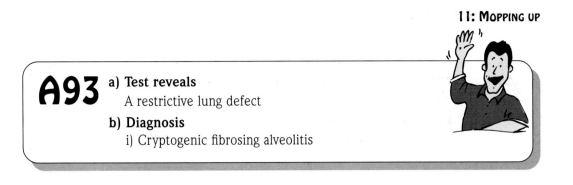

**A93** a) **Test reveals**
    A restrictive lung defect
  b) **Diagnosis**
    i) Cryptogenic fibrosing alveolitis

A number of classic patterns of pulmonary function appear in the MRCP examination. To understand these requires you to know the meaning of the various types of lung volume.

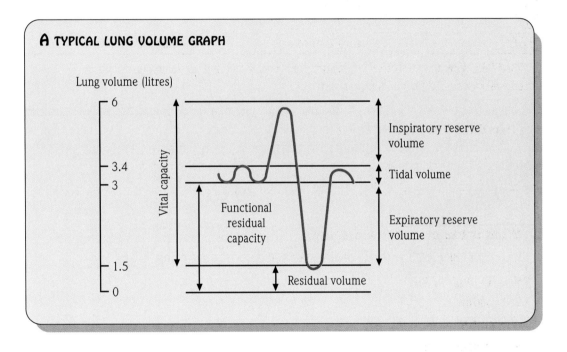

**A TYPICAL LUNG VOLUME GRAPH**

A restrictive pattern results in the reduction in both forced expiratory volume in 1 second ($FEV_1$) and forced vital capacity (FVC) with a normal $FEV_1$/FVC ratio. These diseases result in a significant reduction in total lung capacity, with a parallel reduction in the functional residual capacity, residual volume, and vital capacity. Furthermore, there is a reduction in the carbon monoxide transfer factor (TLCO) (or KCO [transfer coefficient of carbon monoxide] when TLCO is corrected for lung volumes) due to inefficiency of the lungs.

## Causes of a low TLCO

- Emphysema
- Pulmonary emboli
- Pulmonary fibrosis
- Ageing
- Pulmonary oedema
- Low cardiac output states

## Causes of a raised TLCO

- Asthma (although TLCO can also be normal)
- Pulmonary haemorrhage (Wegener's granulomatosis, Goodpasture's syndrome)
- Left-to-right cardiac shunting

An obstructive pulmonary function test pattern results in a reduction in the peak expiratory flow rate and $FEV_1$ with a reduction in the $FEV_1/FVC$ ratio. Typically, the FVC is normal in early disease, but is reduced in more severe disease as the residual volume is increased as a consequence of air trapping.

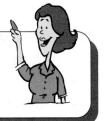

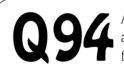 **Q94** A 36-year-old man has a cardiac catheterisation as part of his investigation for breathlessness. The following data are obtained.

| CAVITY | PRESSURE (MMHG) |
| --- | --- |
| Right atrial end diastolic | 8 |
| Right ventricular end diastolic | 4 |
| Pulmonary wedge | 19 |
| Pulmonary artery | 64/32 |
| Left ventricular end diastolic | 12 |

### a) What are the most likely valve abnormalities?

i) mitral regurgitation and tricuspid regurgitation

ii) aortic stenosis and mitral stenosis

iii) tricuspid stenosis and mitral stenosis

iv) aortic regurgitation and mitral regurgitation

v) pulmonary stenosis and tricuspid stenosis

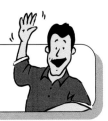

**A94** a) Likely abnormalities

iii) Tricuspid stenosis and mitral stenosis

## MEAN (RANGE) NORMAL CARDIAC PRESSURES (MMHG)

| | | | |
|---|---|---|---|
| Right atrial | Mean | 4 | (0–8) |
| Right ventricular | Systolic | 25 | (15–30) |
| | Diastolic | 4 | (0–8) |
| Pulmonary artery | Systolic | 25 | (15–30) |
| | Diastolic | 10 | (5–15) |
| | Mean | 15 | (10–20) |
| Left atrial | Mean | 7 | (4–12) |
| Left ventricular | Systolic | 120 | (90–140) |
| | Diastolic | 7 | (4–12) |
| Aortic | Systolic | 120 | (90–140) |
| | Diastolic | 70 | (60–90) |
| | Mean | 85 | (70–105) |

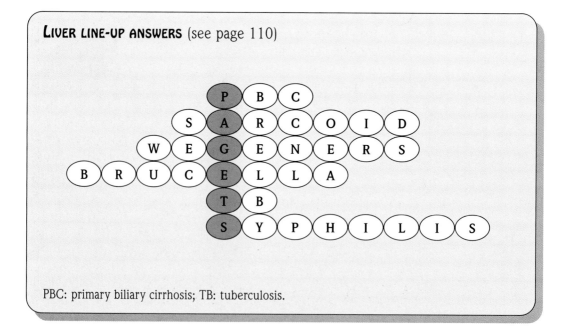

**LIVER LINE-UP ANSWERS** (see page 110)

PBC: primary biliary cirrhosis; TB: tuberculosis.

# QUIZ SPOT!

**Q:** What are the causes of cerebrospinal fluid lymphocytosis?

A: See page 41 for our list.

**SOLUTION TO SIADH PUZZLE** (see page 213)

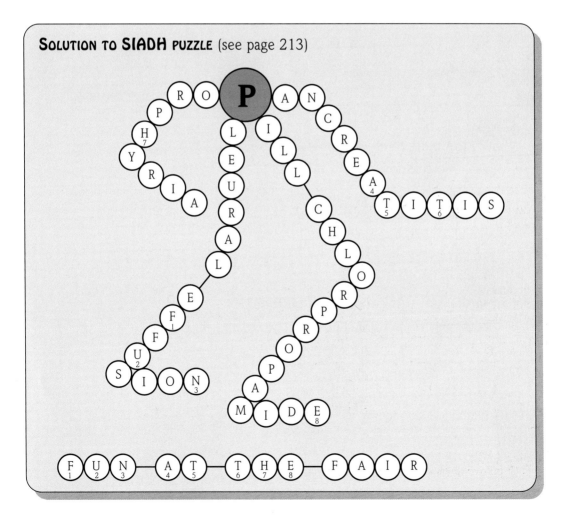

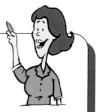

# Q95

A 32-year-old man presents to the emergency department with a decreased level of consciousness. He was well until 3 hours previously when he complained of feeling cold. He was driven home from work by a friend, but seemed increasingly lethargic, became confused, and then rapidly lost consciousness. Previously, he has been relatively fit except for an episode of pneumonia as a child. He is not receiving any medication, drinks only a moderate amount of alcohol, and smokes 10 cigarettes per day.

| INVESTIGATIONS | RESULTS |
|---|---|
| Temperature | 38.5°C |
| Blood pressure | 90/50 mmHg |
| Pulse | 110 beats/min |
| Kernig's sign | Negative |
| Meningism | Negative |
| Glasgow Coma Scale | 8 |
| Lower limbs | Diffuse, nonblanching, petechial rash |

### a) What is the most likely diagnosis?

i) meningococcal meningitis

ii) scarlet fever

iii) staphylococcal toxic-shock syndrome

iv) meningococcal septicaemia

v) toxoplasmosis

### b) What is the first thing that you would do?

i) urgent lumbar puncture

ii) high-dose intravenous benzylpenicillin

iii) urgent CT scan

iv) high-dose intravenous ceftriaxone

v) endotracheal intubation

c) **Give two tests to confirm your diagnosis.**

    i)       blood cultures and lumbar puncture

    ii)     serology and fundoscopy

    iii)    blood cultures and CT scan

    iv)    serology and CT scan

    v)     blood cultures and urine cultures

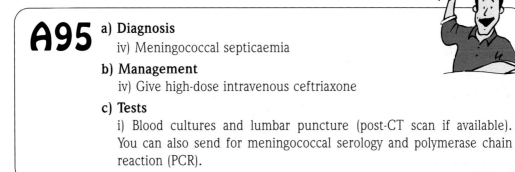

**A95**   a) **Diagnosis**
        iv) Meningococcal septicaemia

       b) **Management**
        iv) Give high-dose intravenous ceftriaxone

       c) **Tests**
        i) Blood cultures and lumbar puncture (post-CT scan if available). You can also send for meningococcal serology and polymerase chain reaction (PCR).

This question often graced the pages of the MRCP written examination, when it existed. In the newer best-of-five format, it is highly likely that the same question will appear in its new incarnation. However, it is important to choose the correct answer. For example, meningococcal meningitis would not score any marks, but meningococcal septicaemia would. In part b, the correct answer according to the latest guidelines would be ceftriaxone as opposed to penicillin. This exemplifies the importance of being up-to-date with the guidelines for common conditions that you might see as a medical registrar.

The issue of serology and PCR is important. In the past, physicians have erroneously held off antibiotics (especially in those with meningitis) in the hope of sending cerebrospinal fluid/blood to the laboratory for culture first. Always treat first; you can send off cerebrospinal fluid or blood for meningococcal antigen testing many hours after the event.

Always watch out for other complications – your examiners will. Apart from shock, these patients almost all get a coagulopathy, whether or not this is frank disseminated intravascular coagulation. Remember to correct this; there is evidence that provision of protein C (an anti-clotting factor) may improve prognosis, especially in children. This form of meningitis can be complicated by acute haemorrhagic adrenal failure and is known as the Waterhouse–Friderichsen syndrome. In meningitis and in proven septicaemia, remember to treat contacts with rifampicin or ciprofloxacin – Carter got his residency in *ER* for remembering that!

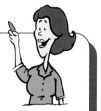

**Q96** A 34-year-old man presents with a deep vein thrombosis of his right leg. He had a similar episode affecting his left leg 3 years ago, for which he received warfarin for 3 months with no complications. At the age of 31 years he presented with an acutely painful eye, which was diagnosed as an anterior uveitis. In addition, he has suffered from recurrent episodes of knee and arm pain and has been investigated by rheumatologists for this, but no diagnosis has been made. He also admits to suffering from mouth ulcers, for which he takes over-the-counter remedies.

| INVESTIGATIONS | RESULTS |
|---|---|
| Haemoglobin | 12.4 g/dl |
| White cell count | 6.8 (normal differential) × $10^9$/l |
| Platelets | 253 × $10^9$/l |
| Erythrocyte sedimentation rate | 25 mm in first hour |
| Plasma sodium | 134 mmol/l |
| Plasma potassium | 4.2 mmol/l |
| Plasma urea | 4 mmol/l |
| Plasma creatinine | 89 μmol/l |
| Liver function tests | Normal |
| Urinalysis | NAD |
| Chest X-ray | Normal |
| Doppler ultrasound right leg | Extensive DVT |
| ANCA | Negative |
| Anti-nuclear antibodies | Negative |
| Anti-double-stranded DNA | Negative |
| Rhesus factor | Negative |
| Ham's acid lysis/acidified serum test | Negative |

ANCA: anti-neutrophilic cytoplasmic antibodies; DVT: deep vein thrombosis;
NAD: no abnormality detected.

### a) What is the most likely diagnosis?

i) anti-phospholipid syndrome

ii) Behçet's syndrome

iii) Reiter's syndrome

iv) hyperhomocysteinaemia

v) ulcerative colitis

## b) How would you confirm the diagnosis?

i)     anti-phospholipid antibody

ii)    human leucocyte antigen (HLA)-B27 testing

iii)   serum homocysteine levels

iv)    colonoscopy

v)     clinical grounds only

## c) What is the inheritance pattern?

i)     autosomal dominant

ii)    autosomal recessive

iii)   X-linked dominant

iv)    X-linked recessive

v)     unknown

This requires knowledge of a number of lists: the causes of recurrent oral ulceration, anterior uveitis, recurrent deep vein thrombosis, and polyarthropathy (write this last list down or cheat and look it up in the list of lists at the end of the book).

## CAUSES OF RECURRENT ORAL ULCERATION

- Aphthous ulcers
- Inflammatory bowel disease (IBD) (ulcerative colitis/Crohn's disease)*
- Behçet's syndrome*
- Reiter's syndrome*
- Seronegative arthritis
- Coeliac disease
- Other causes of malabsorption (see earlier list, page 185)
- Pemphigus (and, rarely, pemphigoid)
- SLE

*These cause both oral and genital ulcers.

## CAUSES OF AN ANTERIOR UVEITIS

- infectious: cytomegalovirus, toxoplasmosis, syphilis, tuberculosis
- neoplastic conditions: lymphomas
- systemic diseases: ankylosing spondylitis, Reiter's syndrome, Behçet's syndrome, sarcoidosis, IBD, psoriatic arthropathy, juvenile arthritis, Kawasaki's disease
- others: drug-induced (e.g. rifabutin)

## CAUSES OF RECURRENT DEEP VEIN THROMBOSIS

- thrombophilia: antithrombin III deficiency, protein S or protein C deficiency, factor V Leiden mutation
- dysfibrinogenaemia
- factor XII deficiency
- malignancy
- surgery and trauma
- post-operative
- drugs: oral contraceptive pill
- hyperhomocystinaemia
- Behçet's syndrome
- anti-phospholipid syndrome
- paroxysmal nocturnal haemoglobinuria
- nephrotic syndrome

## CAUSES OF POLYARTHROPATHY (WHICH YOU KNOW)

If you can remember the first two lists, have a working knowledge of the third, and know the fourth then this question is an absolute gift.

**A96**

a) **Diagnosis**

ii) Behçet's syndrome

b) **Test**

v) Clinical grounds only! There are no specific tests for Behçet's syndrome.

c) **Inheritance pattern**

v) Unknown. A genetic basis has been suggested, with an increased prevalence of histocompatibility class HLA-B5. Affected children of patients with Behçet's syndrome may have an earlier age of onset, which is termed genetic anticipation. In many genetic disorders, this characteristic has been linked to an increased number of nucleotide repeats within each successive generation.

## CLINICAL FEATURES OF BEHÇET'S SYNDROME

- Predominantly affects males – HLA-B5
- Predominates along the old trade routes – Japan, China, Iran, Turkey, and the Mediterranean
- Oral, gastrointestinal, and genital ulceration (nasty!)
- Skin: pustules (at venepuncture sites ++), papules, erythema nodosum
- Eyes: anterior/posterior uveitis/cataracts
- Neurological: aseptic meningitis, cranial nerve palsies
- Vascular: recurrent venous and arterial thromboses
- Arthritis
- Renal: usually mild proteinuria, can get amyloidosis
- Treatment: topical or systemic steroids with or without colchicine; treat neurological/ocular symptoms with immunosuppressants

Behçet's syndrome is often a mimic of other arthritides, other autoimmune syndromes such as SLE/IBD, multiple sclerosis, or more commonly *Reiter's syndrome*. The single major difference between Behçet's syndrome and Reiter's syndrome is that the latter may be caught in the context of pleasure, while sufferers of the former have no such luck. More conventionally, Reiter's syndrome is chronologically related to infections, has different skin and genito-urinary manifestations (no erythema nodosum or pathergy, but balanitis is present), has different HLA associations, and less in the way of systemic side effects.

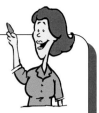

# Q97

A 34-year-old man is admitted to the emergency department with central chest pain of 2 hours, duration. The pain started initially in his back and was of great severity. He vomited three times and felt dizzy at the onset of the pain. In the past, he has suffered from repeated right-sided pneumothoraces, requiring a pleurodesis 2 years ago. He has also had a number of eye problems and was diagnosed last year with a lens dislocation and blue sclerae. He also has mild asthma for which he takes salbutamol and beclometasone inhalers.

On examination, he is a tall, thin man who appears unwell. He is sweating and has a pulse of 120 beats per minute in sinus rhythm. His blood pressure is 121/82 mmHg. He has a right thoracotomy scar. His abdomen is soft, but not tender.

| INVESTIGATIONS | RESULTS |
| --- | --- |
| Serial electrocardiograms | Sinus tachycardia only |
| Chest X-ray | No focal lung lesion |
| | Prominent mediastinum |
| Creatinine kinase | 120 IU/l (normal: 0–200 IU/l) |
| Plasma sodium | 135 mmol/l |
| Plasma potassium | 4.8 mmol/l |
| Plasma urea | 3.2 mmol/l |
| Plasma creatinine | 89 μmol/l |
| Liver function tests | Normal |

## a) What is the most likely underlying diagnosis?

i) Noonan's syndrome

ii) Klinefelter's syndrome

iii) Aicardi syndrome

iv) Kallmann's syndrome

v) Marfan's syndrome

**b) What two diagnostic tests would you do next?**

   i)     blood pressure in both arms and CT scan

   ii)    CT scan and transoesophageal echocardiogram

   iii)   blood pressure in both arms and MRI scan

   iv)    MRI scan and transthoracic echocardiogram

   v)     blood pressure in both arms and transthoracic echocardiogram

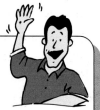

**A97**  **a) Diagnosis**

v) Marfan's syndrome. He has now presented with a dissecting thoracic aneurysm.

**b) What two diagnostic tests would you do next**

iii) Check the blood pressure in both arms. An MRI scan is superior to a CT scan of the chest, which is superior to a transoesophageal echocardiogram, which in turn is superior to a transthoracic echocardiogram.

This patient has a fairly classical case of Marfan's syndrome. He is tall and thin, and has experienced a number of well-recognised complications of this condition. Again, it is a case of recognising the syndrome and then the answer is obvious.

Answering the question requires the knowledge of a list that we haven't yet given you – causes of blue sclerae.

### CAUSES OF BLUE SCLERAE

Remember the POKEMon craze?

   •    Pseudoxanthoma elasticum

   •    Osteogenesis imperfecta

   •    Kongenital

   •    Ehlers–Danlos syndrome

   •    Marfan's syndrome

## Marfan's syndrome

"The only way is up" – this song describes the condition beautifully, in particular the way that the lens dislocates (compare it with homocystinuria, in which dislocation occurs downwards). Marfan's syndrome has multiple complications that may appear in the written or clinical parts of the examination:

- lung: repeated pneumothoraces
- cardiac: aortic dissection, aortic regurgitation, mitral valve prolapse, regurgitation
- eyes: 'upward' lens dislocation, blue sclera, retinal detachment

It has to be said, at this point, that one of the authors has fond memories of a patient with Marfan's who was seen as his MRCP long case. He failed the case and was given a score of 2 out of 6 because he was unable to tell the examiners what the patient's brother did for a living. One of the examiners was heard to tell another candidate who saw the patient later (as a short case) that this patient's brother bred pigs for valve replacements, and they had been failing candidates earlier that day for not telling them this as part of the social history. You have been warned: take a full social history in the examination.

## For the record

EJA Marfan (1858–1942), French paediatrician.

**Q98** A 43-year-old woman presents to the endocrinology outpatient clinic with recurrent episodes of dizziness with collapse. She is admitted to the hospital for further investigation. During one of these episodes her blood glucose is noted to be 1 mmol/l. A serum sample is sent with the following results – serum glucose 1.3 mmol/l. She has never suffered from diabetes and nor has any member of her family. She is not on any routine medication. In the past, she was investigated for hypercalcaemia and a parathyroid adenoma was discovered that was successfully resected with no long-term problems.

### a) What two investigations would you next perform?

    i)    serum insulin level and MRI scan of the abdomen

    ii)   insulin C-peptide level and CT scan of the abdomen

    iii)  serum insulin level and insulin C-peptide level

    iv)   oral glucose tolerance test and insulin levels

    v)    serum glucagon level and CT scan of the abdomen

### b) What is the relationship between hypoglycaemia and a parathyroid adenoma?

    i)    multiple endocrine neoplasia (MEN) type I

    ii)   MEN type IIa

    iii)  MEN type IIb

    iv)   polyglandular autoimmune syndrome type I

    v)    polyglandular autoimmune syndrome type II

**A98** **a) Investigations**
    ii) Insulin C-peptide levels
    CT scan of the abdomen looking for an insulinoma

**b) Hypoglycaemia and parathyroid adenoma**
    i) MEN type I

This patient is under investigation for a cause of her dizziness. Clearly the patient has become hypoglycaemic. The important part of this case is to recognise the link between hypoglycaemia and her pituitary adenoma.

## MEN TYPE I (THE THREE Ps) – WERMER SYNDROME
- Parathyroid adenoma
- Pancreatic adenoma: insulinoma, Zollinger–Ellison syndrome/gastrinoma and glucagonoma, Cushing's syndrome, and carcinoids are also recognised
- Pituitary tumour

Note: glucagonoma is an islet α-cell-derived pancreatic tumour. The clinical features include necrolytic erythema migrans, diabetes mellitus, weight loss, anaemia, cheilitis, stomatitis, thromboembolism, gastrointestinal disturbances, and neuropsychiatric disturbances.

Glucagon, liver disease, aberrant fatty acids, and zinc deficiency states may also contribute to the pathogenesis of the eruption in some cases – hence the zinc treatment. It is often caught late and is treated with cytotoxic drugs and palliative care.

## MEN TYPE II SYNDROMES
These are characterised by their predisposition to medullary thyroid carcinomas, which are seen in 70%–80% of cases, and phaeochromocytomas (seen in 60% of cases).

## MEN TYPE IIA (SIPPLE'S SYNDROME)
- Phaeochromocytoma
- Medullary cancer of the thyroid
- Parathyroid hyperplasia
- Hirschsprung's disease

## MEN TYPE IIB
- Phaeochromocytoma
- Medullary cancer of the thyroid plus skin (neuromas, pigmentation) plus marfanoid habitus plus intestinal ganglioneuromatosis

---

**TIP**

It is important to note that, in the MRCP examination, if hypoglycaemia occurs in a healthcare professional then the examiners may be thinking of insulin or sulphonylurea self-administration. In the latter, the C-peptide level will also be raised, as in insulinoma. Thus, a measure of urinary sulphonylurea must be performed.

---

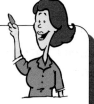

**Q99** A 56-year-old man presents with a 3-hour history of central crushing chest pain associated with sweating, nausea, and vomiting. He admits to being unwell, and has been vomiting for the last 7 days following a prolonged alcoholic binge. He has not vomited any blood. He usually drinks a bottle of vodka a day plus several cans of strong lager. He has been investigated for possible angina in the past, and had a 30% stenosis of the right coronary artery on an angiogram 2 years ago. He does not usually take any medication, although he took aspirin for a few weeks following the angiogram, but failed to attend for follow-up. He had an over-sew of a bleeding duodenal ulcer 10 years ago and has not had any problems since. In addition, he has recently been diagnosed by his GP with chronic obstructive pulmonary disease and is a smoker of 30 cigarettes per day. However, he has not used the inhalers that he was prescribed. He usually works as a labourer on a building site, but has not suffered any recent trauma.

On examination, he appears unwell and has tachycardia with a pulse of 110 beats/min. His blood pressure is 122/80 mmHg and he has pyrexia with a temperature of 38.3°C. He also has surgical emphysema in the right supraclavicular fossa and stigmata of chronic liver disease, including a left Dupuytren's contracture, palmar erythema, and multiple spider naevi on his anterior chest wall. He is cardiovascularly stable and has no murmurs. He has a respiratory rate of 20 breaths/min with an oxygen saturation of 91%.

| INVESTIGATIONS | RESULTS |
| --- | --- |
| Haemoglobin | 12.6 g/dl |
| Mean corpuscular volume | 101 fl |
| White cell count | $14.2 \times 10^9$/l |
| Neutrophils | $12.8 \times 10^9$/l |
| Platelets | $62 \times 10^9$/l |
| Plasma sodium | 131 mmol/l |
| Plasma potassium | 3.2 mmol/l |
| Plasma urea | 3.1 mmol/l |
| Plasma creatinine | 93 μmol/l |
| Serum aspartate aminotransferase | 65 IU/l (normal: 5–15 IU/l) |
| Serum alanine aminotransferase | 32 IU/l (normal: 5–15 IU/l) |
| Serum alkaline phosphatase | 195 IU/l |
| Serum albumin | 32 g/l |
| Serum creatinine kinase | 65 IU/l (normal: 0–190 IU/l) |
| Clotting international normalised ratio | 1.2 |
| Electrocardiogram | Sinus tachycardia, no evidence of acute ischaemia |

## a) What is the most likely diagnosis?

i)    Mallory–Weiss syndrome

ii)   Boerhaave's syndrome

iii)  acute myocardial infarction

iv)   dissecting aortic aneurysm

v)    perforated gastric ulcer

## b) What test will confirm the diagnosis?

i)    electrocardiogram

ii)   MRI scan

iii)  Chest X-ray

iv)   CT scan

v)    endoscopy

This initially appears to be a complex question in which there are a lot of leads. However, as is often the case in the MRCP examination, there is a give-away clue. Again, if you can spot the clue then the diagnosis is obvious. In this case, the fact that the patient has surgical emphysema and has had prolonged vomiting should quickly lead you to the diagnosis of oesophageal perforation (Boerhaave's syndrome).

**A99**

**a) Diagnosis**
   ii) Oesophageal perforation (Boerhaave's syndrome) secondary to recurrent vomiting.

**b) Test**
   iii) Chest X-ray. In this case it showed mediastinal air.
   A Gastrografin swallow may also confirm the diagnosis.

## BOERHAAVE'S SYNDROME

Hermann Boerhaave (1668–1738) was a Dutch physician who was the first to describe oesophageal perforation in a Dutch seaman who presented to him with central chest pain and rapidly died. At autopsy, an oesophageal perforation was diagnosed with the patient's gastric contents within the mediastinum (or so the story goes).

An alternative theory is that all the above is bulls**t and in fact he just decided to have a syndrome named after him, which was a popular pasttime during this era. As many of you are aware, a lot of physical signs have eponymous names.

### ANSWERS TO PRESENTATION PUZZLE (see page 175)

Here are the diseases and presenting features:

| Presenting condition | Carpal tunnel | BHL | Bronchiectasis | Lung fibrosis |
|---|---|---|---|---|
| George | Acromegaly | Sarcoid | Kartagener's | Sarcoid |
| Michael | TB | TB | TB | TB |
| Sarah | Pregnancy | TB | TB | Pigeons |
| Nicole | TB | Phenytoin | *Aspergillus* | TB |
| Peter | Gout | CF | CF | Amiodarone |
| Ruth | RA | EAA | Yellow nail | EAA |

BHL: bilateral hilar lymphadenopathy; CF: cystic fibrosis; EAA: extrinsic allergic alveolitis; TB: tuberculosis.

George and Ruth are the least infected. Neither has an infectious disease. Peter has cystic fibrosis, and thus chronic chest infection. Serum angiotensin-converting enzyme (ACE) levels might be elevated in all of the patients. Although sarcoid classically raises serum ACE levels, so too does lung fibrosis in general. This is perhaps especially true of tuberculous scarring.

# Q100

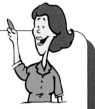

An 80-year-old man presents to the emergency department with erythroderma. The only history that is available is from his elderly wife, who is clearly upset and attributes his acute illness to the GP who had given the patient amoxycillin for his third chest infection of the year. Although the patient had suggested he was allergic to penicillin, he had received (against the wishes of his wife) the drug for the first and third infections and a macrolide for the second infection. His wife is also upset that her husband was recently given the diagnosis of bronchiectasis. He has also recently suffered from cellulitis, for which he was given clindamycin.

On examination, the patient has an exfoliative dermatitis with scaling erythematous dermatitis involving 90% or more of the surface area. He is confused and scratching himself uncontrollably. He also has periorbital inflammation, splenomegaly, and retromandibular lymphadenopathy.

| INVESTIGATIONS | RESULTS |
| --- | --- |
| Haemoglobin | 12.6 g/dl |
| White cell count | 35.8 × 10⁹/l |
| Neutrophils | 12.8 × 10⁹/l |
| Platelets | 62 × 10⁹/l |
| Plasma sodium | 131 mmol/l |
| Plasma potassium | 3.2 mmol/l |
| Plasma urea | 15.0 mmol/l |
| Plasma creatinine | 300 μmol/l |
| Serum aspartate aminotransferase | 12 IU/l (normal: 5–15 IU/l) |
| Serum alanine aminotransferase | 12 IU/l (normal: 5–15 IU/l) |
| Serum alkaline phosphatase | 195 IU/l |
| Serum albumin | 20 g/l |
| Creatinine kinase | 300 IU/l (normal: 0–190 IU/l) |
| Clotting international normalised ratio | 1.0 |

## a) What is the cause of this man's acute illness?

i)  allergic reaction to penicillin

ii)  infectious mononucleosis

iii)  psoriasis

iv)  chronic lymphocytic leukaemia

v)  atopic dermatitis

Despite the obvious red herring of the drug-induced erythroderma (who said the examiners were subtle!), clearly the patient has had cellulitis, bronchiectasis, and recurrent pneumonias – he must be immunocompromised. Furthermore, he has splenomegaly and lymphadenopathy. Thus, he must have chronic lymphocytic leukaemia (CLL).

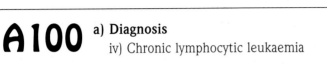

**A100** a) **Diagnosis**
iv) Chronic lymphocytic leukaemia

CLL is a clonal proliferation of mature lymphocytes, normally B-cells, with accumulation in the blood, bone marrow, lymph nodes, and spleen. It is the most common form of leukaemia in adults, predominantly affecting the elderly (mean age 64 years). Its pathogenesis is thought to be linked to abnormal tumour suppressor genes, such as *BCL-1* and the oncogene *C-MYC*. Lymphocyte counts are >10,000 per mm³ of blood. Cells can be identified by their cell surface markers: CD19, CD20, and CD5 (note, CD stands for cluster of differentiation). Clinically, patients are often identified incidentally with an indolent lymphocytosis. Lymphadenopathy, organomegaly, and bone marrow involvement with pancytopenia may also be present. Immunological complications include immunoparesis due to depressed immunoglobulin levels, which result in recurrent respiratory and other infections and bronchiectasis. Other immunological phenomena include direct Coombs-test-positive haemolytic anaemia and immune thrombocytopenia/neutropenia. CLL can also transform into a number of haematological tumours – the most feared of which is large cell lymphoma. Patients also get homme rouge, which is a form of erythroderma. Please don't be caught out – they have warm haemolytic anaemia (i.e. evidence of haemolysis at room temperature), but *also* have cryoglobulins.

The overall 5-year survival is approximately 60%, but depends on the stage of disease, serum levels of $\beta_2$-microglobulin, lactate dehydrogenase levels, the presence or absence of CD23, and cytogenetic abnormalities such as deletions in chromosome 11q and somatic mutations in the immunoglobulin heavy-chain genes. Antileukaemic therapy includes chlorambucil and fludarabine, a purine analogue, steroids, and monoclonal antibodies. Also note the need for antimicrobial therapy.

## RAI STAGING SYSTEM FOR CLL

| Stage 0 | Isolated lymphocytosis (>15,000/mm³) |
| --- | --- |
| Stage I | Lymphocytosis with lymphadenopathy |
| Stage II | Lymphocytosis with splenomegaly |
| Stage III | Lymphocytosis with anaemia (haemoglobin <11 g/dl) |
| Stage IV | Lymphocytosis and thrombocytopenia (<100,000/mm³) |

## CAUSES OF ERYTHRODERMA

| | |
|---|---|
| Dermatoses | Atopic dermatitis, candidiasis, contact dermatitis, dermatophytosis (e.g. tinea), ichthyosis, lichen planus, mastocytosis, nummular eczema, pemphigus, photosensitive eczema, pityriasis, psoriasis, Reiter's syndrome, scabies, seborrhoeic dermatitis, staphylococcal scalded skin syndrome |
| Autoimmune | Systemic lupus erythematosus |
| Malignancies | T-cell lymphomas and other lymphomas, leukaemias, internal visceral malignancies |
| Drugs | Many! |
| Miscellaneous | Hepatitis, HIV, congenital immunodeficiency syndromes (Omenn's syndrome), graft-versus-host disease |

Erythroderma with blood redistribution to the integumentary surface and exfoliation is reminiscent of severe burns. The catabolic state coupled with severe block of hepatic albumin synthesis and surface loss may lead to oedema. The large open wounds may result in sepsis and must be treated with broad-spectrum antibiotics. High-output cardiac failure may result from the massive redistribution of blood to the skin. Management requires close haemodynamic monitoring with covering of wounds to prevent hypothermia and sepsis. Perhaps the most important aspect of treatment is total body coverage with emollients, together with antihistamines for pruritus. Recently, evidence has accumulated for the use of systemic immunosuppression with corticosteroids and cyclosporin.

### ANSWERS TO JIGSAW PUZZLE (see page 316)

| | | | | | | | | | | | |
|---|---|---|---|---|---|---|---|---|---|---|---|
| | A | C | R | O | M | E | G | A | L | Y | |
| | R | E | F | S | U | M | S | | | | |
| T | H | A | L | A | S | S | A | E | M | I | A |
| | F | R | I | E | D | R | E | I | C | H | S |
| | | A | L | P | O | R | T | S | | | |

Acromegaly and thalassaemia are causes of angioid retinal streaks.

# Q101

Just before her fifth attempt at the MRCP examination, a 25-year-old woman presents to the emergency department with vomiting. She admits to taking 30 tablets of paracetamol 4 hours ago with a few glasses of wine at the thought of having to take the exam yet again! She has no other medical problems and takes no medications. She drinks a bottle of wine each night. In the emergency department she weighs 60 kg.

## a) How will you initially manage this woman?

   i)    immediately take blood for a paracetamol level

   ii)   gastric lavage and then take blood for a paracetamol level

   iii)  give activated charcoal

   iv)   start N-acetylcysteine

   v)    discharge once she has been seen by the psychiatrist

## b) 24 hours after treatment, which of the following is the strongest indicator of toxic liver damage from the paracetamol overdose?

   i)    an international normalised ratio of >1.5 at 24 hours

   ii)   agitation

   iii)  hyperglycaemia

   iv)   an alanine aminotransferase level of 830 IU/l

   v)    renal failure, with a creatinine level of 600 μmol/l

It is important to establish whether the patient has taken a single or staggered dose. In patients who have taken a single dose, establish the time the paracetamol was taken and whether patient is in the high-risk group for liver damage. A significant overdose is >10 g, or ≥75 mg/kg if the patient is in the high-risk group or ≥150 mg/kg if they are in the low-risk group.

## THE HIGHS AND LOWS OF LIFE

Have you ever wondered why we are concerned about whether the patient is above (low risk) or below (high risk) the treatment line?

Let's look at the pharmacology of paracetamol... Normally, paracetamol is metabolised in the liver by conjugation with glucuronide, sulphate, and cysteine into nontoxic metabolites. A small amount is metabolised via cytochrome P450 into N-acetyl p-benzoquinone imine (NAPQI), which is toxic to the liver. Glutathione inactivates the small amounts of NAPQI to make it harmless. In paracetamol overdose, glutathione becomes depleted and the excess NAPQI leads to toxic liver damage.

We can now work out who is in the high-risk group for liver damage from a lower level of plasma paracetamol:

- Patients on enzyme-inducing drugs such as phenytoin or carbamazepine can have increased production of NAPQI via cytochrome P450.

- Patients who are malnourished (e.g. anorexia nervosa, alcoholism) or who are HIV-positive are often glutathione depleted.

## MANAGEMENT OF OVERDOSE

- Within 1 hour of ingestion of a significant overdose, give activated charcoal. Unfortunately, our patient presented 4 hours post-ingestion, and therefore activated charcoal should not be used.

- Wait until 4 hours post-ingestion before taking the paracetamol level (paracetamol has a half-life of 1–4 hours).

- Patients who have taken a significant overdose, but present 8–24 hours post-ingestion, should have N-acetylcysteine while you wait for the paracetamol level. N-acetylcysteine and methionine replenish glutathione stores.

- Patients who have taken a significant overdose should have their clotting profile, renal and liver function, and venous bicarbonate level checked.

The criteria for liver transplantation in paracetamol-induced acute liver failure, based on the

*King's College Hospital* criteria and additional recent evidence, are:

- arterial pH <7.3, or arterial blood lactate concentration >3.0 mmol/l after adequate fluid resuscitation
- OR if all 3 of the following within a 24 hour period:
    1. creatinine >300 μmol/l
    2. INR >6.5
    3. grade III/IV encephalopathy

Evidence also suggests that a patient should be referred for transplantation if their arterial blood lactate concentration is >3.5 mmol/L after early fluid resuscitation.

### Did you know?

...in staggered overdose, paracetamol level is not interpretable on the nomogram because the measurement was derived from a single overdose

...a nomogram is less reliable if the patient presents late, especially after 15 hours, because the data is extrapolated beyond 15 hours

...management in these patients can be difficult, and should be guided by the paracetamol dose ingested, biochemical markers, risk assessment, and comorbidities

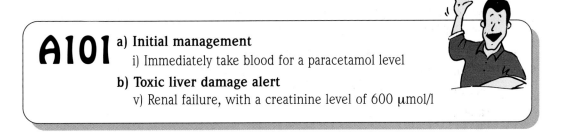

**A101**
a) **Initial management**
   i) Immediately take blood for a paracetamol level
b) **Toxic liver damage alert**
   v) Renal failure, with a creatinine level of 600 μmol/l

# Q102

A 65-year-old patient attends your outpatient clinic with a 4-week history of pain and stiffness in the shoulders, neck, thighs, and hips. Her symptoms are worse in the morning. At times, the pain is so severe that she finds it hard to carry out her normal daily tasks. Examination does not reveal any synovitis. There is pain on movement, but there is no weakness or alteration in sensation.

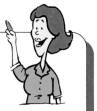

| INVESTIGATIONS | RESULTS |
| --- | --- |
| Haemoglobin | 9.7 g/dl |
| White cell count | 7.4 × 10⁹/l |
| Platelets | 189 × 10⁹/l |
| Plasma sodium | 138 mmol/l |
| Plasma potassium | 4.5 mmol/l |
| Plasma urea | 7.0 mmol/l |
| Plasma creatinine | 87 μmol/l |
| Creatine kinase | 100 U/l |
| Bilirubin | 12 μmol/l |
| Serum alkaline phosphatase | 180 IU/l |
| Serum alanine aminotransferase | 20 IU/l |
| Total protein | 72 g/l |
| Serum albumin | 34 g/l |
| Erythrocyte sedimentation rate | 60 mm/hour |
| Anti-nuclear antibodies | Weakly positive |
| Rheumatoid factor | Negative |
| X-rays of the shoulders, cervical spine, and hips | Normal |

## a) What is the most likely diagnosis?

i) polymyositis

ii) early-onset rheumatoid arthritis

iii) Paget's disease

iv) chronic inflammatory demyelinating polyneuropathy

v) polymyalgia rheumatica

Let's look at each of our options, one at a time...

## Polymyositis

The major feature of polymyositis is proximal muscle weakness, which this patient does not have. Patients with polymyositis often have difficulty rising from a chair or going up stairs. Dysphagia and dysphonia are important symptoms to elicit. The respiratory muscles can be affected, particularly in patients who are positive for anti-Jo-1 antibodies.

Patients can have cutaneous features in dermatomyositis, including a heliotrope rash on the cheeks and eyelids, and periorbital oedema. Polymyositis is associated with autoimmune disease and malignancy (lung, ovary, breast, and stomach cancer), particularly in males with dermatomyositis.

Creatine kinase is usually raised in polymyositis. The diagnosis requires electromyography and muscle biopsy.

## Early-onset rheumatoid arthritis

The most typical presentation is a progressive symmetrical polyarthropathy, with pain, swelling, and stiffness in the metacarpophalangeal, proximal interphalangeal, and distal interphalangeal joints of the hands and feet, as well as of the wrists, elbows, shoulders, knees, and ankles. The stiffness is worse in the morning and after inactivity. A small proportion of patients present with monoarthritis of the large joints (shoulders and knees). The hips are rarely affected early in the disease.

X-rays may be normal, or show periarticular osteopenia or erosions. Rheumatoid factor is positive in 70%–80% of people with rheumatoid arthritis. Approximately 30% of patients with rheumatoid arthritis also have positive anti-nuclear antibodies. But watch out – anti-nuclear antibodies are also weakly positive in up to 10% of healthy people.

*More about rheumatoid factor*

- Rheumatoid factor is not diagnostic of rheumatoid arthritis – up to 80% of patients with rheumatoid arthritis have positive rheumatoid factor, but 20% are seronegative.
- Rheumatoid factor has a low specificity for rheumatoid arthritis. It can be positive in other conditions, including mixed connective tissue disease, Sjögren's syndrome, SLE, systemic sclerosis, subacute bacterial endocarditis, tuberculosis, sarcoidosis, and chronic liver disease.
- In rheumatoid arthritis, seropositive patients with persistently high rheumatoid factor titres in early disease have a poor prognosis. They are more likely to have erosive joint damage, greater functional disability, and extra-articular manifestations.

## PAGET'S DISEASE

Paget's disease is a bone remodelling disorder with excessive resorption and formation of structurally abnormal bone. Many patients are asymptomatic, but presenting features can include bone pain (most often of the spine and pelvis), joint pain due to cartilage damage, cranial nerve compression, high-output cardiac failure, a pathological fracture, or sarcoma.

Alkaline phosphatase levels are markedly raised in Paget's disease, but calcium and phosphate levels are normal. Characteristic changes on X-rays (most often in the skull, pelvis, and spine) include osteolytic lesions, sclerosis, and thickening of trabeculae in the long bones and vertebrae.

## CHRONIC INFLAMMATORY DEMYELINATING POLYNEUROPATHY

Chronic inflammatory demyelinating polyneuropathy causes progressive weakness and impaired sensory function, which this patient does not have. As a result of demyelination of the peripheral nerves, this polyneuropathy has a relapsing and remitting course. It is more common in young adults, who often present with symptoms of tingling or numbness (beginning in the toes and fingers), weakness of the arms and legs, areflexia, and fatigue.

## POLYMYALGIA RHEUMATICA

That only leaves us with polymyalgia, which fits this patient's symptoms perfectly. Beware of the patient with polymyalgia rheumatica (usually aged >50 years) who complains of headache, scalp or temporal artery tenderness (pain on combing their hair), jaw claudication, or loss of vision. They may have giant cell arteritis, the most serious complication of polymyalgia rheumatica.

Temporal artery biopsy is the definitive diagnostic test and should be done before or within 36 hours of starting high-dose steroids. Giant cell arteritis requires high-dose prednisolone, usually 40–60 mg daily. Polymyalgia rheumatica requires a lower steroid dose. Steroids should be continued until remission of disease activity and weaned gradually. Most patients require at least 2 years of treatment.

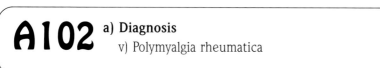

**A102** a) Diagnosis
v) Polymyalgia rheumatica

## FINAL THOUGHTS

All the authors hope you have enjoyed your foray through some of the important questions for MRCP. By now you should be armed with a large number of useful lists that you should use in other MRCP books. We strongly recommend that you go through the book again and practice all that you have learnt. The next chapter deals with some eponymous MRCP syndromes and this is then followed by a chapter on the important lists for the exams. Carry this around with you and practice at your leisure.

Good Luck.

*Victoria Campbell*

*Neil Goldsack*

*Dorothy Ip*

*Hugh Montgomery*

*Vivek Sivaraman*

# 12

## MORE ON EPONYMOUS CONDITIONS IN THE MRCP EXAMINATION

To finish our quick trawl through the MRCP examination, here is a list of some of the eponymous syndromes that may appear. We have also given a brief line on what these eminent doctors actually did.

## BERNARD–SOULIER SYNDROME

- Congenital condition with large platelets, associated with prolonged bleeding time
- Thrombocytopenia
- Due to a specific lack of glycoprotein 1b

Jean Bernard (1907–2006), French physician; Jean-Pierre Soulier (born 1915), French haematologist.

## BROWN-SÉQUARD'S SYNDROME

- Hemisection of the spinal cord
- Contralateral loss of pain and temperature (spinothalamic tracts)
- Ipsilateral flaccid paralysis (corticospinal tracts) and loss of touch, conscious proprioception, and vibration (dorsal columns)

Charles Brown-Séquard (1817–1894), French physiologist and neurologist.

## CHAGAS' DISEASE

- Caused by *Trypanosoma cruzi*
- Acute: fevers, rash, and meningisms
- Chronic: megaoesophagus and cardiomegaly

Carlos Chagas (1879–1934), Brazilian physician.

## CHÉDIAK–HIGASHI SYNDROME

- Neutrophil granule abnormality
- Albinism, recurrent bacterial infections

Moisés Chédiak (born 1903), Cuban physician; Otokata Higashi, 20th century Japanese paediatrician.

## CHRISTMAS DISEASE

- Sex-linked factor IX deficiency

Christmas: a patient with this disease. Not actually named after Santa Claus.

## DARIER'S DISEASE

- Pseudoxanthoma elasticum
- Keratosis

Jean Darier (1856–1938), French dermatologist.

## DRESSLER'S SYNDROME

- Pericardial or pleural chest pain 4–6 weeks after myocardial infarction or cardiac surgery
- May have pleural/pericardial effusion
- Associated with the presence of anti-cardiolipin antibodies
- May present with associated systemic symptoms

William Dressler (1890–1969), US physician.

## EATON–LAMBERT SYNDROME

- Myasthenic syndrome
- Associated with lung cancer

Lee Eaton (1905–1958), US neurologist; Edward Lambert (1915–2003), US neurologist.

## EHLERS–DANLOS SYNDROME

- Collagen disorder
- Hyperextensibility
- Thin, elastic skin
- Repeated pneumothoraces
- Aortic dissection and aortic regurgitation
- Mitral valve prolapse

Edward Ehlers (1863–1937), Danish dermatologist; Henri Danlos (1844–1912), French dermatologist.

## FANCONI'S ANAEMIA

- Congenital aplastic anaemia
- Multiple skeletal abnormalities
- Increased risk of leukaemia

Guido Fanconi (1892–1979), Swiss paediatrician.

## FRIEDREICH'S ATAXIA

- High-arched palate
- Cerebellar signs
- Cardiomyopathy
- Dementia
- Diabetes
- Optic atrophy

Nikolaus Friedreich (1825–1882), German neurologist.

## FROIN'S SYNDROME

- Spinal block
- Highly raised levels of cerebrospinal fluid protein levels

Georges Froin (1874–1932), French neurologist.

## GAUCHER'S DISEASE

- Defect of β-glucocerebrosidase
- Marked hepatosplenomegaly
- Pancytopenia

Philippe Gaucher (1854–1918), French physician.

## GUILLAIN–BARRÉ SYNDROME

- Post-viral polyneuropathy
- Ascending motor neuropathy
- High levels of cerebrospinal fluid protein

Georges Guillain (1876–1961), French neurologist; Jean Barré (1880–1967), French neurologist.

## HEERFORDT'S SYNDROME

- Seen in patients with sarcoidosis
- Triad of parotid and lacrimal swelling with uveitis
- May be associated with systemic features

Christian Heerfordt (1871–1953), Danish ophthalmologist.

## KAWASAKI'S SYNDROME

- Most common childhood vasculitis
- Unknown aetiology
- Systemic illness with conjunctivitis, lymphadenopathy, and rash
- 25% of patients develop coronary artery aneurysms
- Treated with intravenous γ-globulin

Tomisaku Kawasaki, 20th century Japanese paediatrician.

## PRINZMETAL'S ANGINA

- Coronary artery spasm
- Associated with transient ST elevation

Myron Prinzmetal (1908–1987), US cardiologist.

## Reiter's syndrome

- An MRCP examination favourite
- Keratoderma blenorrhagica (looks like psoriasis on palms and feet)
- Genital ulceration and conjunctivitis
- Seronegative arthritis
- Balanitis circinata
- Human leucocyte antigen-B27 associated
- Follows sexually transmitted diseases or enteric infections

Hans Reiter (1881–1969), German bacteriologist. His reputation was tainted over the years: he joined Hitler before the Second World War as a physician and remained a staunch supporter throughout the course of the war. He was convicted of war crimes at Nuremberg.

## Shy–Drager syndrome

- Autonomic neuropathy
- Parkinsonism

George Milton Shy (1919–1967), US neurologist; Glenn Drager (1917–1967), US neurologist.

## Waldenström's macroglobulinaemia

- Often appears in the MRCP examination as a differential diagnosis for multiple myeloma
- Patients are not anaemic, and do not have immunosuppression
- Usually characterised by a monoclonal increase in immunoglobulin M

Jan Waldenström (1906–1996), Swedish physician.

## Weil's disease

- Spread by contact with rat urine
- In the MRCP examination, it may occur in laboratory workers
- Caused by leptospirosis icterohaemorrhagica
- May present with jaundice, fever, oliguria, and haemorrhage

Adolf Weil (1848–1916), German physician.

# 13

# THOSE INFAMOUS
# LISTS AGAIN

A SUMMARY OF THE MRCP EXAMINATION LISTS

# 1. THE STRATEGY

## POLYARTHRALGIA

- rheumatoid arthritis, Still's disease
- Henoch–Schönlein purpura
- pseudogout (pyrophosphate)
- systemic lupus erythematosus
- infectious: hepatitis, gonorrhoea, group A β-haemolytic *Streptococcus*, chicken pox, parvovirus, tuberculosis, rubella, varicella zoster virus, Lyme disease
- familial Mediterranean fever
- Behçet's syndrome
- chronic active hepatitis
- ulcerative colitis/Crohn's disease
- Whipple's disease
- sarcoidosis
- sickle cell disease
- seronegativity
- subacute bacterial endocarditis
- widespread malignancy

# 2. NERVOUS TICKS ON THE LIST: THE NEUROLOGICAL MRCP LISTS

## THIRD NERVE PALSY

- damage to the nerve origin in the midbrain (e.g. midbrain amyloid, multiple sclerosis, Weber's syndrome)
- damage to the nerve vasculature (e.g. diabetes, vasculitis due to systemic lupus erythematosus, rheumatoid arthritis, polyarteritis nodosa)
- nerve compression and stretch (e.g. posterior cerebral artery aneurysm, tumours)
- migraine (transient and repetitive paroxysmal third nerve palsies)

## PAPILLOEDEMA

- benign intracranial pressure
- malignant hypertension or tumour
- mass lesions in or around the brain
- hypercapnia
- central retinal vein, sagittal sinus, or cavernous sinus thrombosis
- hydrocephalus including postsubarachnoid haemorrhage
- lead poisoning, optic neuritis, and vitamin A toxicity

## OPTIC ATROPHY

- congenital Friedreich's ataxia, Leber's optic atrophy, Wolfram's syndrome (DIDMOAD – diabetes insipidus, diabetes mellitus, optic atrophy, deafness)
- papilloedema (longstanding)
- pressure (e.g. compression by tumour and glaucoma)
- poisons (quinine overdose, tobacco amblyopia, wood alcohol)
- Paget's disease

- pernicious anaemia and poor diet (vitamin $B_{12}$ deficiency)
- pulselessness (retinal artery ischaemia)
- syphilis
- multiple sclerosis

## ANGIOID RETINAL STREAKS

- Paget's disease
- sickle cell anaemia
- Ehlers–Danlos syndrome
- pseudoxanthoma elasticum
- thalassaemia
- acromegaly

## CHOROIDORETINITIS

- sarcoidosis
- syphilis
- tuberculosis
- cytomegalovirus
- toxoplasmosis
- toxocariasis

## RETINITIS PIGMENTOSA

- hereditary ataxias, such as Friedreich's ataxia
- Refsum's disease
- Lawrence–Moon–Biedl syndrome
- Alport's syndrome
- Kearns–Sayre syndrome
- Usher's syndrome
- abetalipoproteinaemia and vitamin E deficiency

## CEREBELLAR SYNDROMES: FAT CAT SCAN FOR MS

- Friedreich's ataxia
- alcohol
- tumours: primary (cerebellar haemangioblastomas and von Hippel–Lindau syndrome) or secondary (especially lung cancer as a paraneoplastic syndrome)
- congenital: ataxia telangiectasia, Arnold–Chiari malformations
- strokes
- multiple sclerosis

## SPASTIC PARAPARESIS

- transverse myelitis complicating a viral infection, multiple sclerosis, or a paraneoplastic syndrome
- sudden vascular occlusion
- tropical spastic paraparesis

### ABSENT ANKLE JERKS, EXTENSOR PLANTARS

- syringomyelia
- taboparesis (syphilis)
- Friedreich's ataxia
- cervical spondylosis, peripheral neuropathy
- motor neurone disease
- subacute combined degeneration of the cord

### CEREBROSPINAL FLUID LYMPHOCYTOSIS

- viral or tuberculous meningitis
- encephalitis
- tumour
- cerebral abscess
- cerebral lymphoproliferative disease
- partially treated bacterial meningitis
- Whipple's disease
- multiple sclerosis
- systemic lupus erythematosus
- Behçet's syndrome
- sarcoidosis
- viruses (including HIV)
- fungi
- syphilis
- *Rickettsia*, *Listeria*, *Brucella*, *Coxiella*, *Mycoplasma*

### CEREBROSPINAL FLUID (CSF) PROTEIN (RAISED) WITH NORMAL CSF CELLS

- Guillain–Barré syndrome
- lead poisoning
- cord compression
- spinal block (Froin's syndrome)
- cord malignant deposits
- syphilis
- subacute sclerosing panencephalitis

### PERIPHERAL POLYNEUROPATHY

- born unlucky: Friedreich's ataxia, Refsum's disease, Charcot–Marie–Tooth disease
- three dejected: alcoholics due to alcohol; vitamin $B_1$, $B_6$, and $B_{12}$ deficiencies; isoniazid for tuberculosis
- two infected: leprosy, Guillain–Barré syndrome
- two injected: cancer-associated paraneoplasia or the effects of its treatment, such as vincristine and isoniazid; diabetes mellitus
- one connected: connective tissue disease (e.g. rheumatoid arthritis, systemic lupus erythematosus, polyarteritis nodosa)

- granuloma suspected: sarcoidosis, Churg–Strauss syndrome
- hypothyroid

## Motor neuropathy (alone)

- diabetic amyotrophy
- diphtheria
- porphyria (acute intermittent)
- polymyositis
- lead poisoning
- Guillain–Barré syndrome
- cancer-associated paraneoplasia

## Axonal neuropathies

- hereditary sensory and motor neuropathy type I
- diabetes mellitus
- vitamin $B_{12}$ deficiency
- folate deficiency
- renal failure
- carcinomatous neuropathy
- porphyria
- amyloidosis
- toxins (e.g. phenytoin, isoniazid, nitrofurantoin, dapsone, organophosphate, vincristine, alcohol, heavy metals)
- HIV infection
- critical care neuropathy

## Demyelinating neuropathies

- hereditary sensory and motor neuropathy type II
- diabetes mellitus
- vitamin $B_{12}$ deficiency
- paraprotein neuropathy
- inflammation: Guillain–Barré syndrome and chronic inflammatory demyelinating neuropathy

## Mononeuritis multiplex

- diabetes mellitus
- leprosy
- connective tissue diseases (e.g. polyarteritis nodosa, systemic lupus erythematosus, rheumatoid arthritis, giant cell arteritis)
- sarcoidosis
- malignancy
- amyloidosis
- neurofibromatosis
- HIV infection/AIDS
- Churg–Strauss syndrome

### CARPAL TUNNEL SYNDROME: HAVE GOUT TB P²R²A²M

- gout
- tuberculosis (TB)
- pregnancy/oral contraceptive pill
- rheumatoid arthritis, renal disease
- acromegaly, amyloidosis
- myxoedema
- also, diabetes mellitus may be associated through amyloidosis

## 3. PANTS: RESPIRATORY MRCP LISTS

### BILATERAL HILAR LYMPHADENOPATHY: TWO PAIRS ARE C²HEAP²

- sarcoidosis and tuberculosis
- lymphoma and cancers
- cystic fibrosis, Churg–Strauss syndrome, HIV, extrinsic allergic alveolitis (hypersensitivity pneumonitis), phenytoin treatment, pneumoconioses (especially berylliosis)

### LUNG FIBROSIS

- tuberculosis
- drugs (e.g. amiodarone, bleomycin, busulphan)
- pneumoconioses: silicosis, asbestosis
- acute rheumatic disease (e.g. rheumatoid arthritis, systemic lupus erythematosus)
- radiation
- sarcoidosis
- hypersensitivity pneumonitis (e.g. pigeon breeders' lung)
- paraquat
- pulmonary haemosiderosis
- histiocytosis X

Remember: Pigeon CRA²PS: cryptogenic fibrosing alveolitis, radiation, amiodarone, (extrinsic) allergic alveolitis, pigeon breeders' lung, sarcoidosis

### EOSINOPHILIA: EoS⁴I³N³oP⁶HI⁵LIA

- skin: rheumatoid arthritis with cutaneous manifestations, dermatitis herpetiformis, scabies, atopic eczema
- immune: asthma, atopy, any drug reactions
- neoplastic: Hodgkin's lymphoma, acute lymphoblastic lymphoma, all solid malignancies
- pulmonary eosinophilia (see Bronchopulmonary eosinophilia)
- infective: nematodes, cestodes, trematodes, *Schistosoma* and other parasites, Whipple's disease

### BRONCHOPULMONARY EOSINOPHILIA

- adult asthma
- allergic bronchopulmonary aspergillosis
- Churg–Strauss syndrome
- Löffler's syndrome

- drugs
- tropical (ascariasis, ankylostomiasis, toxocariasis, strongyloidiasis, filariasis)

## BRONCHIECTASIS: TACKY HI²P

- post tuberculosis
- aspergillosis
- cystic fibrosis/bronchial compression
- Kartagener's syndrome (dysmotile cilia with situs inversus and infertility)
- yellow nail syndrome
- hypogammaglobulinaemia
- idiopathic
- inhalation of foreign body
- postchildhood infection (whooping cough/pertussis, measles)

## PLEURAL EFFUSION

- transudates: congestive heart failure, renal failure, nephrotic syndrome, liver failure, hypoalbuminaemia, peritoneal dialysis, protein-losing enteropathy
- exudates: lung cancer, infection (pneumonia, tuberculosis), vasculitic diseases, yellow nail syndrome, mesothelioma, pulmonary embolism, uraemia, lymphoma, Meigs' syndrome, Dressler's syndrome, subphrenic abscess, pancreatitis, hypothyroidism, connective tissue diseases (systemic lupus erythematosus, rheumatoid arthritis), local trauma

## CAVITATION ON A CHEST X-RAY

- cancers (particularly squamous cell)
- tuberculosis
- Wegener's granulomatosis
- rheumatoid nodules, progressive massive fibrosis
- pulmonary embolism
- histoplasmosis, coccidioidomycosis, aspergillosis
- abscesses (think *Staphylococcus*, *Klebsiella*, amoebiasis, aspiration)

## SINGLE WELL-ROUNDED LARGE OPACITY ON A CHEST X-RAY

- neoplasms: primary malignant or metastases; hamartomas
- infections: bacterial, abscesses; tuberculoma; fungal, mycetoma; parasites, hydatid cyst
- vascular: arteriovenous malformations; haematoma (posttraumatic)

## MULTIPLE WELL-ROUNDED LARGE OPACITIES ON A CHEST X-RAY

- sarcoidosis
- metastases
- hydatid cysts
- abscesses
- septic emboli

### Multiple small (<5 mm) opacities on a chest X-ray

- miliary tuberculosis
- sarcoidosis
- pneumoconioses
- interstitial fibrosis
- extrinsic allergic alveolitis

### Localised radiolucencies

- cavitation in an abscess/carcinoma/tuberculosis
- bullae
- pneumatoceles (think of cystic fibrosis)
- cystic bronchiectasis

## 4. Metabollocks: the metabolic MRCP lists

### Hypercalcaemia

- excess parathyroid hormone (PTH): primary and tertiary hyperparathyroidism, ectopic PTH/PTH-related protein (e.g. from oat cell carcinoma of the lung), multiple endocrine neoplasias type I/II
- vitamin D toxicity
- high hormone levels (COAT): Cushing's disease/Addison's disease, oestrogen excess, acromegaly, thyrotoxicosis
- metastatic malignancy: the five 'b's: bronchus, breast, byroid, brostate, bidney
- multiple myeloma and lymphoma
- sarcoidosis (phosphate often normal)
- tuberculosis
- leprosy
- others: milk-alkali syndrome, iatrogenic, idiopathic infantile (supravalvular aortic stenosis, elfin facies), histoplasmosis, coccidioidomycosis, and Wegener's granulomatosis

### Hypocalcaemia

- hypoparathyroidism and parathyroid gland excision: pseudohypoparathyroidism
- low vitamin D levels
- malabsorption syndromes
- chronic renal failure
- acute pancreatitis (calcium sequestered as 'soaps')
- rhabdomyolysis

### Syndrome of inappropriate antidiuretic hormone secretion (SIADH): CCCP

- chest: infections (abscess, effusions, pneumonia, tuberculosis), tumours (small cell carcinoma especially)
- cerebral: infections (abscess, meningitis, tuberculosis); tumours
- cancers: lung and other sites rarely, such as the pancreas
- Ps: pleural effusions, pancreatitis, porphyria, and pills CCCAN (carbamazepine, chlorpropamide, clofibrate, antipsychotics, nonsteroidal anti-inflammatory drugs)

## Diabetes insipidus

- low production:  posterior pituitary damage: hypothalamic damage, craniopharyngioma, pituitary stalk damage (e.g. Sheehan's syndrome of pituitary stalk infarction complicating postpartum haemorrhagic shock), pituitary tumours, basal meningitis (particularly tuberculous meningitis), sarcoidosis
- resistance to action:  drugs: lithium, amphotericin therapy

    electrolytes: prolonged hypercalcaemia or hyponatraemia, distal tubular disease

    inherited: nephrogenic diabetes insipidus (X-linked)

## Addison's disease

- congenital adrenal hyperplasia
- tuberculosis, fungi (including *Cryptococcus*, coccidioidomycosis, histoplasmosis), *Neisseria meningitidis* (Waterhouse–Frederichsen syndrome)
- drugs such as rifampicin, phenytoin, carbamazepine
- adrenal metastases
- autoimmune adrenal failure

## Hypokalaemic alkalosis: STEROID hormones GIVE VILE Diuresis

- **steroids**: Conn's syndrome, Cushing's disease, corticosteroid treatment, phaeochromocytomas, liquorice, carbenoxolone
- **GI** (gastroinstestinal): vomiting
- villous adenoma
- laxatives
- diuretics (e.g. thiazides)

## Hypokalaemic acidosis: PARADE

- partially treated diabetic ketoacidosis
- acetazolamide
- renal tubular acidosis (type I = proximal, type II = distal)
- diarrhoea plus hypovolaemic shock
- enteric (ureterosigmoidostomy or biliary/pancreatic fistula leading to bicarbonate loss: vipoma with multiple endocrine neoplasia type I)

## Respiratory acidosis

- respiratory depression: raised intracranial pressure, drugs such as opioids and barbiturates, and overdoses
- neuromuscular disease: neuropathy (such as Guillain–Barré syndrome and motor neurone disease), myopathy
- skeletal disease: thoracic cage abnormalities
- severe asthma or chronic obstructive pulmonary disease

## Respiratory alkalosis

- pulmonary embolism
- early stages of salicylate overdose

- hysterical hyperventilation
- any cause of a metabolic acidosis

### METABOLIC ACIDOSIS WITH HIGH ANION GAP

- diabetic ketoacidosis
- lactic acidosis type A (tissue hypoxia): circulatory shock (sepsis, cardiogenic, left ventricular failure, bleeds, severe anaemia)
- lactic acidosis type B (no tissue hypoxia): acute hepatic failure, renal failure (acute and chronic), leukaemias, biguanides (metformin, phenformin)
- poisoning with acids: salicylates, methanol, ethanol

### METABOLIC ACIDOSIS WITH NORMAL ANION GAP

- renal tubular acidosis
- severe diarrhoea (remember villous adenomata, where potassium can be lost in quantity!)
- carbonic anhydrase inhibitors (cause potassium and bicarbonate loss)

### METABOLIC ALKALOSIS

- acid loss: potassium loss, chloride depletion, pyloric stenosis, hyperaldosteronism
- increased alkali: forced alkaline diuresis, excess alkali in chronic renal failure

### RHABDOMYOLYSIS: TEASED

- trauma: ischaemic muscle damage (compartment syndrome), bullet wounds, road traffic accidents
- severe exertion: paratroopers, prolonged epileptic seizures
- alcoholics: via seizures, prolonged immobility, hypophosphataemia
- snake bites
- excessive temperature: malignant hyperthermia or environmental
- drug intoxication: cocaine, ecstasy

### RENAL TUBULAR ACIDOSIS TYPE I

- idiopathic
- congenital: autosomal dominant, autosomal recessive
- secondary: rheumatoid arthritis, systemic lupus erythematosus, Sjögren's syndrome, cirrhosis, sickle cell anaemia, myeloma
- drug-induced: ifosfamide, amphotericin, lithium

### RENAL TUBULAR ACIDOSIS TYPE II

- idiopathic
- congenital: Wilson's disease, cystinosis, galactosaemia, glycogen storage disease type I
- secondary: heavy metals, amyloidosis, paroxysmal nocturnal haemoglobinuria
- drugs: carbonic anhydrase inhibitors, ifosfamide

### UREA/CREATININE RATIO ELEVATED

- urea disproportionately raised compared with creatinine: huge high-protein meal, upper gastrointestinal bleed, dehydration

- increase in creatinine: trimethoprim, cimetidine
- decrease in both: chronic liver disease, malnutrition

## Glucose tolerance test: lag storage

- postgastrectomy
- liver failure

## Hepatomegaly

- biliary cirrhosis
- copper and iron storage diseases
- infections: viral, amoebae, hydatid, Weil's disease
- polycystic disease
- proliferative disease: lymphoproliferative, myeloproliferative, myeloma, Waldenström's macroglobulinaemia
- raised venous pressure: Budd–Chiari syndrome, congestive cardiac failure
- cancer and adenomata
- sarcoidosis, amyloidosis, cirrhosis, Riedel's lobe

## 5.  Have a heart: the cardiological MRCP lists

### Cardiac failure and hepatomegaly

- congestive heart failure (with hepatic engorgement)
- amyloidosis
- lymphoma with cardiac involvement/tamponade
- haemochromatosis
- alcoholic cardiomyopathy
- sarcoidosis

### Tricuspid regurgitation

- valve problems: rheumatic heart disease, bacterial endocarditis, congenital heart disease (Ebstein's anomaly), carcinoid syndrome/slimming tablets, myxomatous change
- secondary to elevated pulmonary artery pressures: mitral valve disease, cor pulmonale, primary pulmonary hypertension
- secondary to right ventricular dilatation: right ventricular infarction, any dilated cardiomyopathy

### Dominant R-waves in V1

- posterior myocardial infarction
- pulmonary embolus
- right ventricular hypertrophy (pulmonary hypertension/cor pulmonale/pulmonary stenosis, Noonan's syndrome, Duchenne's muscular dystrophy)
- right bundle branch block
- Wolff–Parkinson–White syndrome type A
- dextrocardia

### Long QT syndrome
- hereditary: Jervell and Lange–Nielsen syndrome, Romano–Ward syndrome
- electrolytes: hypokalaemia, hypomagnesaemia, hypocalcaemia
- endocrine disorders: hypothyroidism, hyperparathyroidism, phaeochromocytoma
- cardiac conditions: chronic myocardial ischaemia, myocardial infarction, myocarditis, bradyarrhythmia, atrioventricular node block
- intracranial disorders: subarachnoid haemorrhage, encephalitis, head trauma
- nutritional disorders: anorexia nervosa, starvation
- drugs: antiarrhythmics, H1-receptor antagonists, cholinergic antagonists, antibiotics, antifungal agents, psychotropic agents, tricyclic antidepressants

## 6. Skinny dips: a selection of dermatological MRCP lists
### Erythema nodosum
- sarcoidosis
- tuberculosis
- inflammatory bowel disease
- infection: streptococcal, histoplasmosis, coccidioidomycosis, North American blastomycosis
- leprosy
- drugs: oral contraceptive pill, sulphonamides, bromides, iodides, penicillins

### Erythema multiforme
- infection: herpes simplex virus types I/II, *Streptococcus*, *Mycoplasma*, Epstein–Barr virus, varicella zoster virus, adenovirus, hepatitis B/C viruses, fungi
- drugs: sulphonamides, sulphonylureas, nonsteroidal anti-inflammatory drugs, anticonvulsants, barbiturates
- collagen vascular disease: systemic lupus erythematosus
- malignancy: especially adenocarcinoma
- sarcoidosis

### Pyoderma gangrenosum
- inflammatory bowel disease
- haematological: myeloma, acute myeloid leukaemia, polycythaemia rubra vera,    IgA paraproteinaemia
- connective tissue diseases: systemic lupus erythematosus, rheumatoid arthritis, polyarteritis nodosa

### Clubbing
- congenital
- cardiac: subacute bacterial endocarditis, atrial myxoma, congenital cyanotic heart disease
- respiratory: carcinoma of bronchus, bronchiectasis, cystic fibrosis, pulmonary fibrosis, mesothelioma
- gastrointestinal: inflammatory bowel disease, liver cirrhosis, coeliac disease
- endocrine: thyroid acropachy
- lung abscess

## 7. GASTROINTESTINAL TRACTS: THE GI MRCP LISTS

### CIRRHOSIS

- congenital: haemochromatosis and Wilson's disease, $\alpha_1$-antitrypsin (remember early emphysema), galactosaemia, type IV glycogenosis
- infectious: chronic active hepatitis (hepatitis B and C)
- immunological: primary biliary cirrhosis and autoimmune hepatitis
- prolonged cholestasis: secondary biliary cirrhosis
- vascular diseases: congestive heart failure, hepatic vein thrombosis, Rendu–Osler–Weber syndrome
- adverse drug reactions: methotrexate, methyldopa, sulphonamides, isoniazid, carbon tetrachloride, amiodarone
- cryptogenic

### MALABSORPTION

- tropical sprue
- coeliac disease
- infectious diarrhoea
- lymphoma of the small bowel

### LIVER GRANULOMATA

- primary biliary cirrhosis
- classic granulomatous disease: sarcoidosis, tuberculosis, Wegener's granulomatosis, *Brucella*, berylliosis
- other autoimmune disease: inflammatory bowel disease, polyarteritis nodosa, giant cell arteritis
- infections ($T^2AG$ along and $C^4$): tropical (leprosy, schistosomiasis), toxocariasis, ascariasis, giardiasis, and *Coxiella*, cytomegalovirus, coccidioidomycosis, clap (syphilis)
- malignancies, drugs, and the chronic granulomatous diseases

### PRIMARY BILIARY CIRRHOSIS: ASSOCIATED CONDITIONS

- rheumatoid arthritis
- CREST syndrome (calcinosis, Raynaud's disease, oesophageal motility disorder, sclerodactyly and telangiectasia)
- systemic sclerosis
- Sjögren's syndrome
- Hashimoto's disease
- coeliac disease
- dermatomyositis
- renal tubular acidosis

### OSTEOMALACIA: DIFFERENTIAL DIAGNOSIS

- lack of vitamin D: poor diet, low sun exposure
- vitamin D malabsorption: postgastrectomy, small bowel surgery, biliary disease (e.g. primary biliary cirrhosis), coeliac disease
- renal disease: chronic renal failure; vitamin D-resistant rickets (due to reduced renal tubular phosphate reabsorption); all causes of renal tubular acidosis (proximal and distal)

- miscellaneous: phenytoin-induced osteomalacia; sclerosing haemangiomas; hypophosphataemic rickets; end-organ resistance to 1,25 dihydroxy-vitamin D

### ALKALINE PHOSPHATASE, RAISED

- biliary obstruction, cholangiocarcinoma, alcoholic liver disease
- pregnancy
- growing children
- Paget's disease
- temporal arteritis
- metastatic bone or liver disease
- vitamin D deficiency

## 8. A BLOODY HELL: HAEMATOLOGICAL MRCP LISTS

### LEUCOERYTHROBLASTIC BLOOD FILM

- marrow infiltration: metastases, malignancies (myeloma, chronic myeloid leukaemia, and acute myeloid leukaemia), myelofibrosis, myeloproliferative (polycythaemia rarely), mycobacteria (tuberculosis), sarcoidosis, storage (Gaucher's disease, Niemann–Pick disease)
- switch on: massive sepsis, massive haemolysis, massive haemorrhage

### PANCYTOPENIA: VD THAT C²LIM⁴BS² P²RETTY F²AST

- viral infections
- drug reactions
- thymic tumours
- hypersplenism
- alcohol
- tuberculosis
- carcinoma and chemotherapy
- lymphoproliferative disease
- irradiation
- myelofibrosis, multiple myeloma, megaloblastic anaemia, myelodysplasia
- *Brucella*
- systemic lupus erythematosus, sideroblastic anaemia
- paroxysmal nocturnal haemoglobinuria, parvovirus with sickle cell/haemolytic disease
- Fanconi's syndrome, Felty's syndrome

### HYPERSPLENISM

- 6 infections: tuberculosis, *Brucella*, syphilis, malaria, subacute bacterial endocarditis, kala azar
- 5 haematological: lymphoma, chronic lymphocytic leukaemia, chronic myeloid leukaemia, myelofibrosis, thalassaemia/haemoglobinopathies
- 4 connective tissue: rheumatoid arthritis, Still's disease, Felty's syndrome, systemic lupus erythematosus
- 3 other: congestion, sarcoidosis, idiopathic
- 2 metabolic: Gaucher's disease, Niemann–Pick disease

## NEUTROPENIA: PIES[2]

- pancytopenia
- infection: typhoid, typhus, tuberculosis, any type of viral infection, *Brucella*, kala azar, malaria
- endocrine: hypopituitarism, hypothyroidism, hyperthyroidism
- systemic lupus erythematosus, specific drugs (alcohol and alcoholic cirrhosis, thiouracil)

## THROMBOCYTOPENIA

- decreased production: megaloblastic anaemia, liver failure, bacterial or viral infection (tuberculosis, typhoid, typhus, kala azar, malaria, *Brucella*, parvovirus with sickle cell/haemolytic disease), malignancy (lymphoproliferative disease, myelodysplasia, thymic tumours, sideroblastic anaemia, myelofibrosis, multiple myeloma)
- increased destruction: hypersplenism, Felty's syndrome, Fanconi's syndrome, systemic lupus erythematosus, paroxysmal nocturnal haemoglobinuria, thrombotic thrombocytopenic purpura, haemolytic–uraemic syndrome, idiopathic thrombocytopenic purpura
- toxic suppression: chemotherapy, irradiation, drugs
- hypopituitarism, hypothyroidism, hyperthyroidism

## POLYCYTHAEMIA

- relative: dehydration, Gaisböck's syndrome (stress)
- primary: polycythaemia rubra vera (splenomegaly, raised platelets)
- secondary: hypoxia, chronic obstructive pulmonary disease, altitude, abnormal haemoglobin, sleep apnoea
- excess erythropoietin: cerebellar haemangioma, hepatoma, phaeochromocytoma, hypernephroma, polycystic/transplant kidneys, uterine leiomyomata/fibromata

## MACROCYTOSIS: L[3]EG CR[3]A[3]M[4]P[2]S

- liver disease, leucoerythroblastosis, lead poisoning
- cytotoxic chemotherapy
- reticulocytosis, renal failure, respiratory failure
- alcohol ingestion, aplastic anaemia, azathioprine treatment
- megaloblastic anaemia (vitamin $B_{12}$/folate deficiency), myeloma, myxoedema, malaria
- pregnancy, pellagra
- sideroblastic anaemia

## MICROANGIOPATHIC HAEMOLYTIC ANAEMIA

- growths: cancers
  foetuses (eclampsia, abruption, intrauterine death, amniotic fluid embolus)
- renal-failure causes: thrombotic thrombocytopenic purpura
  haemolytic uraemic syndrome
  acute glomerulonephritis
- small vessel damage: disseminated intravascular coagulation, malignant hypertension, vasculitides, burns, sepsis
- drugs: cytotoxic agents, cyclosporin

## Haemolytic anaemia

*Congenital*

- membrane defects: hereditary spherocytosis, hereditary elliptocytosis
- haemoglobinopathies: sickle cell anaemia, thalassaemia
- enzyme defects: glucose-6-phosphate dehydrogenase deficiency, pyruvate kinase deficiency

*Acquired*

- immune: autoimmune (lymphoma, rheumatoid arthritis), drug-induced (methyldopa, penicillin; post transfusion; paroxysmal nocturnal haemoglobinuria)
- microangiopathic haemolytic anaemia
- disseminated intravascular coagulation
- hypersplenism

## Splenomegaly

- massive:      chronic myeloid leukaemia, myelofibrosis, malaria, kala azar, Gaucher's disease
- moderate:   all massive disease causes, cirrhosis with portal hypertension, leukaemia, haemolysis, myeloproliferative disease
- mild:            all the above, infection, lymphoproliferative disease disorders, immunoproliferative disease disorders, *Brucella*, typhoid, tuberculosis, trypanosomiasis, subacute bacterial endocarditis, viral infections (infectious mononucleosis, hepatitis B), sarcoidosis, amyloidosis, systemic lupus erythematosus, Felty's syndrome, idiopathic thrombocytopenic purpura, haemolysis, iron deficiency, pernicious anaemia

## Hepatosplenomegaly with lymphadenopathy

- Waldenström's macroglobulinaemia
- acute lymphoblastic leukaemia
- lymphoma
- lymphoproliferative disorders

## Erythrocyte sedimentation rate, low

- polycythaemia
- afibrinogenaemia
- hypofibrinogenaemia

## Erythrocyte sedimentation rate, very high

- first line: temporal arteritis, polymyalgia rheumatica, systemic lupus erythematosus, multiple myeloma
- second line: carcinoma, chronic infection

## Leucocyte alkaline phosphatase score, high

- myeloproliferative disorders: polycythaemia rubra vera, myelofibrosis, Hodgkin's lymphoma
- steroids: Cushing's disease, treatment with steroids, the pill, pregnancy
- Down's syndrome
- hypoproteinaemia

## LEUCOCYTE ALKALINE PHOSPHATASE SCORE, LOW

- chronic myeloid leukaemia
- pernicious anaemia
- idiopathic membranous nephropathy or Epstein–Barr virus
- paroxysmal nocturnal haemoglobinuria
- rickets
- hypophosphataemia

## GRANULOMATA

- sarcoidosis
- tuberculosis (caseating)
- Langerhans' cell histiocytosis
- Wegener's granulomatosis
- Churg–Strauss disease
- fungal and helminthic infections
- hypersensitivity reactions (e.g. dust)
- malignancy: primary or secondary to colon, kidney, germ-cell, bone, prostate, melanoma

## 9. TAKING THE P**S: RENAL MRCP LISTS

### NEPHROTIC SYNDROME

- glomerulonephritis
- subacute bacterial endocarditis
- systemic lupus erythematosus
- rheumatoid arthritis treatment (e.g. gold and penicillamine)
- polyarteritis nodosa
- malaria (*Plasmodium malariae*)
- amyloidosis
- sickle cell anaemia
- cancer (particularly lymphoma)
- bee stings
- renal vein thrombosis
- nonsteroidal anti-inflammatory drugs
- captopril
- interferon-$\alpha$
- heroin

### NEPHROTIC SYNDROME, COMPLICATIONS: TH²ROMB²otI³c

- thrombosis
- hyperlipidaemia, hyponatraemia
- osteomalacia
- malnutrition
- vitamin $B_{12}$ deficiency, Budd–Chiari syndrome
- iron deficiency, infection, immunodeficiency

### Red cell casts in the urine: Generally Inflammatory And Harmful

- glomerulonephritis
- interstitial nephritis
- accelerated hypertension
- haemolytic uraemic syndrome

### Retroperitoneal fibrosis

- drugs: practolol, methysergide therapy
- aortic aneurysm
- lymphoma
- radiation
- idiopathic

## 10. Sex: the MRCP lists of sexual medicine
### Galactorrhoea

- pregnancy
- excess oestrogens
- hypothalamic/pituitary lesions
- prolactinoma and ectopic prolactin secretion: bronchogenic carcinoma, hypernephroma
- antidopaminergic drugs: phenothiazines, butyrophenones, metoclopramide, methyldopa
- hypothyroidism
- chronic renal failure
- polycystic ovaries

## 11. Mopping up
### Cytoplasmic antineutrophil cytoplasmic antibody associations

- Wegener's granulomatosis

### Perinuclear antineutrophil cytoplasmic antibody associations

- microscopic polyarteritis
- polyarteritis nodosa
- a variety of rheumatic autoimmune diseases, including: rheumatoid arthritis, systemic lupus erythematosus, Sjögren's syndrome, polymyositis, dermatomyositis

### Oral ulceration: recurrent

- aphthous ulcers
- ulcerative colitis/Crohn's disease
- Behçet's syndrome
- coeliac disease
- other causes of malabsorption
- systemic lupus erythematosus
- Reiter's syndrome
- seronegative arthritis
- pemphigus (and, rarely, pemphigoid)

## ANTERIOR UVEITIS

- infectious: cytomegalovirus, toxoplasmosis, syphilis, tuberculosis
- neoplastic conditions: lymphomas
- systemic diseases: ankylosing spondylitis, Reiter's syndrome, Behçet's syndrome, sarcoidosis, inflammatory bowel disease, psoriatic arthropathy, juvenile arthritis, Kawasaki disease
- drug induced: rifabutin

## RECURRENT DEEP VENOUS THROMBOSIS

- thrombophilia: antithrombin III deficiency, protein S/C deficiencies, factor V Leiden mutation
- dysfibrinogenaemia
- factor XII deficiency
- malignancy
- surgery and trauma
- post operative
- drugs: oral contraceptive pill
- hyperhomocystinaemia
- Behçet's syndrome
- antiphospholipid syndrome
- paroxysmal nocturnal haemoglobinuria
- nephrotic syndrome

## BLUE SCLERA: POKEMON

- pseudoxanthoma elasticum
- osteogenesis imperfecta
- k(c)ongenital
- Ehlers–Danlos syndrome
- Marfan's syndrome

## MULTIPLE ENDOCRINE NEOPLASIA TYPE I (WERMER SYNDROME): THE 3 Ps

- parathyroid adenoma
- pancreatic adenoma: insulinoma, Zollinger–Ellison syndrome/gastrinoma, glucagonoma, Cushing's syndrome, carcinoids
- pituitary tumour

## MULTIPLE ENDOCRINE NEOPLASIA TYPE II

- medullary thyroid carcinomas (70%–80% of cases)
- phaeochromocytomas (60% of cases)

## MULTIPLE ENDOCRINE NEOPLASIA TYPE IIA (SIPPLE'S SYNDROME)

- phaeochromocytoma
- medullary cancer of the thyroid
- parathyroid hyperplasia
- Hirschsprung's disease

### MULTIPLE ENDOCRINE NEOPLASIA TYPE IIB

- phaeochromocytoma
- medullary cancer of the thyroid plus skin (neuromas, pigmentation) plus marfanoid habitus plus intestinal ganglioneuromatosis

### ERYTHRODERMA

- Dermatoses: atopic dermatitis, candidiasis, contact dermatitis, dermatophytosis (e.g. tinea), ichthyosis, lichen planus, mastocytosis, nummular eczema, pemphigus, photosensitive eczema, pityriasis, psoriasis, Reiter's syndrome, scabies, seborrhoeic dermatitis, staphylococcal scalded skin syndrome
- Autoimmune: systemic lupus erythematosus
- Malignancies: T-cell lymphomas and other lymphomas, leukaemias, internal visceral malignancies
- Drugs: many!
- Miscellaneous: hepatitis, HIV infection, congenital immunodeficiency syndromes (Omenn's syndrome), graft-versus-host disease

### TLCO (CARBON MONOXIDE TRANSFER FACTOR), LOW

- emphysema
- pulmonary emboli
- pulmonary fibrosis
- ageing
- pulmonary oedema
- low cardiac output states

### TLCO (CARBON MONOXIDE TRANSFER FACTOR), HIGH

- asthma (although KCO can also be normal)
- pulmonary haemorrhage (Wegener's granulomatosis, Goodpasture's syndrome)
- left-to-right cardiac shunting
- polycythaemia

# ALL THE LISTS, IN ALPHABETICAL ORDER:

### ABSENT ANKLE JERKS, EXTENSOR PLANTARS

- syringomyelia
- taboparesis (syphilis)
- Friedreich's ataxia
- cervical spondylosis, peripheral neuropathy
- motor neurone disease
- subacute combined degeneration of the cord

### ADDISON'S DISEASE

- congenital adrenal hyperplasia
- tuberculosis, fungi (including *Cryptococcus*, coccidioidomycosis, histoplasmosis), *Neisseria meningitidis* (Waterhouse–Frederichsen syndrome)
- drugs such as rifampicin, phenytoin, carbamazepine
- adrenal metastases
- autoimmune adrenal failure

### ALKALINE PHOSPHATASE, RAISED

- biliary obstruction, cholangiocarcinoma, alcoholic liver disease
- pregnancy
- growing children
- Paget's disease
- temporal arteritis
- metastatic bone or liver disease
- vitamin D deficiency

### ANGIOID RETINAL STREAKS

- Paget's disease
- sickle cell anaemia
- Ehlers–Danlos syndrome
- pseudoxanthoma elasticum
- thalassaemia
- acromegaly

### ANTERIOR UVEITIS

- infectious: cytomegalovirus, toxoplasmosis, syphilis, tuberculosis
- neoplastic conditions: lymphomas
- systemic diseases: ankylosing spondylitis, Reiter's syndrome, Behçet's syndrome, sarcoidosis, inflammatory bowel disease, psoriatic arthropathy, juvenile arthritis, Kawasaki disease
- drug induced: rifabutin

### AXONAL NEUROPATHIES

- hereditary sensory and motor neuropathy type I
- diabetes mellitus
- vitamin $B_{12}$ deficiency
- folate deficiency
- renal failure
- carcinomatous neuropathy
- porphyria
- amyloidosis
- toxins (e.g. phenytoin, isoniazid, nitrofurantoin, dapsone, organophosphate, vincristine, alcohol, heavy metals)
- HIV infection
- critical care neuropathy

### BILATERAL HILAR LYMPHADENOPATHY: TWO PAIRS ARE $C^2$HEAP$^2$

- sarcoidosis and tuberculosis
- lymphoma and cancers
- cystic fibrosis, Churg–Strauss syndrome, HIV, extrinsic allergic alveolitis (hypersensitivity pneumonitis), phenytoin treatment, pneumoconioses (especially berylliosis)

### BLUE SCLERA: POKEMon

- pseudoxanthoma elasticum
- osteogenesis imperfecta
- kongenital
- Ehlers–Danlos syndrome
- Marfan's syndrome

### BRONCHIECTASIS: TACKY HI$^2$P

- post tuberculosis
- aspergillosis
- cystic fibrosis/bronchial compression
- Kartagener's syndrome (dysmotile cilia with situs inversus and infertility)
- yellow nail syndrome
- hypogammaglobulinaemia
- idiopathic
- inhalation of foreign body
- postchildhood infection (whooping cough/pertussis, measles)

### BRONCHOPULMONARY EOSINOPHILIA

- adult asthma
- allergic bronchopulmonary aspergillosis
- Churg–Strauss syndrome
- Löffler's syndrome
- drugs
- tropical (ascariasis, ankylostomiasis, toxocariasis, strongyloidiasis, filariasis)

### CARDIAC FAILURE AND HEPATOMEGALY

- congestive heart failure (with hepatic engorgement)
- amyloidosis
- lymphoma with cardiac involvement/tamponade
- haemochromatosis
- alcoholic cardiomyopathy
- sarcoidosis

### CARPAL TUNNEL SYNDROME: HAVE GOUT TB P$^2$R$^2$A$^2$M

- gout
- tuberculosis (TB)
- pregnancy/oral contraceptive pill
- rheumatoid arthritis, renal disease
- acromegaly, amyloidosis
- myxoedema
- also, diabetes mellitus may be associated through amyloidosis

### CAVITATION ON A CHEST X-RAY

- cancers (particularly squamous cell)
- tuberculosis

- Wegener's granulomatosis
- rheumatoid nodules, progressive massive fibrosis
- pulmonary embolism
- histoplasmosis, coccidioidomycosis, aspergillosis
- abscesses (think *Staphylococcus*, *Klebsiella*, amoebiasis, aspiration)

### CEREBELLAR SYNDROMES: FAT CAT SCAN FOR MS
- Friedreich's ataxia
- alcohol
- tumours: primary (cerebellar haemangioblastomas and von Hippel–Lindau syndrome) or secondary (especially lung cancer as a paraneoplastic syndrome)
- congenital: ataxia telangiectasia, Arnold–Chiari malformations
- strokes
- multiple sclerosis

### CEREBROSPINAL FLUID LYMPHOCYTOSIS
- viral or tuberculous meningitis
- encephalitis
- tumour
- cerebral abscess
- cerebral lymphoproliferative disease
- partially treated bacterial meningitis
- Whipple's disease
- multiple sclerosis
- systemic lupus erythematosus
- Behçet's syndrome
- sarcoidosis
- viruses (including HIV)
- fungi
- syphilis
- *Rickettsia*, *Listeria*, *Brucella*, *Coxiella*, *Mycoplasma*

### CEREBROSPINAL FLUID (CSF) PROTEIN (RAISED) WITH NORMAL CSF CELLS
- Guillain–Barré syndrome
- lead poisoning
- cord compression
- spinal block (Froin's syndrome)
- cord malignant deposits
- syphilis
- subacute sclerosing panencephalitis

### CHOROIDORETINITIS
- sarcoidosis
- syphilis
- tuberculosis
- cytomegalovirus
- toxoplasmosis
- toxocariasis

### CIRRHOSIS
- congenital: haemochromatosis and Wilson's disease, $\alpha_1$-antitrypsin (remember early emphysema), galactosaemia, type IV glycogenosis
- infectious: chronic active hepatitis (hepatitis B and C)
- immunological: primary biliary cirrhosis and autoimmune hepatitis

- prolonged cholestasis: secondary biliary cirrhosis
- vascular diseases: congestive heart failure, hepatic vein thrombosis, Rendu–Osler–Weber syndrome
- adverse drug reactions: methotrexate, methyldopa, sulphonamides, isoniazid, carbon tetrachloride, amiodarone
- cryptogenic

### CLUBBING
- congenital
- cardiac: subacute bacterial endocarditis, atrial myxoma, congenital cyanotic heart disease
- respiratory: carcinoma of bronchus, bronchiectasis, cystic fibrosis, pulmonary fibrosis, mesothelioma
- gastrointestinal: inflammatory bowel disease, liver cirrhosis, coeliac disease
- endocrine: thyroid acropachy
- lung abscess

### CYTOPLASMIC ANTINEUTROPHIL CYTOPLASMIC ANTIBODY ASSOCIATIONS
- Wegener's granulomatosis

### DEMYELINATING NEUROPATHIES
- hereditary sensory and motor neuropathy type II
- diabetes mellitus
- vitamin $B_{12}$ deficiency
- paraprotein neuropathy
- inflammation: Guillain–Barré syndrome and chronic inflammatory demyelinating neuropathy

### DIABETES INSIPIDUS
- low production:
  - posterior pituitary damage: hypothalamic damage, craniopharyngioma, pituitary stalk damage (e.g. Sheehan's syndrome of pituitary stalk infarction complicating postpartum haemorrhagic shock), pituitary tumours, basal meningitis (particularly tuberculous meningitis), sarcoidosis
- resistance to action:
  - drugs: lithium, amphotericin therapy
  - electrolytes: prolonged hypercalcaemia or hyponatraemia, distal tubular disease
  - inherited: nephrogenic diabetes insipidus (X-linked)

### DOMINANT R-WAVES IN V1
- posterior myocardial infarction
- pulmonary embolus
- right ventricular hypertrophy (pulmonary hypertension/cor pulmonale/pulmonary stenosis, Noonan's syndrome, Duchenne's muscular dystrophy)
- right bundle branch block
- Wolff–Parkinson–White syndrome type A
- dextrocardia

### EOSINOPHILIA: EoS⁴I³N³oP⁶HI⁵LIA
- skin: rheumatoid arthritis with cutaneous manifestations, dermatitis herpetiformis, scabies, atopic eczema
- immune: asthma, atopy, any drug reactions
- neoplastic: Hodgkin's lymphoma, acute lymphoblastic lymphoma, all solid malignancies
- pulmonary eosinophilia (see Bronchopulmonary eosinophilia)

- infective: nematodes, cestodes, trematodes, *Schistosoma* and other parasites, Whipple's disease

## Erythema multiforme

- infection: herpes simplex virus types I/II, *Streptococcus*, *Mycoplasma*, Epstein–Barr virus, varicella zoster virus, adenovirus, hepatitis B/C viruses, fungi
- drugs: sulphonamides, sulphonylureas, nonsteroidal anti-inflammatory drugs, anticonvulsants, barbiturates
- collagen vascular disease: systemic lupus erythematosus
- malignancy: especially adenocarcinoma
- sarcoidosis

## Erythema nodosum

- sarcoidosis
- tuberculosis
- inflammatory bowel disease
- infection: streptococcal, histoplasmosis, coccidioidomycosis, North American blastomycosis
- leprosy
- drugs: oral contraceptive pill, sulphonamides, bromides, iodides, penicillins

## Erythrocyte sedimentation rate, low

- polycythaemia
- afibrinogenaemia
- hypofibrinogenaemia

## Erythrocyte sedimentation rate, very high

- first line: temporal arteritis, polymyalgia rheumatica, systemic lupus erythematosus, multiple myeloma
- second line: carcinoma, chronic infection

## Erythroderma

- Dermatoses: atopic dermatitis, candidiasis, contact dermatitis, dermatophytosis (e.g. tinea), ichthyosis, lichen planus, mastocytosis, nummular eczema, pemphigus, photosensitive eczema, pityriasis, psoriasis, Reiter's syndrome, scabies, seborrhoeic dermatitis, staphylococcal scalded skin syndrome
- Autoimmune: systemic lupus erythematosus
- Malignancies: T-cell lymphomas and other lymphomas, leukaemias, internal visceral malignancies
- Drugs: many!
- Miscellaneous: hepatitis, HIV infection, congenital immunodeficiency syndromes (Omenn's syndrome), graft-versus-host disease

## Galactorrhoea

- pregnancy
- excess oestrogens
- hypothalamic/pituitary lesions
- prolactinoma and ectopic prolactin secretion: bronchogenic carcinoma, hypernephroma
- antidopaminergic drugs: phenothiazines, butyrophenones, metoclopramide, methyldopa
- hypothyroidism
- chronic renal failure
- polycystic ovaries

## Glucose tolerance test: lag storage

- postgastrectomy
- liver failure

## Granulomata

- sarcoidosis
- tuberculosis (caseating)
- Langerhans' cell histiocytosis
- Wegener's granulomatosis
- Churg–Strauss disease
- fungal and helminthic infections
- hypersensitivity reactions (e.g. dust)
- malignancy: primary or secondary to colon, kidney, germ-cell, bone, prostate, melanoma

## Haemolytic anaemia

*Congenital*

- membrane defects: hereditary spherocytosis, hereditary elliptocytosis
- haemoglobinopathies: sickle cell anaemia, thalassaemia
- enzyme defects: glucose-6-phosphate dehydrogenase deficiency, pyruvate kinase deficiency

*Acquired*

- immune: autoimmune (lymphoma, rheumatoid arthritis), drug-induced (methyldopa, penicillin; post transfusion; paroxysmal nocturnal haemoglobinuria)
- microangiopathic haemolytic anaemia
- disseminated intravascular coagulation
- hypersplenism

## Hepatomegaly

- biliary cirrhosis
- copper and iron storage diseases
- infections: viral, amoebae, hydatid, Weil's disease
- polycystic disease
- proliferative disease: lymphoproliferative, myeloproliferative, myeloma, Waldenström's macroglobulinaemia
- raised venous pressure: Budd–Chiari syndrome, congestive cardiac failure
- cancer and adenomata
- sarcoidosis, amyloidosis, cirrhosis, Riedel's lobe

## Hepatosplenomegaly with lymphadenopathy

- Waldenström's macroglobulinaemia
- acute lymphoblastic leukaemia
- lymphoma
- lymphoproliferative disorders

## Hypercalcaemia

- excess parathyroid hormone (PTH): primary and tertiary hyperparathyroidism, ectopic PTH/PTH-related protein (e.g. from oat cell carcinoma of the lung), multiple endocrine neoplasias type I/II
- vitamin D toxicity
- high hormone levels (COAT): Cushing's disease/Addison's disease, oestrogen excess, acromegaly, thyrotoxicosis
- metastatic malignancy: the five 'b's: bronchus, breast, byroid, brostate, bidney

- myeloma and lymphoma
- sarcoidosis (phosphate often normal)
- tuberculosis
- leprosy
- others: milk-alkali syndrome, iatrogenic, idiopathic infantile (supravalvular aortic stenosis, elfin facies), histoplasmosis, coccidioidomycosis, and Wegener's granulomatosis

### HYPERSPLENISM
- 6 infections: tuberculosis, *Brucella*, syphilis, malaria, subacute bacterial endocarditis, kala azar
- 5 haematological: lymphoma, chronic lymphocytic leukaemia, chronic myeloid leukaemia, myelofibrosis, thalassaemia/haemoglobinopathies
- 4 connective tissue: rheumatoid arthritis, Still's disease, Felty's syndrome, systemic lupus erythematosus
- 3 other: congestion, sarcoidosis, idiopathic
- 2 metabolic: Gaucher's disease, Niemann–Pick disease

### HYPOCALCAEMIA
- hypoparathyroidism and parathyroid gland excision: pseudohypoparathyroidism
- low vitamin D levels
- malabsorption syndromes
- chronic renal failure
- acute pancreatitis (calcium sequestered as 'soaps')
- rhabdomyolysis

### HYPOKALAEMIC ACIDOSIS: PARADE
- partially treated diabetic ketoacidosis
- acetazolamide
- renal tubular acidosis (type I = proximal, type II = distal)
- diarrhoea plus hypovolaemic shock
- enteric (ureterosigmoidostomy or biliary/pancreatic fistula leading to bicarbonate loss: vipoma with multiple endocrine neoplasia type I)

### HYPOKALAEMIC ALKALOSIS: STEROID HORMONES GIVE VILE DIURESIS
- steroids: Conn's syndrome, Cushing's disease, corticosteroid treatment, phaeochromocytomas, liquorice, carbenoxolone
- GI (gastroinstestinal): vomiting
- villous adenoma
- laxatives
- diuretics (e.g. thiazides)

### LEUCOCYTE ALKALINE PHOSPHATASE SCORE, HIGH
- myeloproliferative disorders: polycythaemia rubra vera, myelofibrosis, Hodgkin's lymphoma
- steroids: Cushing's disease, treatment with steroids, the pill, pregnancy
- Down's syndrome
- hypoproteinaemia

### LEUCOCYTE ALKALINE PHOSPHATASE SCORE, LOW
- chronic myeloid leukaemia
- pernicious anaemia
- idiopathic membranous nephropathy or Epstein–Barr virus

- paroxysmal nocturnal haemoglobinuria
- rickets
- hypophosphataemia

### LEUCOERYTHROBLASTIC BLOOD FILM
- marrow infiltration: metastases, malignancies (myeloma, chronic myeloid leukaemia, and acute myeloid leukaemia), myelofibrosis, myeloproliferative (polycythaemia rarely), mycobacteria (tuberculosis), sarcoidosis, storage (Gaucher's disease, Niemann–Pick disease)
- switch on: massive sepsis, massive haemolysis, massive haemorrhage

### LIVER GRANULOMATA
- primary biliary cirrhosis
- classic granulomatous disease: sarcoidosis, tuberculosis, Wegener's granulomatosis, *Brucella*, berylliosis
- other autoimmune disease: inflammatory bowel disease, polyarteritis nodosa, giant cell arteritis
- infections ($T^2AG$ along and $C^4$): tropical (leprosy, schistosomiasis), toxocariasis, ascariasis, giardiasis, and *Coxiella*, cytomegalovirus, coccidioidomycosis, clap (syphilis)
- malignancies, drugs, and the chronic granulomatous diseases

### LOCALISED RADIOLUCENCIES
- cavitation in an abscess/carcinoma/tuberculosis
- bullae
- pneumatoceles (think of cystic fibrosis)
- cystic bronchiectasis

### LONG QT SYNDROME
- hereditary: Jervell and Lange–Nielsen syndrome, Romano–Ward syndrome
- electrolytes: hypokalaemia, hypomagnesaemia, hypocalcaemia
- endocrine disorders: hypothyroidism, hyperparathyroidism, phaeochromocytoma
- cardiac conditions: chronic myocardial ischaemia, myocardial infarction, myocarditis, bradyarrhythmia, atrioventricular node block
- intracranial disorders: subarachnoid haemorrhage, encephalitis, head trauma
- nutritional disorders: anorexia nervosa, starvation
- drugs: antiarrhythmics, H1-receptor antagonists, cholinergic antagonists, antibiotics, antifungal agents, psychotropic agents, tricyclic antidepressants

### LUNG FIBROSIS
- tuberculosis
- drugs (e.g. amiodarone, bleomycin, busulphan)
- pneumoconioses: silicosis, asbestosis
- acute rheumatic disease (e.g. rheumatoid arthritis, systemic lupus erythematosus)
- radiation
- sarcoidosis
- hypersensitivity pneumonitis (e.g. pigeon breeders' lung)
- paraquat

- pulmonary haemosiderosis
- histiocytosis X

Remember: Pigeon CRA$^2$PS: cryptogenic fibrosing alveolitis, radiation, amiodarone, (extrinsic) allergic alveolitis, pigeon breeders' lung, sarcoidosis

## MACROCYTOSIS: L$^3$EG CR$^2$A$^3$M$^4$P$^2$S
- liver disease, leucoerythroblastosis, lead poisoning
- cytotoxic chemotherapy
- reticulocytosis, renal failure, respiratory failure
- alcohol ingestion, aplastic anaemia, azathioprine treatment
- megaloblastic anaemia (vitamin B$_{12}$/folate deficiency), myeloma, myxoedema, malaria
- pregnancy, pellagra
- sideroblastic anaemia

## MALABSORPTION
- tropical sprue
- coeliac disease
- infectious diarrhoea
- lymphoma of the small bowel

## METABOLIC ACIDOSIS WITH HIGH ANION GAP
- diabetic ketoacidosis
- lactic acidosis type A (tissue hypoxia): circulatory shock (sepsis, cardiogenic, left ventricular failure, bleeds, severe anaemia)
- lactic acidosis type B (no tissue hypoxia): acute hepatic failure, renal failure (acute and chronic), leukaemias, biguanides (metformin, phenformin)
- poisoning with acids: salicylates, methanol, ethanol

## METABOLIC ACIDOSIS WITH NORMAL ANION GAP
- renal tubular acidosis
- severe diarrhoea (remember villous adenomata, where potassium can be lost in quantity!)
- carbonic anhydrase inhibitors (cause potassium and bicarbonate loss)

## METABOLIC ALKALOSIS
- acid loss: potassium loss, chloride depletion, pyloric stenosis, hyperaldosteronism
- increased alkali: forced alkaline diuresis, excess alkali in chronic renal failure

## MICROANGIOPATHIC HAEMOLYTIC ANAEMIA
- growths:
  - cancers
  - foetuses (eclampsia, abruption, intrauterine death, amniotic fluid embolus)
- renal-failure causes:
  - thrombotic thrombocytopenic purpura
  - haemolytic uraemic syndrome
  - acute glomerulonephritis
- small vessel damage:
  - disseminated intravascular coagulation, malignant hypertension, vasculitides, burns, sepsis
- drugs:
  - cytotoxic agents, cyclosporin

## MONONEURITIS MULTIPLEX
- diabetes mellitus
- leprosy
- connective tissue diseases (e.g. polyarteritis nodosa, systemic lupus erythematosus, rheumatoid arthritis, giant cell arteritis)
- sarcoidosis
- malignancy
- amyloidosis
- neurofibromatosis
- HIV infection/AIDS
- Churg–Strauss syndrome

## MOTOR NEUROPATHY (ALONE)
- diabetic amyotrophy
- diphtheria
- porphyria (acute intermittent)
- polymyositis
- lead poisoning
- Guillain–Barré syndrome
- cancer-associated paraneoplasia

## MULTIPLE ENDOCRINE NEOPLASIA TYPE I (WERMER SYNDROME): THE 3 Ps
- parathyroid adenoma
- pancreatic adenoma: insulinoma, Zollinger–Ellison syndrome/gastrinoma, glucagonoma, Cushing's syndrome, carcinoids
- pituitary tumour

## MULTIPLE ENDOCRINE NEOPLASIA TYPE II
- medullary thyroid carcinomas (70%–80% of cases)
- phaeochromocytomas (60% of cases)

## MULTIPLE ENDOCRINE NEOPLASIA TYPE IIA (SIPPLE'S SYNDROME)
- phaeochromocytoma
- medullary cancer of the thyroid
- parathyroid hyperplasia
- Hirschsprung's disease

## MULTIPLE ENDOCRINE NEOPLASIA TYPE IIB
- phaeochromocytoma
- medullary cancer of the thyroid plus skin (neuromas, pigmentation) plus marfanoid habitus plus intestinal ganglioneuromatosis

## MULTIPLE SMALL (<5 MM) OPACITIES ON A CHEST X-RAY
- miliary tuberculosis
- sarcoidosis
- pneumoconioses
- interstitial fibrosis
- extrinsic allergic alveolitis

## MULTIPLE WELL-ROUNDED LARGE OPACITIES ON A CHEST X-RAY
- sarcoidosis
- metastases
- hydatid cysts
- abscesses
- septic emboli

## NEPHROTIC SYNDROME
- glomerulonephritis
- subacute bacterial endocarditis
- systemic lupus erythematosus
- rheumatoid arthritis treatment (e.g. gold and penicillamine)
- polyarteritis nodosa
- malaria (*Plasmodium malariae*)
- amyloidosis
- sickle cell anaemia
- cancer (particularly lymphoma)
- bee stings
- renal vein thrombosis
- nonsteroidal anti-inflammatory drugs
- captopril
- interferon-$\alpha$
- heroin

## NEPHROTIC SYNDROME, COMPLICATIONS: TH²ROMB²OTI³C
- thrombosis
- hyperlipidaemia, hyponatraemia
- osteomalacia
- malnutrition
- vitamin $B_{12}$ deficiency, Budd–Chiari syndrome
- iron deficiency, infection, immunodeficiency

## NEUTROPENIA: PIES²
- pancytopenia
- infection: typhoid, typhus, tuberculosis, any type of viral infection, *Brucella*, kala azar, malaria
- endocrine: hypopituitarism, hypothyroidism, hyperthyroidism
- systemic lupus erythematosus, specific drugs (alcohol and alcoholic cirrhosis, thiouracil)

## OPACITIES ON A CHEST X-RAY, MULTIPLE SMALL (<5 MM)
- miliary tuberculosis
- sarcoidosis
- pneumoconioses
- interstitial fibrosis
- extrinsic allergic alveolitis

## OPACITIES ON A CHEST X-RAY, MULTIPLE WELL-ROUNDED LARGE
- sarcoidosis
- metastases
- hydatid cysts
- abscesses
- septic emboli

## OPACITY ON A CHEST X-RAY, SINGLE WELL-ROUNDED LARGE
- neoplasms: primary malignant or metastases; hamartomas
- infections: bacterial, abscesses; tuberculoma; fungal, mycetoma; parasites, hydatid cyst
- vascular: arteriovenous malformations; haematoma (posttraumatic)

## OPTIC ATROPHY
- congenital Friedreich's ataxia, Leber's optic atrophy, Wolfram's syndrome (DIDMOAD – diabetes insipidus, diabetes mellitus, optic atrophy, deafness)

- papilloedema (longstanding)
- pressure (e.g. compression by tumour and glaucoma)
- poisons (quinine overdose, tobacco amblyopia, wood alcohol)
- Paget's disease
- pernicious anaemia and poor diet (vitamin $B_{12}$ deficiency)
- pulselessness (retinal artery ischaemia)
- syphilis
- multiple sclerosis

## ORAL ULCERATION: RECURRENT
- aphthous ulcers
- ulcerative colitis/Crohn's disease
- Behçet's syndrome
- coeliac disease
- other causes of malabsorption
- systemic lupus erythematosus
- Reiter's syndrome
- seronegative arthritis
- pemphigus (and, rarely, pemphigoid)

## OSTEOMALACIA: DIFFERENTIAL DIAGNOSIS
- lack of vitamin D: poor diet, low sun exposure
- vitamin D malabsorption: postgastrectomy, small bowel surgery, biliary disease (e.g. primary biliary cirrhosis), coeliac disease
- renal disease: chronic renal failure; vitamin D-resistant rickets (due to reduced renal tubular phosphate reabsorption); all causes of renal tubular acidosis (proximal and distal)
- miscellaneous: phenytoin-induced osteomalacia; sclerosing haemangiomas; hypophosphataemic rickets; end-organ resistance to 1,25 dihydroxy-vitamin D

## PANCYTOPENIA: VD THAT C²LIM⁴BS² P²RETTY F²AST
- viral infections
- drug reactions
- thymic tumours
- hypersplenism
- alcohol
- tuberculosis
- carcinoma and chemotherapy
- lymphoproliferative disease
- irradiation
- myelofibrosis, multiple myeloma, megaloblastic anaemia, myelodysplasia
- *Brucella*
- systemic lupus erythematosus, sideroblastic anaemia
- paroxysmal nocturnal haemoglobinuria, parvovirus with sickle cell/haemolytic disease
- Fanconi's syndrome, Felty's syndrome

## PAPILLOEDEMA
- benign intracranial pressure
- malignant hypertension or tumour
- mass lesions in or around the brain
- hypercapnia
- central retinal vein, sagittal sinus, or cavernous sinus thrombosis

- hydrocephalus including postsubarachnoid haemorrhage
- lead poisoning, optic neuritis, and vitamin A toxicity

### PERINUCLEAR ANTINEUTROPHIL CYTOPLASMIC ANTIBODY ASSOCIATIONS

- microscopic polyarteritis
- polyarteritis nodosa
- a variety of rheumatic autoimmune diseases, including: rheumatoid arthritis, systemic lupus erythematosus, Sjögren's syndrome, polymyositis, dermatomyositis

### PERIPHERAL POLYNEUROPATHY

- born unlucky: Friedreich's ataxia, Refsum's disease, Charcot–Marie–Tooth disease
- three dejected: alcoholics due to alcohol; vitamin $B_1$, $B_6$, and $B_{12}$ deficiencies; isoniazid for tuberculosis
- two infected: leprosy, Guillain–Barré syndrome
- two injected: cancer-associated paraneoplasia or the effects of its treatment, such as vincristine and isoniazid; diabetes mellitus
- one connected: connective tissue disease (e.g. rheumatoid arthritis, systemic lupus erythematosus, polyarteritis nodosa)
- granuloma suspected: sarcoidosis, Churg–Strauss syndrome
- hypothyroid

### PLEURAL EFFUSION

- transudates: congestive heart failure, renal failure, nephrotic syndrome, liver failure, hypoalbuminaemia, peritoneal dialysis, protein-losing enteropathy
- exudates: lung cancer, infection (pneumonia, tuberculosis), vasculitic diseases, yellow nail syndrome, mesothelioma, pulmonary embolism, uraemia, lymphoma, Meigs' syndrome, Dressler's syndrome, subphrenic abscess, pancreatitis, hypothyroidism, connective tissue diseases (systemic lupus erythematosus, rheumatoid arthritis), local trauma

### POLYARTHRALGIA

- rheumatoid arthritis, Still's disease
- Henoch–Schönlein purpura
- pseudogout (pyrophosphate)
- systemic lupus erythematosus
- infectious: hepatitis, gonorrhoea, group A β-haemolytic *Streptococcus*, chicken pox, parvovirus, tuberculosis, rubella, varicella zoster virus, Lyme disease
- familial Mediterranean fever
- Behçet's syndrome
- chronic active hepatitis
- ulcerative colitis/Crohn's disease
- Whipple's disease
- sarcoidosis
- sickle cell disease
- seronegativity
- subacute bacterial endocarditis
- widespread malignancy

### POLYCYTHAEMIA

- relative: dehydration, Gaisböck's syndrome (stress)
- primary: polycythaemia rubra vera (splenomegaly, raised platelets)
- secondary: hypoxia, chronic obstructive pulmonary disease, altitude, abnormal haemoglobin, sleep apnoea

- excess erythropoietin: cerebellar haemangioma, hepatoma, phaeochromocytoma, hypernephroma, polycystic/transplant kidneys, uterine leiomyomata/fibromata

### PRIMARY BILIARY CIRRHOSIS: ASSOCIATED CONDITIONS

- rheumatoid arthritis
- CREST syndrome (calcinosis, Raynaud's disease, oesophageal motility disorder, sclerodactyly and telangiectasia)
- systemic sclerosis
- Sjögren's syndrome
- Hashimoto's disease
- coeliac disease
- dermatomyositis
- renal tubular acidosis

### PYODERMA GANGRENOSUM

- inflammatory bowel disease
- haematological: myeloma, acute myeloid leukaemia, polycythaemia rubra vera, IgA paraproteinaemia
- connective tissue diseases: systemic lupus erythematosus, rheumatoid arthritis, polyarteritis nodosa

### RADIOLUCENCIES, LOCALISED

- cavitation in an abscess/carcinoma/tuberculosis
- bullae
- pneumatoceles (think of cystic fibrosis)
- cystic bronchiectasis

### RECURRENT DEEP VENOUS THROMBOSIS

- thrombophilia: antithrombin III deficiency, protein S/C deficiencies, factor V Leiden mutation
- dysfibrinogenaemia
- factor XII deficiency
- malignancy
- surgery and trauma
- post operative
- drugs: oral contraceptive pill
- hyperhomocystinaemia
- Behçet's syndrome
- antiphospholipid syndrome
- paroxysmal nocturnal haemoglobinuria
- nephrotic syndrome

### RED CELL CASTS IN THE URINE: GENERALLY INFLAMMATORY AND HARMFUL

- glomerulonephritis
- interstitial nephritis
- accelerated hypertension
- haemolytic uraemic syndrome

### RENAL TUBULAR ACIDOSIS TYPE I

- idiopathic
- congenital: autosomal dominant, autosomal recessive
- secondary: rheumatoid arthritis, systemic lupus erythematosus, Sjögren's syndrome, cirrhosis, sickle cell anaemia, myeloma
- drug-induced: ifosfamide, amphotericin, lithium

### RENAL TUBULAR ACIDOSIS TYPE II

- idiopathic
- congenital: Wilson's disease, cystinosis, galactosaemia, glycogen storage disease type I
- secondary: heavy metals, amyloidosis, paroxysmal nocturnal haemoglobinuria
- drugs: carbonic anhydrase inhibitors, ifosfamide

### RESPIRATORY ACIDOSIS

- respiratory depression: raised intracranial pressure, drugs such as opioids and barbiturates, and overdoses
- neuromuscular disease: neuropathy (such as Guillain–Barré syndrome and motor neurone disease), myopathy
- skeletal disease: thoracic cage abnormalities
- severe asthma or chronic obstructive pulmonary disease

### RESPIRATORY ALKALOSIS

- pulmonary embolism
- early stages of salicylate overdose
- hysterical hyperventilation
- any cause of a metabolic acidosis

### RETINITIS PIGMENTOSA

- hereditary ataxias, such as Friedreich's ataxia
- Refsum's disease
- Lawrence–Moon–Biedl syndrome
- Alport's syndrome
- Kearns–Sayre syndrome
- Usher's syndrome
- abetalipoproteinaemia and vitamin E deficiency

### RETROPERITONEAL FIBROSIS

- drugs: practolol, methysergide therapy
- aortic aneurysm
- lymphoma
- radiation
- idiopathic

### RHABDOMYOLYSIS: TEASED

- trauma: ischaemic muscle damage (compartment syndrome), bullet wounds, road traffic accidents
- severe exertion: paratroopers, prolonged epileptic seizures
- alcoholics: via seizures, prolonged immobility, hypophosphataemia
- snake bites
- excessive temperature: malignant hyperthermia or environmental
- drug intoxication: cocaine, ecstasy

### SINGLE WELL-ROUNDED LARGE OPACITY ON A CHEST X-RAY

- neoplasms: primary malignant or metastases; hamartomas
- infections: bacterial, abscesses; tuberculoma; fungal, mycetoma; parasites, hydatid cyst
- vascular: arteriovenous malformations; haematoma (posttraumatic)

### SPASTIC PARAPARESIS

- transverse myelitis complicating a viral infection, multiple sclerosis, or a paraneoplastic syndrome
- sudden vascular occlusion

- tropical spastic paraparesis

### SPLENOMEGALY

- massive:
  - chronic myeloid leukaemia, myelofibrosis, malaria, kala azar, Gaucher's disease
- moderate:
  - all massive disease causes, cirrhosis with portal hypertension, leukaemia, haemolysis, myeloproliferative disease
- mild:
  - all the above, infection, lymphoproliferative disease disorders, immunoproliferative disease disorders, *Brucella*, typhoid, tuberculosis, trypanosomiasis, subacute bacterial endocarditis, viral infections (infectious mononucleosis, hepatitis B), sarcoidosis, amyloidosis, systemic lupus erythematosus, Felty's syndrome, idiopathic thrombocytopenic purpura, haemolysis, iron deficiency, pernicious anaemia

### SYNDROME OF INAPPROPRIATE ANTIDIURETIC HORMONE SECRETION (SIADH): CCCP

- chest: infections (abscess, effusions, pneumonia, tuberculosis), tumours (small cell carcinoma especially)
- cerebral: infections (abscess, meningitis, tuberculosis); tumours
- cancers: lung and other sites rarely, such as the pancreas
- Ps: pleural effusions, pancreatitis, porphyria, and pills CCCAN (carbamazepine, chlorpropamide, clofibrate, antipsychotics, nonsteroidal anti-inflammatory drugs)

### THIRD NERVE PALSY

- damage to the nerve origin in the midbrain (e.g. midbrain amyloid, multiple sclerosis, Weber's syndrome)
- damage to the nerve vasculature (e.g. diabetes, vasculitis due to systemic lupus erythematosus, rheumatoid arthritis, polyarteritis nodosa)
- nerve compression and stretch (e.g. posterior cerebral artery aneurysm, tumours)
- migraine (transient and repetitive paroxysmal third nerve palsies)

### THROMBOCYTOPENIA

- decreased production: megaloblastic anaemia, liver failure, bacterial or viral infection (tuberculosis, typhoid, typhus, kala azar, malaria, *Brucella*, parvovirus with sickle cell/haemolytic disease), malignancy (lymphoproliferative disease, myelodysplasia, thymic tumours, sideroblastic anaemia, myelofibrosis, multiple myeloma)
- increased destruction: hypersplenism, Felty's syndrome, Fanconi's syndrome, systemic lupus erythematosus, paroxysmal nocturnal haemoglobinuria, thrombotic thrombocytopenic purpura, haemolytic–uraemic syndrome, idiopathic thrombocytopenic purpura
- toxic suppression: chemotherapy, irradiation, drugs
- hypopituitarism, hypothyroidism, hyperthyroidism

### TLCO (CARBON MONOXIDE TRANSFER FACTOR), HIGH

- asthma (although KCO can also be normal)
- pulmonary haemorrhage (Wegener's granulomatosis, Goodpasture's syndrome)
- left-to-right cardiac shunting
- polycythaemia

## TLCO (CARBON MONOXIDE TRANSFER FACTOR), LOW

- emphysema
- pulmonary emboli
- pulmonary fibrosis
- ageing
- pulmonary oedema
- low cardiac output states

## TRICUSPID REGURGITATION

- valve problems: rheumatic heart disease, bacterial endocarditis, congenital heart disease (Ebstein's anomaly), carcinoid syndrome/slimming tablets, myxomatous change
- secondary to elevated pulmonary artery pressures: mitral valve disease, cor pulmonale, primary pulmonary hypertension
- secondary to right ventricular dilatation: right ventricular infarction, any dilated cardiomyopathy

## UREA/CREATININE RATIO ELEVATED

- urea disproportionately raised compared with creatinine: huge high-protein meal,
  upper gastrointestinal bleed, dehydration
- increase in creatinine: trimethoprim, cimetidine
- decrease in both: chronic liver disease, malnutrition

# INDEX

Note: Page references in **bold** refer to figures and those in *italics* refer to tables or boxed material.